SHADOW OF SWORDS

A Biography of Elsie Inglis

SHADOW OF SWORDS

A Biography of Elsie Inglis

MARGOT LAWRENCE

'Paradise is under the shadow of swords'—Mahomet
(quoted in Emerson's essay, 'On Heroism')

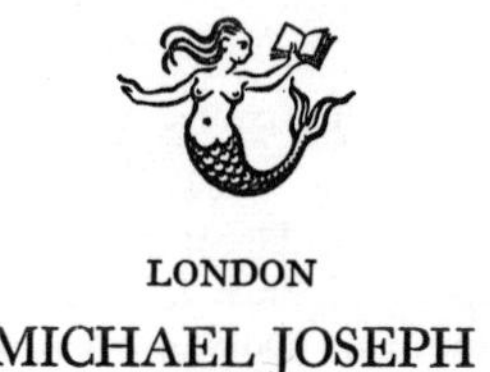

LONDON
MICHAEL JOSEPH

First published in Great Britain by
MICHAEL JOSEPH LTD
52 Bedford Square
London, W.C.1
1971

7181 0871 x

Printed in Great Britain by
Northumberland Press Limited, Gateshead
and bound by Dorstel Press, Harlow

To the Happy Few
who remember the days of the
Scottish Women's Hospitals

CONTENTS

LIST OF ILLUSTRATIONS

[9]

ACKNOWLEDGEMENTS

[11]

NOTE ON THE SPELLING OF PROPER NAMES

[13]

SHADOW OF SWORDS

[17]

APPENDIX

[283]

BIBLIOGRAPHY

[287]

NOTES

[291]

INDEX

[313]

LIST OF ILLUSTRATIONS

Inglis family group, taken about 1879 (*The Rev. R. S. MacNicol*) *facing* 64

Horace, Eva and Elsie Inglis, 1885 (*Mrs E. T. Maddox*) 64

Sophia Jex-Blake (*Fawcett Library*) 64

Elsie Inglis with her two sisters, about 1912 (*Mrs E. T. Maddox*) 65

Suffrage March leaving King's Park, Edinburgh, 1913 (*Fawcett Library*) 65

Mrs Eveline Haverfield (*Fawcett Library*) 65

Dr Alice Hutchison (*Illustrated Newspapers Ltd*) 65

The fountain built as a tribute to Dr Elsie Inglis and the Scottish Women's Hospitals in Serbia (*Illustrated Newspapers Ltd*) 128

Nurses making the retreat from Serbia, December 1915 (*Illustrated Newspapers Ltd*) 128

Elsie Inglis and three other members of the Scottish Women's Hospitals in Zurich after their release as prisoners of war, February 1916 (*Fawcett Library*) 129

Elsie Inglis in 1916 (*Mrs E. T. Maddox*) 192

Elsie Inglis and companions during the retreat in Roumania (*Fawcett Library*) 193

Elsie Inglis riding, May 1917 (*The Rev. R. S. MacNicol*) 193

Elsie Inglis, drawn in the late summer of 1917 (*private picture*) 224

Elsie Inglis, a photograph of the same date (*Fawcett Library*) 224

The front page of the *Daily Mirror*, 1st December, 1917 (*Daily Mirror*) 225

MAPS

Serbia, 1914-15 *page* 147
Roumania and South-East Russia, 1916-17 201

ACKNOWLEDGEMENTS

The unstinted help, kindness and encouragement which I have received from everyone to whom I have applied, has been an impressive and inspiring testimony to the affection and respect which the name of Dr Elsie Inglis still evokes.

To the members of her family, Miss Violet Inglis, the Rev. and Mrs R. S. MacNicol, and Mrs E. T. Maddox, I am indebted for many kindnesses, much valuable personal recollection and the loan of treasured family papers, photographs and books, with permission to quote from these and reproduce the photographs. Miss Amy MacNicol and Mr Moray McLaren also assisted greatly with valuable personal recollection.

The Trustees of the Fawcett Society have most kindly afforded me unlimited access to the records of the Scottish Women's Hospitals at the Fawcett Library and I have to thank them for permission to quote from these, and for permission to reproduce photographs in their possession. To Miss Vera Douie, O.B.E. and Mrs Horton I owe especial thanks for much help and kind encouragement.

Mr R. A. Dickson, B.L., F.H.A., Secretary of the Board of Management for Edinburgh Southern Hospitals, very kindly allowed me to consult the minute books of The Hospice and the Bruntsfield Hospital. Dr H. B. Tait, M.D. F.R.C.P., D.P.H., most generously made available to me the results of his own researches into the founding of the School of Medicine for Women and of The Hospice and I am also grateful for his advice on professional aspects of these events. My handling of this and all the rest of the available material is, of course, entirely my own responsibility.

I am indebted to the Librarian of the Foreign Office for permission to study certain Foreign Office records at a time when these were not publicly available, and to the Controller of H. M. Stationery Office for permission to quote from Crown Copyright material; the kind and able help of the staff of the Public Record Office greatly facilitated my researches there.

Thanks are due in large measure to Miss R. E. B. Coombs, Librarian, and the staff of the Imperial War Museum; to Miss A. M. C. Thompson, Librarian of the Royal College of Nursing; Mr E. M. Evans, Deputy Librarian of the Royal Society of

Medicine; Dr Joan Laurie and the Librarian of the Medical Women's Federation; Dame Beryl Oliver, archivist of the British Red Cross Society; Miss E. M. Sugden, librarian of the Elizabeth Garret Anderson Hospital; the Naval Librarian of the Ministry of Defence; Lieutenant-Colonel Neave Hill of the Central and Army Library of the Ministry of Defence; and the Librarians and staffs of the National Library of Scotland, the British Museum Reading Room and Newspaper Library, Westminster Public Libraries and the Reference Library of Hendon Public Libraries. Mr A. B. Piechoviak most kindly allowed me to study the records of the Serbian Relief Fund at the School of Slavonic Studies and Professor Hugh Seton Watson very kindly helped me with certain of his father's papers.

Many who were personally associated with Dr Inglis have very generously given me their recollections, answered questions and afforded me the benefit of personal discussion and for this I am indeed grateful to Miss Elizabeth Arbuthnot, Mrs Carlile, Dame May Curwen, Miss Gertrude Herzfeld, F.R.C.S., Miss Vera Holme, Dr Joan Rose, Mrs Sherry and Dr Gillian Ward.

Mr K. St. Pavlowitch was kind enough to help and advise on some aspects of Serbian life and Mrs Lula Evans helped me with the translation and interpretation of Serbian sources. For help and encouragement in other ways great and small I owe thanks to Mr Arnold Beevers, Mr H. G. Castle, Mr Charles Curran, Miss Alison Downie, Mrs Wyn Gibbons, Dr Douglas Guthrie, Dr Kate Harrower, Miss Rosemary Heaward, Marian Holbourn, Mr and Mrs David Holloway, Dr Margaret Lawton, Mr A. L. Lloyd, Miss Isabella McCarten, Mr Stevan Majstorovic, Mrs Radmila Petrovic, Mr Willard Rosenquist, Miss Margaret Stephens, the Rev. Edward Vernon, Miss Mildred Warburton, and Sir Frederick Whyte, K.C.S.I., and also to my sister Barbara Burrows and my daughter Alison Harrop.

It is a matter of real sorrow that the late Mrs E. Cochrane Shanks, the late Miss May Simson, the late Miss Lena Yovitch-itch, the late Miss Geraldine Hedges, and the late Sir Harold Nicolson are no longer alive to receive the small tribute of my thanks.

For permission to quote from published sources I must thank the following: the late Lieutenant-Colonel F. C. C. Balfour, C.I.E., C.V.O., C.B.E., M.C., for *Dr Elsie Inglis* by Lady Frances Balfour; Messrs. Collins, for *Paper Boats* by E. M. Butler; the Proprietors of the *Guardian,* and Mr Arthur Johnson, for an extract from an article; Mrs A. S. Strachey and Chatto and Windus Ltd., for *Eminent Victorians* by Lytton Strachey; Lieutenant-General Sir Thomas Hutton, K.C.I.E., C.B., M.C., for *With a Women's Unit in Serbia, Salonika and Sebastopol* by I. Emslie Hutton; and Messrs. John Murray Ltd., for *With the Scottish Nurses in Rumania* by Yvonne Fitzroy.

My dear Laurence Thompson not only helped with characteristic patience and insight in innumerable practical ways, great and small, but throughout has given infinitely generously of enthusiasm and encouragement, without which I should not have undertaken or completed this book, and for which I can never be sufficiently grateful to him.

A note on the spelling of Serbian, Russian and Roumanian proper names:

To the expected difficulties of a writer trying to render in English nouns normally written in Cyrillic script, has been added in this case the fact that much of the manuscript material upon which this book is based was written by women totally unfamiliar with the Slavonic languages who simply spelled every name phonetically and often varied their usage from page to page of a single letter. This was not unusual at the time: in one single edition in 1915 the *Manchester Evening News* spelled Kragujevatz in seven different ways, none of them that which is adopted in this book.

It seemed simplest, therefore, to avoid tampering unnecessarily with the spelling of quoted source material, to adopt the versions most commonly used in the letters and diaries consulted.

This has the twofold advantage that the spelling, being roughly phonetic, will convey to the non-linguist reader the actual sound of the name; and that it approximates to the spellings in earlier published material about Dr Inglis and the Scottish Women's Hospitals.

The principal exception is the name of Dr Curcin: since he later became fairly well known in England I have retained the spelling under which he is most easily recognisable.

This system is an uneasy compromise, but anyone seriously interested in the question of transliteration of proper names should have no real difficulty in knowing how the names should be rendered according to the Cyrillic or Croatian methods of spelling.

SHADOW OF SWORDS

A Biography of Elsie Inglis

CHAPTER 1

All day the retreat went on.

Along the main road, a track by English standards, soldiers of three nations trudged eastwards. Russians, Serbians, Roumanians, disorganised, dirty, dazed from the five-day battle, hunted for their units through villages crowded with refugees. In springless, slow-moving ox carts, the wounded were brought painfully back. The less badly injured struggled along on foot, their field dressings untouched for days, their uniforms filthy and verminous.

In the barrack hospital on the hill, in the little shell-torn town of Megidia, thirty British women worked. They were the only doctors and nurses remaining to help the retreating thousands.

All day they moved their wounded out of the wards; loaded men barely fit to travel into the springless ox carts, *Serbische automobile*[1] the orderlies called them; or, the luckier ones, into the hospital's own Ford ambulances with their English girl drivers, en route for the railway and safety. As fast as the stretcher parties moved men out, more walking wounded struggled in. Everyone knew by now of the help one could rely upon from the English sisters; and that their *doktoritza,* when appealed to by the Russian commander-in-chief the day before, had quietly told him, that of course her party of women would stay where it could be most useful.

It was Saturday, October 21st, 1916. The Battle of the Somme, then in its one hundred and thirteenth day, has, by its enormous scale of pity and terror, blinded western observers to much that was happening elsewhere.

On the Eastern Front, Russia had, in the summer of 1916, taken advantage of Germany's engagement with England and France at Verdun and on the Somme to launch the Brusilov Offensive, a brilliant ten-weeks' campaign, the success of which encouraged neutral Roumania to back what seemed the winning horse and enter the war on the side of the Allies at the end of August.[2]

On September 2nd the Dobruga, that marshy, poverty-stricken tract of Roumanian territory lying between the Danube's south bank and the Black Sea, was invaded by a mixed army of Germans, Bulgarians and Turks. Farther north the Russian steam-roller had run out of steam, and the German Ninth Army was slowly pushing back through the mountains of Transylvania a Roumanian peasant army, stoutly manned but inefficiently officered, and having only nominal support from her great Russian ally.

Also fighting with the Allies on the Eastern Front were two Serbian Divisions and it is their story which concerns us. Recruited from former Austrian subjects of Slav race, taken prisoner by Russia earlier in the war, they now considered themselves and fought as Serbians. With nearly 18,000 men, this was then the largest 'volunteer army' known,[3] its creation in March 1916 having preceded by several months that of the better-publicised Czech Divisions in Russia.

To one of these Serbian Divisions was attached a Scottish Women's Hospital Unit of seventy-six women doctors, nurses, drivers and orderlies, commanded by a woman, Dr Elsie Maud Inglis. The melting pot of war had brought together two small but electric forces in improbable alliance: the tough and virile soldiers of resurgent Serbian nationalism, and the insular, British, unfeminine and determinedly practical representatives of the women's suffrage campaign.

Elsie Inglis, whose destiny it was to be the catalyst of these wildly dissimilar forces, was at this time fifty-two years old. Small and ramrod straight, she was impeccable with the neatness of a self-discipline both physical and mental. Her wispy hair, the colour of an autumn leaf, was smooth-combed almost despite itself, her eyes were the blue grey of an autumn bonfire that seems to be dying yet may at any moment crackle into blazing, all-consuming life; her slight, skinny figure was tense, animated with that vitality which is stoked only by the fires of the spirit. Indeed, she knew herself at this moment to be a dying woman. A martinet to her staff, a mother to her patients, to those who risked opposing her on low or selfish grounds Elsie Inglis was a mysterious force which somehow, strangely, inevitably, ruthlessly, bore down all their resistance.[4]

A Victorian born and bred, rigidly dutiful, un-intellectual; no more artistic than the run of her fellow countrymen, and as inarticulate as the best of them about her own deeper feelings; rigidly principled to a point that would have been well the far side of priggishness had it not been for a certain remarkable quality of selflessness that accompanied her disciplined views, Elsie Inglis in her own words was 'British and muddle-headed and insular',[5] an 'old maid who could not stand dirt and muddle'.[6] In the words of one of her staff, she was 'will power incarnate'.[7]

Temperamentally a fighter, her inclination to the unconventional had led her as a young woman to adopt a career in medicine, then only recently open to girls. In her twenties she had brought about the founding of a medical school for women, in her thirties she had opened a hospital of her own. Twenty years of general practice in the Edinburgh slums had tempered her spirit to steel; ten years of stumping the country as a women's suffrage leader had won her hundreds of personal adherents who would follow without question where she led.

When war broke out in 1914, nothing had been farther from Elsie Inglis's thoughts than that she would devote the rest of her life to a small nation in Eastern Europe. She was the average patriotic British person; and the average Briton of the day hardly knew where Serbia *was*, even though he might know that, by getting herself invaded by Austria, Serbia had changed the course of his own life. Elsie Inglis had had one idea when she founded the Scottish Women's Hospitals for service in the war: to show that women could give service to the nation, which would prove them worthy of the vote.

By 1916 her hospitals were serving in France, in the Mediterranean, and on the Eastern Front. They were drawing support and personnel from all over Britain. So the Serbians and Russians who limped painfully in to the little hospital at Megidia in the Dobruga, and to whom Scotland even more than England was a faraway country of which they knew nothing, were not so wrong in labelling these puzzling, brisk creatures, whose womanly compassion took such an *unfeminine* form, the 'English sisters'.[8]

Dr Inglis and her staff had sailed to join the 1st Serbian Division in Russia—whose only hospital they would be—at the end of August 1916. While they were en route, the Division had been assigned to a central part of the line in Roumania by the Russian War Minister, Alexeyev, who hated the Roumanian alliance and determined to waste no Russian life for it.[9] Left unsupported by the collapse of the Roumanians and the withdrawal of the

Russians, the Serbs fought on alone. The immense natural courage of their nation, praised by every military writer without exception, was on this occasion reinforced by the certainty of atrocities if captured by Turks and Bulgars, and the knowledge that the more legalistic Germans would spare scant sympathy for any prisoners who turned out to be Austrian subjects fighting for the other side; and when after twenty-four hours the Serbian Division was withdrawn, out of fifteen thousand men who had gone into battle, four thousand remained.[10] 'No one can imagine what the condition of the Serbs was after that battle,' said the British Consul at Galatz in Roumania. He had never, he added, been so thankful for anything in his life as for the arrival of Dr Elsie Inglis and her hospital.[11]

When she arrived on October 1st at Megidia, the little town at the main road junction of the Dobruga, she found the town partly demolished, still smoking from bombardment and filled with an indescribable desolation.[12] Her first task was to see that the hospital cesspools were empty, her second to organise the cleaning of the barracks inside, for they were filthy. Her Unit, most of them well-bred and well-connected young ladies totally unaccustomed to such work, scrubbed hard and cheerfully for the best part of two days.[13] Some 'gorgeous brigands' of Serbian orderlies arrived to help with the whitewashing, and by the evening of the third day the ground floor ward looked 'lovely' to the girls.[14] It was without beds, having only straw mattresses on the floor and, for furniture, packing cases draped in sheets. The boilers, sterilisers and disinfectors which they had brought with them were working, however, and there was a tiny operating theatre. The Serbian commander was lavish with compliments, but, 'It was not really up to our standard, begun in such a scramble and carried on in such a rush,' was Dr Inglis's own dry assessment.[15]

The rush indeed began at once. At 7.30 a.m. on October 4th the first patients arrived and there was no let up till well past midnight. Between wounds and filth the men's condition beggared description and they were pouring back in hundreds.

In the neat ward, mattresses were pushed ever closer to make room for more patients. The weather was warm, and flies, dirt, the crawling uniforms and the smell of sepsis made a background to the groans, or the more terrible silences, of the men. In the Russian military hospital next door, things were even worse, and the dead sometimes lay side by side with the living for hours. But among the English nurses training triumphed; every man—if he lived long enough—was washed and his wounds were dressed.[16]

The nights were fine, and almost at once Dr Inglis got tents put up for the staff, to make more room for the wounded. There was talk of permanent winter quarters, for an Allied offensive was planned, and reinforcements were streaming up to the front past the hospital doors. Each evening its large sheds filled with men fallen out for the night, while others pitched tiny tents, their camp fires twinkling through the dark. By mid-October the hospital was running smoothly. By now, however, air raids had begun, with anything up to twelve machines taking part.* Fires were lit round the town to make a smoke screen; in one raid two soldiers were killed in the Scottish Women's Hospital yard, and an orderly wounded. Sickness and diarrhoea among the staff added to the difficulties, for it was impossible to keep dust and flies off food; and cholera was rampant in the town—on October 15th one victim was buried in lime just below the hospital grounds.[17]

On October 6th Dr Elsie Inglis sent her chief assistant, Dr Lilian Chesney, a determined woman who could be trusted with any task however formidable, to form a casualty clearing station near the front line, with twelve nurses and girl orderlies. The hospital's motor transport, under the Hon. Mrs Haverfield, had already gone out there to bring back the wounded. 'It has', Elsie Inglis wrote, 'done magnificent work . . . They were out at all hours, never too tired to turn out, always gentle and careful and always cheerful.'[18] Bringing in the wounded, especially by night, in strange country and over the truly appalling roads which seem to have been one of the Turks' chief legacies to any country which had once been under their domination was, as one girl said, 'no joke'. 'It is no wonder England is a great nation, if the women are like that,' a Roumanian official told the *Daily News* correspondent, the young Arthur Ransome.[19]

In mid-October there was a lull in the fighting and Dr Inglis seized the chance to improve her hospital; now even she was

* Germany sent a few first-class aeroplanes to every side show, mainly for reconnaissance but small bombs were also dropped over the side. A 70 h.p. engine gave a speed of 70 m.p.h. Successes were obtained mainly because the opposition was poor.

almost satisfied, she said. 'I hardly like to mention names where everyone did so well,' she wrote on October 25th. 'The theatre and dressing room were nearly perfect . . . and the wards, kitchen and laundry all running well. But I must mention Miss Lewis who was in charge of the uniforms and who stuck to her dirty work with indomitable spirit and organised it so well.'[20] The strongest, indeed, will always be wanted at the washtub.

Elsie Inglis was not long to enjoy this modest satisfaction. On October 17th Mrs Haverfield's cars and Dr Chesney's little field hospital fell back half way to Megidia. It was Dr Inglis's first indication that things were serious, and she began to be anxious about moving her forty-five tons of equipment if a retreat were ordered. But another rush of wounded forced her to put her anxiety aside. As fast as patients could be moved to the rear, more were brought in to the hospital, and two days later she learned that the 1st Serbian Division had been so badly cut up that it was to withdraw beyond the Danube to re-form.

'It was terrible to have those broken men pouring in,' she wrote. 'One of the saddest things was a Serb boy brought in and laid in the hall until there was room for him in the bath-room. I roused him looking to see where his wound was, and he half opened his eyes and murmured "Serbie, Serbie". He died a few hours afterwards, without ever quite gaining consciousness, for Serbia.'

Four officers among the wounded told her they believed Russia would not mind, would even be glad, if Serbia were wiped out. 'Their despair was dreadful,' she wrote. ' "You can save Serbia," one of them said, "but what about the Serbian nation?" Their Division had gone into action so gallantly and so hopefully and only a wreck was left. My German wasn't good enough to even try and comfort them so I could only sympathise. They do love their country so.'[21]

By Friday, October 20th, it was clear things were desperate; but even after a despatch rider brought orders from Col. Hadjitch, commanding the Serbian Division, to remove her equipment by train to Galatz, seventy-five miles to the rear, she spent almost all that day admitting new patients and evacuating others. On the following day, in their spare moments, the women began to pack the equipment, according to a plan Dr Inglis had drawn up in anticipation of just such an emergency. By early afternoon all was ready. But the sixty carts promised her by the Russians to get her equipment away had not arrived; the Serbians produced five and with these and the hospital's own motor transport, clearing to the station began. An hour later an urgent message arrived from Mrs Haverfield with the ambulances: she needed every vehicle to move wounded men from the battle area.

Dr Inglis sent out everything but one ambulance and the Studebaker which served her as a staff car. She made several stormy raids on Russian headquarters before, at ten that evening, the carts materialised, and along unlit roads the moving of equipment could begin again. The vehicles were rickety, the tracks rough and crowded. The blackness was lit only by the incessant flash of guns and an occasional flare of weird green light from a rocket. Carts overturned in the road and had to be re-loaded. Few of the women thought it even worth while to bother Dr Inglis with their problems; they knew by now that she never cared *how* a job was accomplished, so long as it *was* accomplished. One girl who went to her with a tale of woe got no sympathy, only a firm 'That's right, dear child, *stick* to the equipment.'[22]

Stick to the equipment. If some Serb doctors, more used to the rudimentary hospitals of their own still-primitive land, thought the Scottish Women's Hospital unnecessarily comfortable, luxurious even, with its sheets, sterilisers, modern instruments and anaesthetics,[23] Dr Elsie Inglis knew that the most devoted doctors and nurses were helpless without good tools. Her hospitals always had superb equipment; and nothing, even in the most headlong retreat, was allowed to justify the loss of one single box of hypodermic needles, case of drugs, or motor ambulance spares. A murmured 'stick to the equipment' can even today raise a reminiscent smile on the faces of old ladies who were spirited girls in the days of the Dobruga Retreat.

By three next morning all was finished, and the tons of equipment safely aboard a train due to leave at seven. Elsie Inglis made one final trip to the station to see the commandant. The place was crowded with refugee families fleeing before the enemy with their boxes, their bundles and their children. On a step, oblivious of its hardness, a child slept. Against the wall farther along, lay a row of exhausted soldiers. A doctor in a white overall snatched a few minutes' sleep on a hard wood bench during a lull of work at the station dressing-room. Everyone was dropping with fatigue.

A Roumanian officer approached her. He had, he said politely by way of introduction, once been in Scotland. Yes, in Glasgow. He knew something of English customs.

At his words, nostalgia flooded the doctor's mind. The English customs—hot water for baths, breakfasts coming regularly, clean clothes, everything in order and as it should be ... and as it had *not* been since she had landed at Archangel those six weeks before that seemed like as many years.

Homesickness was not a word, nor an emotion, that Elsie Inglis allowed herself to recognise. All the same, it was *something* to her to reflect that somewhere in this world, civilisation and sanity still held sway. 'It was probably absurd', she wrote later, 'but it came like a great wave of comfort to feel that England was there, quiet and strong and invincible behind everything and everybody.' Returning to her deserted hospital on its deserted hill, she found there a fresh problem. It was now clear that nobody could remain at Megidia long. Keeping seventeen, the minimum nucleus of a small hospital in any emergency, she sent everyone else to the station. They must go with the equipment back to Galatz. She and the seventeen would take their chance of getting away by road and work with the Army as they went, setting up temporary little field hospitals wherever they found themselves.

She had little or no sleep that night, for at 4.30 a.m. the Unit was aroused from where they had dropped asleep on straw palliasses in the empty ward. Hardly a chimney smoked in Megidia, and the town, shrouded in the blue morning mist from the marshes, was silent but for the sound of guns. The steppe seemed to stretch away endlessly as a flaming sunrise gave way to the cool late October daylight. The barracks behind the hospital which a few days earlier had teemed with soldiers, dogs, pigs and cattle in characteristically Russian confusion, were now deserted. The Russians had slipped quietly away, saving themselves, giving no notice to Dr Inglis.[25]

The ancient earthwork of Trajan's Wall, bulwark once against barbarism, stretched across the steppe from horizon to horizon two hundred yards from the hospital door. Some of the women may have reflected that barbarity appeared now to have won the day—but probably few did, for introspective spirits were unwelcome as recruits for the Scottish Women's Hospitals, and a university education was positively frowned upon. 'Hard-working, conscientious, good-tempered, plucky, cheerful and the better bred they are the better they stand roughing it' was Elsie Inglis's own recipe for recruits.[26] Like Miss Nightingale before her, she had found that only ladies are truly reliable in the nastiest situations. One of the girls at Megidia was daughter of the Clerk to the Privy Council. The Hon. Mrs Haverfield, who ran the transport, was the daughter of the 3rd Lord Abinger, a woman equally well known in the suffrage movement and in the hunting field, who had organised a horses' rescue camp in the Boer War, as well as horse-caravan speaking tours for the suffrage cause.[27]

True, one girl orderly *had* taught in North London, and another sung in the D'Oyly Carte chorus, but they were exceptions; apart from the trained nurses, most younger volunteers had done no paid work in their lives.[28] A spirited, energetic, confident bunch, they had a sanguine vitality and courage, fruit of the long, secure, Victorian golden age into which they had been born.

Left in Megidia on this Sunday they were all exhausted; but there was that stillness, that freedom from responsibility which, as an oasis in horror, can be strangely delightful. The train party was believed to be on its way to safety (in fact the train did not leave for several hours more, and then only after two of the women had frustrated a most determined effort by station staff to 'lose' the valuable equipment vans).[29] There were no patients left. For the moment, Dr Inglis and her Unit were responsible for no one but themselves.

In mid-morning Dr Kostitchi, their Serbian liaison officer, arrived; he had only just discovered, to his dismay, that they were still in the town—who could have thought that women would not have fled, terrified, long before?—and he brought orders that they must leave at once. The enemy was expected hourly.

Only the staff car and an ambulance remained for them. However, Kostitchi turned out to be (as did a truly surprising number of people who had the advantage of contact with Dr Inglis) 'the kind of man who gets things done'.[30] He procured her a lorry from a Russian air squadron; the last bits of equipment were loaded amid gathering rain clouds. Kostitchi, now extremely alarmed, constantly urged speed upon them. The Bulgarians, he said excitedly, were as good as in the town already. Dr Inglis, unmoved, continued to demand the whereabouts of the Ludgate boiler they had brought from England; that, and one case of ambulance spares, were the only things she had eventually to abandon, reluctantly, to the enemy.

The first drops of rain fell, and soon the roads were turning to rivers of mud. *'Cette diable de pluie, la première fois de ma vie que j'ai fait une acte de bienfaisance, la pluie m'empêche,'* grinned the boyish Russian air officer in charge of the lorry; but he could not get away from Elsie Inglis so easily.[31] She would lend him wheel chains, she said promptly (and even in the chaos of the retreat, she did not fail to note later that she had not got them back). By mid-afternoon, the little party was ready: four women with Dr Inglis in the staff car, driven by Miss Onslow whose private car it actually was; five more in the ambulance, and seven perched atop the equipment in the Russian lorry; with Kostitchi in solitary state in his own quaint little horse carriage. At the last moment, one of the women noted, someone arrived 'with a huge open barrel of treacle which could not possibly be left to a German—oh dear, how we laughed'.[32]

They were all making for a village where they could rejoin the Serbian H.Q., but there was confusion over the route and the vehicles soon became separated. The debonair Russian officer had decided anyway that his own headquarters would be safer for the young ladies. He drove there despite their protest. It was to be next day before Elsie found them, sitting by the road laughing and doling out treacle and courage impartially to all who passed.

On the roads, the whole countryside was in retreat. The glow of burning villages lit the darkening sky, and a vaster glow to the east showed the fate of the Black Sea port of Constanza.[33]

'One reads of refugees, but never could one imagine such a sight,' Elsie wrote home four days later. 'The whole road was one continuous stream of carts loaded up with luggage, on which were children. Men and women tramped along beside them. Every now and then there was a regular Roumanian cart with boards stretched across measuring about 10 or 12 feet piled up with household goods. They filled the whole roadway. Against the stream we tried to go, and through it barged cannon and ammunition wagons and squadrons of cavalry; loose foals and dogs ran about everywhere; and when we turned on our headlights the whole thing became unreal, seemed like a well-staged piece at the theatre. At one point we came on a flock of sheep, and for a minute we saw only red lights reflected from ours in their eyes—no sheep at all. One foal got quite mesmerised by our lights and danced about in front of them.'[34]

Progress was slow; often they were halted for half an hour at a time while the yelling mob sorted itself into order. Guns, cavalry, infantry, ambulances, carts and wounded on foot jostled among the peasants.

It was late that night before Dr Inglis reached her destination, having taken six hours for the journey of a little over ten miles. The village, Caromarat, was a scene of confusion and despair; troops, refugees, livestock, mingled in the dark muddy lanes between the houses; the hooting of cars and the noise of frightened animals added to the babel.

A hunt through the village revealed two of the transport women, but none of Dr Inglis's nurses or orderlies, and she began to be exceedingly anxious, remembering one of her best nurses who had been killed during a retreat in Serbia in 1915. Her anxiety increased when she got a message from Kostitchi, two miles away, asking if everyone was safe with her. But the best she could do was to arrange with the Serb adjutant to send two horsemen to look for her girls.[35]

Meanwhile, her own party of five, cold, hungry, weary, was found a room. It was in a mean cottage having, like most in that poverty-stricken district, only a trodden earth floor. Over half the room straw was spread for the women to rest on, and they managed to borrow some blankets. When they inquired for food, however, they were told none was to be had.

Dr Inglis slipped away. What orders she gave, or to whom, none of them ever found out. But almost at once, a party of soldiers arrived bearing bortsch, roast turkey, bread and tea. 'The most beautiful meal I ever ate; it was like a fairy tale,' said one of the women later. 'When Dr Inglis said she must have a thing, she always got it; and it was never for herself, always for others.' Dr Inglis's own recorded comment was characteristic: 'There now, isn't that better than having to start and cook a meal?' It did not seem to cross her mind that the cook might *not* have managed to prepare a meal, even when food was reported unobtainable.[36]

When they had all eaten, and were warm and drowsy, Dr Inglis, still anxious over the missing women, went out to speak to someone at the garden gate.

Standing there, she wrote later, 'I heard those girls' voices laughing and chattering, and I thought there might be something in what a Russian woman said to me *a propos* of the great cheerfulness of the Unit. "There is certainly something great in the British character which the continental nations don't possess" and when I said "I don't know, we all have our strong points and our weak ones" she said "There is no other nation that goes into trouble laughing." '[37]

CHAPTER 2

At the time of the Dobruga Retreat of 1916, Elsie Maud Inglis was already a veteran of war and suffering. In Serbia itself the previous year she had won, in the words of Dame Rebecca West, 'an imperishably glorious name'.*

One year of life was now left to her. It was to be perhaps the most remarkable single year of a woman's life in this century. The officers who had said despairingly, 'You may save Serbia, but what about the Serbian nation?' had underestimated her. If her personal weight was slight, it was to be the straw that turned the scales of destiny for close on twenty thousand men; men who one year later, in Franchet d'Esperey's brilliant Balkan campaign, 'went through the opposition like a scythe through grass.... It was a marvellous victory. One must doubt whether any leader or any troops other than Franchet d'Esperey and the Serbians who played the major part could have won it.'[1] The influence of Elsie Inglis was certainly decisive in bringing those Serbians to d'Esperey's command. Personally negligible she might, indeed, be; a mere doctor in a field hospital, a mere woman at that. But at a critical moment in its history, she determined the fate of a nation.

The final years of Elsie Inglis's life were passed with the guns of the Great War sounding the knell of the old secure order of society. The epoch into which she was born, on August 16th, 1864, at Naini Tal in the Himalayan foothills, found that old order at its securest and, briefly, at its best. It was the brilliant morning of the British Raj in India, of an order unique in history for its combination of personal authority and privilege with devotion to an ideal of trusteeship and service for others; of ingrained allegiance to strong religious tradition combined with all the assurance to be drawn from the certainty of one's importance in the world. This was the life, the memory of which could even after fifty years still warm the heart of one of its children, on a night of chaos, danger and near-anarchy in Eastern Europe, with the

* Rebecca West, *Black Lamb and Grey Falcon.*

thought that 'England was there'; that could breed a nation of such confident souls that even its womenfolk faced trouble laughing.

The Inglis family had a tradition of service and achievement in India. Both Elsie's grandfathers had held important posts in the East India Company; a great-grandfather was secretary to Warren Hastings. John Inglis, Elsie's father, had gone to Calcutta from Haileybury in 1840 with his way to make, and at his marriage in 1846 was an assistant magistrate on £500 a year and described as 'active, energetic, conciliating to natives, fine-tempered and thoroughly honest ... as good a man as you can have'.[2]

His wife matched him. Harriet Thompson had arrived the year before, aged 17, in Bengal, where her father George Thompson, also of the East India Company, was famous in hunting circles as a man with 'nerve enough for anything.... He never stopped to calculate the chances of a fall.... I can safely say I never saw his heart fail for an instant,' to quote the *Bengal Sporting Magazine* of 1834. Harriet inherited his courage, and passed it to her children. She herself shrank from nothing life faced her with: the adventures of camp life in tiger-infested jungles that were part of Indian official routine; the nine pregnancies in days when each birth was a confrontation with death; or worst of all perhaps to a woman of loving temper, the prolonged separations in family life that service in India then involved.[3]

Unusual in a girl of beauty and charm, for the chance of a dance with whom young men would drive fifty miles, Harriet Thompson's outstanding characteristic was a strong religious faith. It was the real affinity between her and John Inglis, whose family had a similar tradition; in all their doings, the dynamic was always practical religion. John Inglis was, like many of his contemporaries in India, an avowed man of God, dedicated to the uplift of the Indian peoples and with Britain sincerely seen as the chosen instrument of God's purpose.[4] He was a subordinate and devoted disciple of the 'great proconsul', the 'saviour of India', John Lawrence; and had shared, during his early years, in 'the most successful experiment in the art of civilising turbulent millions which history presents'.[5]

When the Mutiny broke out in 1857, the Inglises were on the way to England with their five children and the hope of a long furlough. Harriet was pregnant and, even with a devoted ayah, the four months' trek to Bombay in relays of hired bullock wagons, followed by four months in a sailing ship, must have been arduous for her. The voyage was round the Cape, for though a canal through Suez was under discussion, another twelve years were to pass before it would be open—and tip the balance in favour of the development of steam navigation.

At Southampton, the Inglises learned of the Mutiny and that John was recalled. He stayed only to see Harriet safely through her confinement and the family settled.[6] The subsequent separation, during the earlier part of which Harriet must have suffered great anxiety for her husband's safety, was to last seven years.

When the reunion came, it was at the cost of prolonged separation between Harriet and her children. The eldest three were at Eton, another at Uppingham; the girl Amy, with whom Harriet had a particular bond, was left in England with relations, as was the youngest child, Ernest.[7] Letters took months to travel; there was no possibility of personal meetings.

It was in these circumstances that a girl was born on August 16th, 1864, the first child of her parents' reunion after years of separation, danger and difficulty. Christened, in the fashion for Anglo-Saxon names set by Tennyson and endorsed by the age's confident sense of national identity, Elsie Maud, she was an attractive baby with a ready laugh, an intelligence lively rather than profound, and a strong will of her own modified by an equable temper of mind.[8] Two further children, Eva and Horace, were born, but from the beginning, Elsie, so like himself, so much a symbol of a hopeful new era in his own life, had a special place in her father's heart. Harriet was a dutiful and affectionate mother, but a large part of *her* heart had been left behind in England.[9]

Elsie's was a sunny, happy childhood, spent at first at Allahabad and Naini Tal, later in Calcutta, Lucknow and Simla. She was her father's constant companion when he was at home; when duties took him away, they corresponded daily from the time she was about eleven. Some of his letters have been preserved, letters full of affectionate homely banter—'How are you all after mulligatawny for tea? I never heard of such a thing'—and plans for picnics and outings on his return.[10] As she grew, serious topics were discussed: politics, religion, advice on difficult situations. Until his death when she was twenty-nine Elsie Inglis was in daily sympathetic communication with one of the most gifted and industrious administrators of a period unrivalled in its opportunities for the development of such talents. Whatever her own gifts, they received direction and nourishment from him.

As eldest of the 'second family' she was the recognised leader in nursery and schoolroom with the small privileges and responsibilities of the oldest. She it was who organised nursery games, who was expected to set an example of keeping awake in church,[11] who was charged with seeing that all the children supervised the native syces who cared for their ponies.[12] She had much to live up to, but seems to have been a conscientious child perfectly content to do those things she ought to do and exclude from her mind all those things she ought not to do.

Life, whether at Bareilly, Calcutta, Lucknow, or the bungalow 'Snow View' in Naini Tal, the beautiful hill station which was the summer seat of government for the United Provinces, was full of hope, purpose and happiness. In 1858 the British Crown had replaced the Company as governors of India and John Inglis's career in what was now the Indian Civil Service advanced steadily. The whole family moved easily in exalted circles, filled with their personal friends. The Foreign Secretary of India, Sir William Muir, sent the boy Horace a sailing-boat for his birthday; at eleven Elsie was embroidering, with her sister, slippers for the Commander-in-Chief of the Army, Lord Napier of Magdala, and receiving his lordship's affectionate thanks for them and for 'your pretty little note which is so well written'.[13]

Not for these children the segregation and relegation to the care of servants (there was a staff of thirty for the Inglis household) which often fell to children of officials. Even at her writing table, soon after Elsie's birth, Harriet insisted upon having the cradle beside her, and later the child was not banished to a nursery but given a corner for her playthings in the drawing-room. At home the distinguished administrator became the adored papa, tucking up nine dolls for the night, mixing the children's cocoa in 'exactly equal shares', planning surprise parcels for birthdays, helping the children pick flowers for Harriet's breakfast table.[14]

As they grew, Elsie, Eva and Horace had to learn to say 'Amy' and be told of the other family at home in England, while Amy at home worked baby dresses and later doll's clothes for the little sisters in India.[15] When Elsie was four, Amy travelled to India to be married to Robert Simson of H.M. Bengal Service* and the little sisters were bridesmaids;[16] and in 1871 we find Elsie writing in a large round hand to Amy, 'Thursday will be your birthday, so we are to have a holiday and children's party next week ... Papa says you will be 43. I know he means 23. When is Robert's birthday? We wish to have a party.'[17] At seven she was already adept at finding cogent reasons to do the thing she had determined upon.

The life surrounding and nourishing the Inglis children was at once opulent yet simple, privileged yet inescapably dedicated to service. It was a time when the even balance of world forces freed Englishmen for a few brief decades from considerations of security and enabled them to give rein to that native strain of often inarticulate idealism and service which viewed from outside can be so easily mistaken for mere hypocrisy. It was a life which fostered in Elsie from her earliest years a supreme self-confidence which was never later to fail her; just as the outlook to the majestic eternal snows gave the young girl a vision of nobility which was to shape for ever her attitude to the things of the spirit.

Holiday or not, almost every day at Naini Tal, 6,000 feet up in the hills, was happy. Around the small placid lake with its picturesque temple, wooded slopes rise another 2,000 feet, colourful with exotic flowers and rich in rare wild life. Every day he was at home there was a morning walk with Papa, who would have been at his desk since five. Shortly before seven, the children were dressed and taken to Harriet for prayers and a Bible reading. Then to the verandah with its view to the mountains. 'Father made three cups of cocoa, one for each of us, and then the glorious walk!' recalled Eva in after years. 'Three ponies followed behind, each with their attendant grooms, and two or three red-coated *chaprasis*, father stopping all along the road to talk to every native who wished to speak to him, while we three ran about, laughing and interested in everything. Then at night, the shouting for him after we were in bed and Father's step bounding up the stair in Calcutta or coming along the matted floor of our hill home. All order and quietness was flung to the winds while he said goodnight to us.

'It was always understood that Elsie and he were special chums, but that never made any jealousy. Father was always just! ... We

* Their son, Sir Henry J. F. Simson, was one of the doctors in charge at the birth of H.M. Queen Elizabeth II.

got equal shares of his right and his left hand in our walks, but Elsie and he were comrades, inseparables from the day of her birth.'[18]

The morning walks had a serious function, that of making Inglis Sahib informally available to the people he governed. In pursuance of Lawrence's ideal of India as a country 'thickly cultivated by a fat contented yeomanry, each man riding his own horse, sitting under his own fig tree and enjoying his rude family comforts',[19] John Inglis developed many schemes. One was to improve livestock breeding by an annual Agricultural Show. The natives, Harriet wrote, could not understand being rewarded with money *and* being allowed to take their animals away. They must have been equally puzzled at the second show, when John Inglis took the opportunity to address them on the subjects of Infanticide and Female Education.[20] A more receptive hearer on this last, one may suppose, was his daughter Elsie.

Elsie's own education was that of girls of her class and era. English, especially the Bible, Prayer Book, and Shakespeare, came into the normal activities and recreations of family life. For schoolroom work, there was a governess. 'Elsie is getting on very well; it comes easy enough to her to learn,' wrote her mother at first; but when Eva, two years younger, joined the lessons, Harriet modified her opinion. Elsie, she saw then, was 'very plodding and persevering over her studies and so keeps quite in advance of Eva notwithstanding the latter's extra quickness'. But Eva was 'sure to be the inventor of some piece of mischief', while Elsie, though 'a very cheery and happy child' liked 'quiet play by herself more'.[21]

The children's religious instruction was handled by Harriet, whose outlook is expressed in a letter to Amy, written when Herbert, one of those left in England, was ill.

'It is at such times of trouble that one feels not only the need, but the nearness, of the Lord, His loving kindness and his truth. One of the texts I have been thinking over lately is "the eyes of the Lord thy God are always upon thee from the beginning of the year even unto the ending of the year". And thinking of it in connection with God as a loving Father, what an amount of comfort we may draw from it. The eyes of our Covenant God and Father watching over us for good, succouring in time of temptation, strengthening in time of weakness and comforting in time of sorrow and trial. Take God in Christ as your Covenant

God, dear Amy, whether in times of rejoicing or sorrow, and then you need fear nothing, for God keeps all His saints as the apple of His eye.'[22]

This religious philosophy Elsie absorbed and carried with her, only a little modified, to the end of her life.

Did the child, this early, fix her sights upon a medical career? Years later, someone recalled that she had once organised an epidemic among the doll family and insisted upon playing the doctor herself. But all children sublimate their fears in such games. Had Elsie expressed any serious idea of becoming a doctor, John and Harriet would have been bound to tell her that no means existed for a woman to do this.

In the year after Elsie's birth, Miss Elizabeth Garrett had qualified as a doctor in England; but after that, medical prejudice effectively blocked the way and twelve years of bitter struggle were needed to open it again.

This struggle must have been discussed in the Inglis family circle, for agitation was growing in India for the medical education of native women.[23] No Indian woman could consult a male doctor, and circuitous methods of passing information and advice through the old women and old men of the patient's family had to be resorted to. It was a convention imposing fearful preventable suffering upon Britain's Indian subjects. The situation was similar, if less acute, in Britain itself, especially in Catholic, prudish Ireland. Not all medical men were of refined character. Even the Queen was not protected by her position: on July 11th, 1860, she wrote to her daughter on the subject of childbirth: 'What suffering—what humiliation to the delicate feelings of a poor woman, above all a young one—especially with those nasty doctors.'[24] Thousands of Victoria's subjects endured a lifetime of pain rather than risk an encounter with a nasty doctor.

The question of women as doctors had been precipitated by the Medical Act of 1858 requiring practitioners to be registered, which, by leaving the administration of the provisions to existing professional bodies, had quite unintentionally left medicine virtually a male monopoly. After Elizabeth Garrett's success a blanket of prejudice had descended, so that when in 1869 Sophia Jex-Blake decided to study medicine she had first had to fight an eight-year battle against vested interests, entrenched opinion, the universities, the law and a section of the press.[25]

The would-be medical women had allies in other sections of

the 'women's movement'. Moreover, neither Government nor opposition wished to exclude women as doctors; while the ordinary prudish Victorian husband and father, though probably disapproving of votes for women or higher education for women, did agree that medical attention should be available from one of their own sex. A Bill to allow women to qualify became law in August 1876, when Elsie Inglis was twelve.

Some of this she must have heard discussed in far away Naini Tal. Was it now that her aggressively courageous temperament first felt the attraction of a life in medicine? Could there have been any premonition that the great ones of the struggle, Miss Jex-Blake, Mrs Garrett Anderson, would one day be her own teachers? It seems possible.

All this, however, lay in the future. In the meantime there was the serene untroubled childhood, with Papa a great man and likely to be a greater. By 1875 he was Chief Commissioner of Oudh and was being spoken of as the probable next Lieutenant-Governor of the United Provinces.[26] Life for the children was dominated by love, religion, duty; set amid a happy household and—for seven of Harriet's eight sisters had married into the I.C.S.[27]—a wide circle of relations and friends all full of the overflowing vitality and enthusiasm for well-doing of the mid-Victorians.

Some of the atmosphere of this life, which lingered to illuminate the entire lives of those who shared it, is reflected in a simple little letter of old Sona, the ayah who in 1857 had made the long journey to England with Harriet, had become a Christian through her influence, and with her husband and sons had served the family for over thirty years. When they left India she was given a pension and placed with missionaries and years later, on May 5th, 1883, Sona wrote to Elsie, then nineteen.

> My dear Missibaba, I got your dear letter and it made my old heart very happy to hear from you again. It makes me very proud to think that the little baby I held in my arms is a young lady now and that she does not forget her old nurse but writes her such beautiful letters. Give my love and salaam to Evababa and believe that I love and thank you both for writing to me and telling me all about your schools and holidays and everything. If Horacebaba still wants to be a carpenter tell him to learn to make ships and he will get very rich and then he can

come on one of them and see me.

I am not strong and never very well, for I am growing very old now, but my heart is glad for I know my Saviour will take me to heaven. He gives me great peace now. Your loving nurse, Sona.[28]

In 1876 the shadow of swords fell for the first time over this life and its hopes for the future. The gradual crumbling of the Turkish Empire was leaving a growing power vacuum at which Russia was directing thoughtful glances. Lawrence's 'close border' and 'buffer state' policies had been criticised even before his own term of office ended in 1869,[29] and British policy in India entered an even more strongly imperialist phase with the appointment, in November 1875, of Lord Lytton as Governor-General. His instructions were to clarify, peacefully if possible, but otherwise by any suitable means, the situation vis-à-vis Afghanistan, where Shere Ali was showing a regrettable tendency to entertain Russian overtures.

John Inglis had all along believed with Lawrence that the first duty of Englishmen in India was to the native peoples. He was opposed to the new and tough imperialist line, and it lost him both position and recognition. He was passed over for the expected promotion to Lieutenant-Governor, and Lytton's letter to the Secretary of State for India, Lord Salisbury, was diplomatic but uncompromising. 'I have met with much valuable assistance from Mr Inglis.... Of his character and abilities I have formed so high an opinion that had there been an available vacancy I should have been glad to secure to my government his continued services.'[30]

John Inglis was still only fifty-six. He had been toiling unremittingly in India for thirty-six years, but there was now no future for him there. He decided to retire and live in Edinburgh where Amy and her husband were planning to settle. Not least of the attractions of the scheme must have been the fact that good day schools were by now becoming socially acceptable in Britain for girls of the middle classes. Edinburgh had several. That Female Education whose desirability he had impressed upon the Indians would be available to his own girls. Elsie and Eva should go to school.

CHAPTER 3

Before returning to Britain, one responsibility remained to John Inglis: the setting up in life of his sons Hugh and Cecil.

Most families, in those days of large families, had their less satisfactory members. Hugh and Cecil had never been satisfactory. In the letter home announcing Elsie's birth, John Inglis had inquired in exasperation when Hugh meant to get into the upper school. 'If he delays taking his remove much longer, I shall begin to think he is of the opinion held by some members of the Public Schools Commission, that the only things learnt at Eton are cricket and football.'[1] Cecil was at Uppingham and the letters of his and Hugh's that have survived show they must both have left school virtually illiterate.

The Australian colonies offered a happy solution to such problems. (Newson Garrett, the elder brother of Elizabeth Garrett, was another; he was shipped off to New South Wales.[2]) In particular, under-populated Tasmania had golden opportunities for a hard-working man. Thither in 1876 went the Inglis family.

To the younger children, knowing only the teeming life, ancient cities, obsequious service and rigid social structures of India, Tasmania must have seemed another universe. In place of the large Indian homes with huge staffs, there was Prospect Lodge, Davie Street, in the pleasant little early nineteenth-century town of Hobart; a house small by Inglis standards and so cramped that large items of furniture could not be got upstairs without dismantling.

Money was tighter. When the children were taken to a bootmaker to be measured, the man complimented John Inglis: 'Happy is the man who has a host of them.' Harriet said later with asperity that he should have added 'Lucky is the bootmaker that he brings them to.'[3]

Hugh and Cecil were difficult. Two years were needed before the parents could depart feeling all was well. And Hugh at least was rebellious against the warm family feeling. When the younger ones coaxed him into writing, unwillingly, to Amy he complied, then threw the letter on the fire. 'Is not he naughty?' asked Eva.[4]

For Elsie and the little ones, however, life was still full of laughter, optimism, enthusiasm. Papa was still a Personage, attending the opening of Parliament,[5] presenting prizes at the Cascade School on the famous model workers' estate, to which the whole family went as guests of honour.[6] There were still romps and fun, and if Eva and Elsie had outgrown dolls, they were not too dignified to grab Horace's school prize and read it before he could, or to watch with interest his regattas with the model boats he rigged himself, for which Elsie sewed him flags.[7]

There were neighbouring children to play with and to join in outings to the Botanical Gardens; if the cabmen were friendly, races on the way home ('once when we nearly past them Alice Stephen grew so excited that she threw her muff in one of our horses' faces', Eva wrote to Amy.[8]) Elsie's letters to her small Simson nephew are full of such details, simple, happy, mischievous, yet fundamentally *good.*

Above all, there was school. Only in two Tasmanian cities, Hobart and Launceston, was there in the 1870s compulsory education or the schools to make it possible. Elsie and Eva were sent to a Miss Knott,[9] who with her sister Miss Fanny had gone out from Cheltenham Ladies College where Dorothea Beale, one of the founding mothers of Female Education, was influencing a whole generation of girls who, becoming teachers themselves, spread her ideals in ever-widening circles.

Miss Knott was trying to carry out in the remote colony the principles and practices of Miss Beale, who believed education would form women into a vast army to serve and uplift society.[10] Family tradition had placed Elsie's feet on the path of service. Miss Knott led her decisively along the same road.

Elsie was studying hard now; industry was insisted upon by her parents and John Inglis was a proud father when Miss Knott, who followed Dorothea Beale's system of personally reading each girl's weekly marks before the whole class,[11] complimented Elsie on her work.[12] She must have been the rewarding pupil every teacher dreams of, for Miss Knott, though daunting to Eva and the little ones,[13] was equally gracious when Elsie approached her for permission to organise a system of school colours, a simple bit of ribbon sewn on a pin but of which the children were inordinately proud.[14]

By 1878 George Inglis, the eldest son, having found the Indian climate unhealthy, had also settled in Tasmania with his wife Louisa. They were at Latrobe and the whole family moved there briefly. Photographs preserved by them show a 'frontier' township with wide, unmade streets, timber houses and shops with hitching-posts, peopled by felt-hatted and shirt-sleeved settlers. It was in this setting that the Etonian Hugh and Uppinghamian Cecil were left when in 1878 the family sailed for England.

As a pendant to the story of their more conventional relations, their subsequent moves have an ironic poignancy. Cecil left Tasmania soon and Hugh a few years later, enticed by tales of fortunes in the mainland goldfields. Such tales were indeed alluring. When J. B. Watson the 'Gold digger King' died in 1889 the *Scotsman* reported he was expected to prove worth thirty million pounds;[15] and he had emigrated from Paisley as a butcher's boy. In 1882 the three Morgan brothers bought for £1 an acre a square mile of land from which gold worth £14 million was later extracted.[16]

The Inglis family were indefatigable correspondents. As long as he lived John Inglis wrote to his sons. But the itinerant prospector could drop from a family's ken. In September 1895 Hugh Inglis wrote from Daviesville, N.S.W., to his brother Herbert then in Ceylon. 'It is the first letter I have had from any of you for the last eight or nine years. I got a few when I first came to Sydney but after I left Sydney I could not get any ... I hope you will write again soon and give me all the news ... I went to Queensland about 12 month after I came to Sydney and was working about Warwick for a long time and then I went up to Gympie. I was there for about 18 months when I got the fever and ague ... I am gald (sic) to say I am getting quite well and strong again. I have been prospecting for gold for some time now, just making enough to keep me in clothes and food. I have been in this paddock since last Xmas but have not found any gold yet ... If I do not get any gold in the next shaft that I put down I shall leave this place. I saw Cecil when I first came to Sydney a few times but lost sight of him again.'[17]

Cecil was in fact then on the other side of Australia, at Norsmen, a small township just opened up in the Coolgardie area where three years earlier a gold nugget of 500 oz. had been found. He wrote to Elsie in the following December:

'There are a great many reefs at work. And new ones been

found every day. I am working with a company of six and we have taken up to claims which I think will turn out all right in time... Food and water are both very dear. I am paying ninepence a gallon at present and I am afraid it will go higher as the summer comes on. Flour is sixpence a pound and meat a shillen. Everything is very high a pound goes on distant ... It is always cool here at night I always wont my blankets. It is not like Qnsland were one cannot bear a sheet on.

'You must let me know who to address you. As a Doctor or what,' he added in a postscript.[18] It was three years after Elsie had qualified.

She must have written again. Not to do so would have been uncharacteristic. But of further correspondence there is no record. At this point Hugh and Cecil vanish into vast unknown Australia. It is an ironic sidelight on the reverse aspect of Victorian opportunity, effort and prosperity.

For one cannot forget that with such as Hugh and Cecil Inglis, nineteenth-century moral toughness only took another character. It was such men, and the sons of such men, the failed Etonians, the non-conforming, crock-of-gold-seeking children of worthy Victorian families who, losing themselves somewhere between goldfields and bush, were to re-emerge a generation later as the fighting men whose stubborn valour and heroic fortitude, endurance and boldness, at Gallipoli and on the Western Front, won for them supreme renown and honour.

The disappointment he must have felt over his sons, and his own blighted career, left the father's attention focused more than ever on Elsie. If she could make something of her life, she would never fail for want of help from him.

Early in 1878 the Inglises sailed for England in the steamship *Durham* which, though not reckoned fast, took five weeks instead of the expected six to get to Suez, and that despite strong headwinds. In the Canal they passed the ship taking Ernest, the son born just before the Mutiny recalled John Inglis to India, to serve in the Indian Army after passing out from Sandhurst. Ernest, whom his father had last seen as a 2-week-old baby, was himself a married man and a father before they met again.[19]

On the *Durham*, while the younger two amused themselves with playmates, Elsie sought an outlet for the ideals of service instilled by Miss Knott. Throughout life she kept the simple uncomplicated outlook which can meet young children at their own level; and in later years liked to say, 'Nothing like sitting on the floor for half an hour playing with little children, to prepare you for a strenuous bit of work.' Now on the *Durham* she nursed children who were sick, helped with the care of a tiny baby, took under an authoritative wing some turbulent small boys who lacked supervision and were making themselves a nuisance to everyone on board, already troubled enough by those strong head-winds.

Even in early youth there was nothing dreamy about Elsie Inglis. She was always practical, ready to tackle the work nearest her hand, however simple. Nearly forty years later, Eva was to write with characteristic perception, 'Leaders are of two kinds, "born leaders" and those whose genius lies along the lines of so facing every circumstance, so using every experience, that their life culminates in that character which must inevitably lead.'[20]

From schooldays in Tasmania and on board the *Durham*, on through her sister's entire life, Eva was watching that development in Elsie.

CHAPTER 4

In Edinburgh, the family took a large house, 10 Bruntsfield Place. Some of its neighbours still remain—ample, elegant villas facing the green of Bruntsfield Links. To the north, in the soft air looking close enough to touch, looms the Castle; behind the houses, the town slopes away to the Forth and the Hills of Fife. The Inglises invariably chose a house with a view.

In Edinburgh for the next thirty-six years, with brief interludes, Elsie Inglis was to pass her days. The influence of the place itself upon a developing character must be great. With its views of hills and sea as a constant reminder of man's terrestrial roots, there is also in this city the strongest sense of order, proportion and form, setting a person firmly in relation to the world and demanding his response to the claims of nature and society. It was surely no accident that Edinburgh saw the most vigorous and concerted demands ever made by women for the right to vocational education, and their confronting by the most vigorous opposition.

When the Inglis family arrived, that question had been settled, thanks to Dr Sophia Jex-Blake. The 'woman problem' was now much more open, and in this same year, 1878, London University opened its degrees to women. To this brave new world, Elsie and Eva Inglis were among thousands of hopeful heiresses.

The Edinburgh Institution for the Education of Young Ladies at 23 Charlotte Square, to which they were sent, was a private school adapting itself to the new ideas, satisfying conventional parents with 'accomplishments' and progressive ones with Latin.[1]

Now in a settled home with the prospect of charting a steady course, Elsie's ambitions could crystallise. Many years later a school-mate, Isabella Thornton, was to write of 'the funny little girl with quantities of straight hair, whose favourite lesson was Latin because she meant to be a doctor. A slightly mad idea we considered it in those dim ages though I have often since envied her her fixed idea. She realised what she wanted to do while she was still a little girl, and never changed her mind.'[2]

A little girl? Elsie, now past fourteen, would by the convention of the period remain a child until she put up her red-gold hair and turned overnight into a woman; the illusion of extreme youth was emphasised by her small stature, the quaint old-fashioned plaits[3] looped at the back of her head, and her round blue-eyed face which, to the end of her life, would light up with a smile of infectious, child-like enthusiasm at any prospect of new worlds to conquer.

She was, however, maturing. She held to her ambition despite being considered slightly mad by her friends. They had justification. The 'lady doctor' was a novelty. In all Edinburgh there was only one, the redoubtable Dr Jex-Blake herself who had settled there in the same year as the Inglis family and, by her immediate success, proved irrefutably the wish of women for a woman doctor.[4]

Elsie must have had pointed out to her the formidable lady, who prided herself upon being the most independent person in Edinburgh.[5] Old enough to be venerable to a schoolgirl, Sophia Jex-Blake was only forty-one when in 1881 she went to live at Bruntsfield Lodge,[6] across the Links from the Inglis home, and was to be seen unconventionally driving her own pony carriage on her rounds. She was always a controversial figure, an ardent and prayerful Christian who spent herself untiringly in the dispensary she opened for the women of the city's own slums,[7] yet offended conventional Edinburgh by her lack of interest in missions to the heathen.

She was the sort of character both to fascinate and repel Elsie. Elsie loved anyone who could fight all out in a good cause; Alice Stephen throwing her muff at the horse's head was an opponent she could admire. But she herself had been trained by her father in more conciliatory methods.

One day at Charlotte Square, the history teacher, drawing a moral from the lives of Clive and Hastings, asked how one should deal with calumny. 'Fight it', 'Deny it', said the class.

'Live it down,' was Elsie's confident, eager response.[8]

She must have discussed with her parents the story of Hastings, since Harriet's grandfather had been his secretary. But there is foreshadowed here a remark made by her years later, after a clash with the military mind over setting up a hospital. 'The traditional male disbelief in our capacity cannot be argued away;

it can only be worked away.'[9] All her life she was to hold the belief that a converted opponent is better than a defeated one; and that nobody is converted by argument alone.

By now her plodding perseverance was beginning to tell. Besides the studies useful for a medical career, besides the slog of 'accomplishments' she made time to edit the school magazine and to found and preside over a Literary and Debating Society discussing topical material from W. T. Stead's *Review of Reviews*.[10] The episode which best illustrates her character, however, was her campaign for outdoor exercise for her schoolfellows.

Charlotte Square is an elegant grouping of Robert Adam houses, all then, except for the school, in private occupation, around a central garden; while ladies living there could take a turn in the garden, or tiny children romp under the eyes of nursemaids, the girls of the Edinburgh Institution were cooped up indoors all day.

The health of studious young ladies was always under serious consideration (opponents of Female Education liked to maintain that Latin and mathematics were mysteriously more harmful to girls than to boys) and Elsie sought leave for them all to play in the gardens. The headmistress expressed sympathy, but said the matter lay with the school directors. She did not offer to approach them. Elsie, undaunted, approached each of them herself.

Mr Oliphant, Mr Edmunds and Mr Lichtenstein, the directors, were also disinclined to court neighbourly disapproval. Why, they assured Elsie, any single householder could veto such a project. They themselves were of course in favour, but ...

Elsie had what she wanted. Now with one companion who alone was willing to support her, she set out; rang every bell in the Square and begged an interview with the householder. Such a canvass was imaginative and courageous at a time when all convention allowed a young lady was to accompany her mama on morning calls.

Her demeanour—bright, determined, but still beyond doubt that of a *lady*—reassured every single householder, or at least made it impossible for them to refuse consent. She returned triumphant, she had carried the day.[11] Now she *knew* what she had always felt: difficulties could always be worked away. They might delay, but could not prevent, the accomplishment of a project; one just had to work at it with enough determination.

So the formal dignified square was enlivened by the laughter of the younger girls, while the older ones walked its paths, discussing, no doubt, among other things, the campaign for women's suffrage now well under way, and what they would do with the vote when they got it. An address by Viscountess Harberton, reported in *Review of Reviews,* had stirred the Literary and Debating Society to excitement.[12] That the vote was almost within their grasp was a common belief among feminists of the day, and one which events seemed to justify. After all, the municipal franchise had been extended to women in 1869; and the Liberals, returned to office in 1880, were swinging to the support of votes for women.

So rational seemed their claim, so inevitable the march of progress, that none of those hopeful children could have foreseen that the atmosphere of mild discussion would turn to bitter controversy and even violence; that they would all be over fifty before casting a vote in a Parliamentary election and that Elsie, the one who inspired them all with faith in woman's destiny, would not herself live to do so.

In 1882, not before her parents had made it the subject of earnest prayer, Elsie departed to Paris, to the finishing establishment of a Miss Gordon Brown, a lady whose religious principles were as estimable as her cultural qualifications. Later, after Elsie had returned home, Miss Gordon Brown was to write to her: 'I cannot tell you how much I felt when you all disappeared ... I cannot at all realise that you are now all separated and that we may never meet again on earth. May we meet often at the throne of grace and remember each other there. It is nice to have a French maid to keep up the conversations, and if you will read French aloud, even to yourself, it is of use.'[13]

In Paris, Elsie did the customary things, admired the view from the Arc de Triomphe, visited Notre Dame, heard distinguished preachers, bought herself a Paris hat (it was the year when hats came 'in' and Victorian bonnets, except for old ladies, went 'out' for good); and shopped for French dolls 'with real hair and moveable limbs' for her nieces. There were visits to art galleries, and drawing lessons. 'Why are you drawing heads, my darling?' asked her father. 'I want you to learn landscape painting. You will find this a great resource and amusement hereafter. There is nothing nicer than having sketches of places you have been at at various times to look at afterwards.'[14] A reminder, this, that until in 1888 the Eastman Company with the first portable roll-film camera brought out-door photography to the amateur, drawing was no mere empty 'accomplishment' but had practical value.

She watched Gambetta's funeral procession in January 1883 from a patisserie in the Rue de Rivoli. 'He is a loss to France, I think,' wrote Harriet to her, voicing the customary Victorian view of Abroad: 'Poor France—she always seems to me like a vessel without a helm, driven about where the winds take her. She has no sound Christian principle to guide her. So different from our highly favoured England.'[15]

There were music and singing lessons. Elsie, who had no ear, expressed sympathy for the neighbouring tenant, favoured with two pianos going six hours a day each.[16] She herself laboriously perfected two pieces 'of the regular arpeggio drawing-room style', pieces which later became a family joke enjoyed by her as much as anyone.[17] She was no musician. When years later, she admired the magnificent peasant singing of Serbs or Russians, its appeal was as an expression of national feeling; *that* was something she could understand.

Nor did she ever acquire mastery of languages; perhaps because she could not afford a French maid to keep up the conversations. But if, years later, she was to regret that her German was inadequate to comfort patients, if her French was only just up to routine dealings with Russian officers, she always could make herself understood when really necessary. (Once, in Roumania, her convoy got hopelessly lost. 'I don't think that man is leading us well. I shall speak to him,' she announced. Ignoring a demure 'In what language, Ma'am?' from her girl orderly, she descended, walked over to the guide and harangued him up hill and down dale—in English. She returned shaking with suppressed laughter. 'I don't know what he understood, but it seems to have had an effect.'[18])

Elsie Inglis, it has been put to the present writer by one who worked with her, was in fact one of those who, spiritual in the widest sense of being open to intangible influences, communicate equally well without words.[19] Years later Professor E. M. Butler, too, was to write of an 'extraordinary power she seemed able to exercise, even at distance, over people and events'.[20]

What was this power? In a letter from Paris which has not survived, Elsie asked her father's opinion of such things. He replied, 'As regards the power of communicating our wishes or thoughts to another person, by the exercise of our will, instanced in the game you played at the other night, I believe that this is possible and can be done under certain circumstances. Though we know nothing of the power exercised or of the manner in which it is put forth ... all these things are hidden from us, wisely no doubt. We know that we are in God's hand, that He cares for us and watches over us; and that we have His promise that all things shall work together for good to those who trust in Him.'[21]

He missed her sadly. 'If by any exertion of our will,' he went on, 'we could know what anyone we loved and who was absent from us, was doing, I think I should see you, my darling, every minute of the day.' She sent him a timetable so that he could follow her in thought. 'I shall think of you enjoying your tapioca soup', and, 'I wish I could see you in your Paris hat and jacket', he wrote. 'I should like to see you at your dancing lessons, especially when you are whirling round the room with that talkative French boy.'[22] He sent her regularly *Punch* and *The Spectator* (which she passed around hoping to convert her schoolmates to Liberalism); and wrote that Eva was knitting a comforter for Mr Gladstone, to be sent to him at Christmas by Harriet's sister, who knew him.

Although John Inglis was only sixty-three and Harriet eight years younger, they had settled into a staid routine of mornings devoted to correspondence with the colonies, afternoons of knitting and reading, a routine varied by family visits and attendance at multifarious mission meetings.

In February 1883 came a small omen. Horace, Harriet wrote, was to play football for Merchiston against Fettes. She wanted to collect a party including the Simson children to attend 'but it seems too much of an undertaking'.[23] Harriet at fifty-five was a tired old lady. It was an ageing and failing mother to whom Elsie returned that summer and for the next year and a half this vigorous young woman marked time.

Whether she was satisfied with the family gatherings and mission meetings, the games of croquet, the musical evenings at which her arpeggio drawing-room pieces were regular offerings; whether she hoped that marriage and motherhood might prove her future sphere; or whether she simply held her medical ambitions in check through deference to Harriet, cannot now be known.

In January 1885 this placid interlude ended. Harriet succumbed to a fatal attack of scarlet fever.

'From that day', wrote Eva, 'Elsie shouldered all father's burdens, and they two went on together until his death.'[24]

CHAPTER 5

The family moved, probably to economise, to upper apartments in Melville Street and Elsie kept house. She detested it. She formed written resolutions. 'I must devote my mind more to the housekeeping' is one of a list from this time found in her desk after her death.

Self-criticism was popular with Victorians. Miss Nightingale had stormed at herself for day-dreaming[1] and Miss Beale regularly recorded in her diary failings like 'Thoughtless about Mama' or 'Inattentive twice. Unkind thoughts and words.'[2] Struggling to break the Victorian conventional mould of gentle patience, their ardent vision almost despite themselves fighting to widen woman's horizons, they yet strove conscientiously to discipline their dreams within the pattern the age approved.

Elsie similarly blamed herself. Her self-criticism however looked forward. She preferred forming resolutions to recording failures.

'I *must* give up dreaming—making stories. I must give up getting cross. I must devote my mind more to the housekeeping. I must be more thorough in everything. I *must* be more truthful.

'But the bottom of the whole evil is the habit of dreaming, which must be given up. So help me God.'[3]

It is not clear what Elsie meant by 'dreaming' nor whether her dreams, like Miss Nightingale's, were the romantic ones of the normal girl. Nor is it easy to imagine her untruthful; more often, people found her frank to the point of embarrassment.[4] But her medical ambitions, about which she had earlier spoken freely at school, had now to be kept to herself, dissembled, perhaps dreamed of in private. Edinburgh medical classes were still open only to men, and it would have been difficult, financially, to go away to London to study. Although later her father let her study away from home, he borrowed from his sister Eugenia the cost of Elsie's training was almost certainly the reason, to judge from a letter written by her, after his death, regarding repayment.[5]

'Getting cross' she never eradicated. In later years, the nurse who failed to set out a tray or pack a bag correctly would hear 'I do not consider you *at all* a good nurse' in scathing tones she would remember all her life:[6] and in the war her wrath could be magnificent, sending orderlies scuttling for cover and officers flying to obey. 'Getting cross' was a trait she learned to use constructively.

Clearly, however, these housekeeping years were a strain. She loathed looking after accounts, always saw money not as an end in itself, but rather as a regrettable and uninteresting means. The constant petty domestic interruptions to serious reading or study irked her.

Her main pleasure at this time lay in long walks with her father, during which they discussed everything under the sun but especially politics;[7] and in active political work, now open for the first time to women, since the Corrupt Practices Bill of 1883, meant a vast recruitment of voluntary—hence mainly feminine—political workers. When the Women's Liberal Federation was founded in 1887, she joined. She also organised a discussion group named, naïvely, the Six Sincere Students Society,[8] which studied Emerson on heroism and Emerson on self-reliance, and later grew into a full-scale Debating Society. One of the group remarked with no little surprise that Mr Inglis joined the Sincere Students' discussions on equal terms and without the usual masculine condescension.

In October 1886 Sophia Jex-Blake—having recently founded a small hospital of her own where she could give instruction to students—announced the opening of her Edinburgh School of Medicine for Women.[9]

The entire Medical Register then contained the names of only fifty women. Within one month Dr Jex-Blake received sixteen applications for places at her school. One was from Elsie, who now could speak at home.

'Elsie came in and, sitting down beside father, divulged her plan of "going in for medicine",' Eva described the scene later. 'I still see and hear him, taking it all so perfectly calmly and naturally, and setting to work at once to overcome the difficulties which were in the way.'[10]

He was more realistic than most Victorians. Having no estate to bequeath, he would at least leave Elsie with a career to support her. It was increasingly recognised that a lady might earn her living. Some young women were already wearing what J. M. Barrie was later to label 'the twelve pound look'—an air of independence deriving from the intoxicating knowledge that they could support themselves. 'It is', Miss Jex-Blake had once written of this delightful sensation, 'like oats to a horse that has been a year on hay. I quite laugh at myself to feel how radiant I am.'[11]

It was Elsie's turn now to feel radiant. At twenty-two, small and slender, with red-gold hair and vigorous movements, she created an immediate impression of mental and physical sturdiness, having 'an extremely pleasant face with a finely moulded forehead, soft kind fearless blue eyes and a smile when it came like sunshine; with this her mouth and chin were firm and determined', as a fellow-student described her.[12]

The opening of the new school was providential. She could study there while living at home. The fees were modest—£40 per annum for the full course.[13]

Now the walks of father and daughter were enlivened with another theme, the future when Elsie would be famous. It would be such a joke, she said (only half joking, however) to see 'Dr Elsie Inglis' on a fine brass plate in Walker Street; she would be very grand and keep her carriage as Dr Jex-Blake did. And no matter how busy she was, how much in demand by enormously wealthy and influential patients, Saturday afternoons were to be kept for Father, and the trap sent to bring him to tea.[14]

There was as yet, of course, no idea of women doctors treating male patients, nor even of mixed instruction for men and women students. Before that could come 'professors will have to give up amusing their students with improper stories' an Oxford undergraduate had written in 1870, and Sophia Jex-Blake, just before opening her own school, admitted that she had reluctantly come to agree.[15] She herself had been invited to open a military hospital at Sarajevo during the Balkan risings of the Seventies. She had declined; being known to treat men, might actually damage the cause of all medical women.[16]

Sophia Jex-Blake, dark and handsome with, in her portrait by Samuel Lawrence, the noble and passionate turbulence of a supremely intelligent misfit, had always dreamed of directing a women's college. She had come near it in 1874 when the London School of Medicine was founded on her initiative and that of Mrs Garrett Anderson.[17] She had been defeated then by her own inability to conciliate. Unlike Elizabeth Garrett Anderson who could write 'We are dining with some Enemies tonight ... I shall wear my light silk and appear as rich as I can! This is such an education for low cunning',[18] Sophia Jex-Blake had the unhappy knack of antagonising even possible allies.[19]

For some time, all went well at the Edinburgh School of Medicine for Women. J-B, as the students called her, could teach brilliantly: it was her real métier. The students were exhilarated at finding themselves extended. Some, including Elsie, affected the slovenly dress and short-cropped hair of the emancipated woman of any era. Many lasting friendships were formed. In particular a clever young woman called Jessie MacGregor and two sisters, Grace and Georgina Cadell, became friends of Elsie Inglis.

At the Leith Hospital, too, where some clinical instruction was given, all went well. Nurses were traditionally antagonistic to 'lady medicals' but at Leith J-B's girls were popular; the nurses observed that they were (in contrast perhaps to the male students of the period) kind and considerate to patients.[20]

Then the novelty wore thin. The girls complained that 'the atmosphere had changed'. J-B was hedging them with restrictions, making no allowances for the liveliness of young fillies feeling their oats. She was Victorian enough to fear her girl pupils might collapse through overwork, something else which would disgrace the Cause.

The way in which discontent came to a head, which gave Elsie her first real fight, and in the end was to break the Jex-Blake school of medicine, has been defensively wrapped in mystery by previous biographers of the two women. What happened—it is a common occurrence—was that a trivial event precipitated a serious clash long in brewing.[21]

Among J-B's rules was one that students must leave Leith Hospital promptly at 5 p.m. At first, unknown to her, the rule was disregarded if an interesting case arrived. But in the summer of 1888 the hospital decided to enforce it; there were more students now to get in the way at the patients' tea hour. On Friday, June 8th a head accident came in as the girls were leaving and they turned back to see the house surgeon, Dr Juckes, examine it. The hospital's Lady Superintendent, a Miss Perry, appeared and told Grace Cadell the girls must leave. Miss Cadell made a pert retort, and after sharp exchanges, the students left, noisily affirming their support for her. J-B, when she learned of it from Miss Perry, insisted upon the sisters writing apologies; Georgina subsequently tore her letter up.

The sisters were stormy petrels, Miss Perry petty and fussy, but J-B was not the woman to employ 'low cunning' in handling them. On July 17th another clash came. A Miss Sinclair who had been ill, missed some work, and failed an examination, prevailed upon one of the lecturers, Dr George Gibson, to write to the examiner explaining the circumstances. It was, Dr Gibson later admitted, an error of judgement; but Miss Sinclair got her certificate.

This was precisely the kind of thing over which Sophia Jex-Blake was predictably touchy. Not only was she insistent on the highest standards of achievement and conduct; but also, she herself had once been involved in public argument over failure in an examination, when she had unwisely written to *The Times* accusing examiners of prejudice.[22]

Now she publicly charged Miss Sinclair with dishonourable conduct. The Cadell sisters led applause in support of their fellow-student. J-B's all-too-characteristic reaction was to call for a show of hands and five were raised against her. Three days later she again referred to the matter and again Grace Cadell seized the chance to argue. A few days later the two sisters were informed by the school's Committee that because of insubordination they could not be re-admitted. They brought an action for £500 damages each; a crushing sum in view of the modest fees and the fact that the school was largely dependent upon subscriptions.*

The Action of the Lady Medical Students became the talk of Edinburgh in the summer of 1889, along with such other local excitements as Charles Stewart Parnell's becoming a freeman of the city, and the approaching completion of 'that marvellous structure, the Forth Bridge'.

Whether Elsie Inglis supported the Cadell girls in their original insubordination may never now be known. Certainly her friend and first biographer Lady Frances Balfour† betrays embarrass-

* Accounts for the London School of Medicine for Women may be quoted in comparison. The expenditure for its first three years was £3,267. The outlay, Sophia Jex-Blake wrote, 'seems large', but 'I doubt whether any money was ever better or more usefully spent'.[23]

† The daughter of the 8th Duke of Argyll, widow of Colonel Eustace Balfour, and a friend of Margot Asquith, who described her as 'one of the few women of outstanding intellect that I have known'.

ment in skating over this episode, and many believed that Sophia Jex-Blake's struggles for medical women had earned her more consideration than she now got. The real issue, however, to Elsie, was whether women students were to be recognised as serious individuals with a right to run their own lives and protest about unfair treatment as men did; and for this principle she was ready to be ruthless. Many, even among those who later became her friends, never really forgave her treatment of the lion-hearted old battleaxe that J-B had become.

She allied herself with the insurgents; had 'awful rows' with Jessie MacGregor and others who supported J-B; and enlisted her father's help. Unless *someone* stood up to J-B, whatever the rights and wrongs of the case, the end result would be that no woman who would not accept meekly anything J-B might dictate could get a medical education outside London. This, Elsie could not, would not, accept.

Her father had influential friends. Moreover, Sophia had over the years offended many who might otherwise have rallied to her support now. The woman never went to mission meetings!

The outcome of Elsie's and her father's efforts was the founding of the Scottish Association for the Medical Education of Women, with an imposing list of supporters who knew well how to raise both money and sympathy. Sophia might influence the Leith Hospital to refuse them facilities, the Medical Officer of Health in Edinburgh might oppose them, but by the time judgement was given in November 1889, and reduced damages of £50 awarded to each Miss Cadell, the Association had opened a rival establishment, the Medical College for Women at 30 Chambers Street.

The new college had temporary facilities at the Royal Hospital for Sick Children, and a list of eighteen distinguished lecturers whose subjects, ranging from midwifery to public health, from diseases of children and vaccination to insanity and ophthalmology, throw interesting light upon the branches of medicine it was thought proper for a woman to study in 1889.[24]

In it all, Elsie was the moving spirit. 'Through the stormy and somewhat depressing times of the early career of the Medical College for Women, Edinburgh, her faith and vision never faltered and she helped us all to hold on courageously' wrote a niece, Dr Mary McNicol, who herself studied there.[25]

The new school was a boon to women. Its fees were lower, its committee more influential than that of the Jex-Blake school. Within two years it had endowed with £700 two wards at the Royal Infirmary, the second largest hospital in Britain and a stronghold of anti-feminism, to be set aside for women students. It attracted girls from as far away as Australia, for the Edinburgh degree was a good one and in 1895 an economical girl could live in Edinburgh lodgings for £1 a week.[26]

It cannot, however, be denied that the affair was a tragedy for Sophia Jex-Blake. At a large public meeting she was openly jeered; the lawsuit judge spoke of her 'somewhat excited views' of her position and the 'provocation of her masterful ways'. Her standing never fully recovered and her school of medicine closed in 1898.

Elsie had shown for the first time that determination in over-riding anyone she considered obstructionist or ineffectual which was to become the characteristic her enemies, and even some of her friends, seized upon to criticise. Ruthlessness is not an endearing trait. It is, however, an essential of leadership; and Elsie's had no self-seeking in it. The founding of the Medical College, in which she dragged her elders and betters in her wake, gave her at twenty-five her first success in an important affair. After defeating, more or less single-handed, the legendary Sophia Jex-Blake, would anything ever again seem impossible to her?

She now became a student at the College she had helped to found; stayed for eighteen months, then went to Glasgow to the Royal Infirmary, the third biggest hospital in Britain.

At twenty-six she was for the first time living independently, still a novelty for the period. She boarded at the Y.W.C.A., which had the advantage of being cheap. She knew the sacrifices her father was making. 'I am going to work like *anything*', she wrote to him at the outset, and a few months later, 'The chief reason I tried to get that prize was to pay for those things and not worry you about them. I want to pass awfully well as it tells all one's life through and I mean to be very successful.'[27]

At Glasgow she came under the influence of one of the greatest general surgeons of the day, William MacEwen;* the first to operate for brain disorders, an innovator in bone surgery, one of the earliest men to operate under conditions approaching

* Sir William MacEwen, 1848-1924; Regius Professor of Surgery, Glasgow University, 1892-1924; F.R.S. 1895; knighted 1902.

asepsis, MacEwen did as much as any man to change surgery from a risky craft to a safe science.

At this time forty-three and approaching the peak of his career, MacEwen was young enough to be unprejudiced against women, brilliant enough not to fear their competition even when they *meant* to be very successful, and a good enough teacher to need no help from improper anecdote. Nor, unlike Dr Gibson of Edinburgh, did he make concessions for women. 'He put me through my facings', wrote Elsie of her first prolonged encounter with him on February 9th, 1891. 'It seems it is his way of greeting a new student. Some of them cannot bear him, but I think he is really nice, though he can be abominably sarcastic.'[28] *Mutatis mutandis,* it might in another twenty years be a description of herself.

The women found the pace exhilarating but exhausting. 'I am taking my tonic and my tramp regularly so I ought to keep well', Elsie wrote home. 'I am quite disgusted when girls break down through working too hard. They must remember they are not as strong as men, and then they do idiotic things, such as taking no exercise, into the bargain.'[29]

Work in the slums was an eye-opener; her reaction sometimes struck the slum-dwellers as naïve.

'One [patient] is a shirt finisher. She sews on the buttons and puts in the gores at the rate of 4½d a dozen shirts. We know the shop and they sell the shirts at 4s. 6d. each. Of course political economy is quite true, but I hope that shopkeeper, if ever he comes back to this earth, will be a woman and have to finish shirts at 4½d a dozen and then he'll see the other side of the question. I told the woman it was her own fault for taking such small wages, at which she seemed amused.'[30]

If I don't, there are plenty more who will, was the more usual tart reply to so innocent a remark.[31]

Elsie saw the homes of the poor. Her notions of reform were equally simple and vigorous. 'I went round this morning and saw a few of my patients. I found one woman who ought to have been in bed. I discovered she had been up all night because her husband came in tipsy about eleven o'clock. He was lying there asleep on the bed. I think he ought to have been horse-whipped, and when I have the vote I shall vote that all men who turn their wives and families out of doors at eleven o'clock at night, especially when the wife is ill, shall be horse-whipped. And if they make the excuse that they were tipsy, I should give them double. They would very soon learn to behave themselves.'[32]

In November 1891, having paid their fees, Elsie and the other women students were told by the Royal Infirmary managers that 'mixed classes' could not after all be allowed. Since not all professors would conduct separate sessions for the women, this was a setback.

'So here is another fight,' wrote Elsie to her father, adding, however, 'we cannot be beat here, for the same reason that we cannot beat them in Edinburgh.'

That reason was the support of the local great man. In Glasgow the women had it. 'Were the managers, managers a hundred times over, they cannot turn Mr MacEwen off.'[33] And MacEwen was for the women.

She mentioned to him, only half in jest, her ambition to endow a women's college. MacEwen told her he did not believe in segregation. 'If the women are going to be doctors, equal with the men, they should go to the same school.'

Elsie retorted, 'But when they won't admit you, what are you to do?'

'Leave them alone,' was his advice. 'They *will* admit you in time.'[34]

He was right. The Royal Infirmary obstructionists had to yield. The *Glasgow Herald* might rage that mixed classes were the beginning of the end, leading women to the ballot box and probably even to the pulpit; hidebound professors might threaten to prevent women's attendance at classes 'by physical force';[35] but a new generation, seeing nothing odd about women doctors, was beginning to lead opinion. And meanwhile Elsie Inglis was becoming a bonnie fighter.

MacEwen's teaching kindled in her a life-long devotion to surgery, a devotion which led her into sometimes tactless remarks. She unselfconsciously described to her father an encounter with a medical man.

'[He] has the most absurd way of agreeing with everything you say. He asked me what I would do with a finger. I thought it was past all mending and said "Amputate it". "Quite so, quite so," he said solemnly "but we'll dress it today with such and such a thing." There were two or three other cases in which I recommended desperate measures, in which he agreed but did not follow. Finally he asked Mr B. what he would do with a swelling.

Mr B. hesitated. I said "Open it". Whereupon he went off into fits of laughter, and proclaimed to the whole room my prescriptions, and said I would make a first-rate surgeon for I was afraid of nothing.'[36]

Temperamentally, no doubt, Elsie had the makings of an outstanding surgeon. Certainly surgery was her first love, and those nearest to her were to choose the appellation 'surgeon' for the place of honour on her tombstone. 'She was quiet, calm and collected, and never at a loss, skilful in her manipulations and able to cope with any emergency' was a colleague's assessment.[37]

She was, however, to suffer all her life from a professional disability common to all her generation of medical women: restricted opportunities in the student days, plus the distractions of having to struggle for equality.

Nor are boldness and optimism the only important qualities needed. 'Most of the public imagine', a doctor with the Scottish Women's Hospitals was to write thirty years later, 'that operations are very sanguinary and acrobatic performances, demanding great physical strength ... [They] demand on the contrary great lightness and deftness of touch, in fact the qualities of a good seamstress together with good sight and a young and steady hand are those which are most needed. An operation is as a rule a dainty piece of needlework and as each artery is carefully tied before or immediately after it is cut, there should be only the merest trace of blood ... war surgery and accidents are rather different and may be sanguinary.'[38]

Elsie Inglis's courage equipped her even for war surgery; but by that time, twenty years later, a younger generation of medical women was to assess her theatre work as 'careful and extremely precise, rather slow'.* It was perhaps her only personal tragedy that when war brought her, at last, opportunities of enormously extending her experience, she was over fifty, tired, no longer having the eye and hand of youth, being, indeed, a sick woman.

But now in student days, a golden future loomed ahead, and Elsie freely and gaily forecast for herself a large and paying practice. Even she, however, was not free from pre-examination nerves, and all MacEwen's reassurances could not dispel them; they had to be worked away.

* Personal information, Miss Herzfeld, F.R.C.S.

On August 4th, 1892, when she was twenty-seven, the name of Elsie Inglis, Licentiate of the Royal College of Physicians and Surgeons, Edin., and Licentiate of the Faculty of Physicians and Surgeons, Glasgow, was placed upon the British Medical Register.

CHAPTER 6

The New Hospital for Women* in the Euston Road, London, built by Elizabeth Garrett Anderson in 1890, was the mecca of medical women. There at the end of 1892 went the newly qualified Dr Inglis as Resident Medical Officer at a salary of £25 per annum.[1] It was remarkable that she got the post, for many promising women were now coming out of Mrs Anderson's own London School of Medicine for Women; and besides, the clash with Sophia Jex-Blake had been watched with interest from the Euston Road.

Elizabeth Garrett Anderson, now fifty-six, was the most admired figure in the whole women's movement. Ladylike, serene, beautifully dressed, a happy wife and mother, she was the best possible advertisement for emancipation. At this time, while remaining a consultant, she had just been succeeded as head of the New Hospital by Mrs (later Dame) Mary Scharlieb, the most brilliant of all the early women doctors, who had converted Queen Victoria to the idea of medical women and had worked in India to realise the Nightingale reforms.[2] Years later Dame Mary was to describe Elsie Inglis as 'among the noblest of the noble' and in 1922 as the aged doyenne of medical women would unveil a memorial to Elsie in St Giles Cathedral.[3] But now in 1893 Elsie was merely the new little house surgeon; to her both Mrs Scharlieb and Mrs G. Anderson, as Elsie called her, were kind and encouraging.

They initiated her into responsibility, giving her charge not only of dangerously ill patients but also of the girls, hardly younger than herself, from the Royal Free Hospital who came in as dressers and whose work she supervised. Mrs G. Anderson enlisted Elsie's help with private operations, realising probably how much the half-guinea fee would mean to the impecunious young woman; off duty she was 'jovial and talkative'[4] and showed Elsie a more sophisticated world.

* Now the Elizabeth Garrett Anderson Hospital.

If Elsie was now in authority, it was with a shock that she discovered that neither she, nor Mrs Scharlieb nor even the great Mrs G. Anderson herself, was the real authority the patients acknowledged.

'I have just been so angry!' she wrote to her father. 'A woman came in yesterday very ill. A. took down her case and thought she would have to have an operation. Then her husband arrived and calmly said she was to go home, because he could not look after the children. So I said that if she went she went on her own responsibility, for I would not give my consent ... I gave him my mind pretty clearly, but I went in [to the ward] just now to find she had gone. I said she was stupid. So one woman said "It was not 'er fault, Miss; 'e would have it" ...

'You don't know what trouble we have here with the husbands ... Any idea that anybody is to be thought of but themselves never enters their lordly minds, and the worst of it is, these stupid idiots of women don't seem to think so either ... They don't seem to think they have any right to any individual existence. Well, I feel better now, but I wish I could have scragged that beast.'[5]

The idiots of women were less stupid than she supposed. They knew, what she at first found too iniquitous to credit, that the law did not then allow an operation on a married woman without her husband's consent; and that it was not unusual for a man to withhold approval even though it meant a lifetime of suffering for his wife. What she saw reinforced Elsie's conviction that progress would only come when women had won the right to run their own affairs and had a voice in the counsels of the nation.

She became an active suffrage worker. She had always looked forward confidently to a day 'when I have the vote'. Now she saw that that day was likely to be harder to achieve than she had supposed.

She threw herself into the fight, beginning characteristically with the simple and trivial task lying next to her hand. It was a turning-point in her life, the first easy step along a path of no retreat, a path that was to lead with classic inexorability through years of arduous political campaigning, strenuous back-room work and unobtrusive sacrifice, on to the front-line hospitals, to war and bombardment, retreat and imprisonment, blood and revolution, and ultimately to the saving of half a nation's manhood.

But now the first task nearest her hand was humble and undramatic. 'I got a paper to sign to thank the M.P.s who voted for Sir A. Rollitt's Woman's Suffrage Bill.* I got it filled up in half a minute. I wish she had sent half a dozen. There is no question among women who have to work for themselves about wanting the suffrage. It is the women who are safe and sound in their own drawing-rooms who don't see what on earth they want it for.'[6]

In drawing-rooms or out of them, women were still at the mercy of their menfolk; on women who bore the additional burden of poverty this could be hard indeed.

Although no suffrage supporter could ever be certain of agreement from other people, the New Hospital was a home of the Cause. Not only had the great Mrs G. Anderson carried to Westminster nearly twenty years before the very first suffrage petition; but also, her younger sister Millicent, widow of Henry Fawcett M.P., was now the recognised leader of the campaign. Elsie at the New Hospital soon discovered comrades in arms.

One day a woman arrived at the comfortable, pretty outpatients' room, with a painful breast abscess. Dr Helen Webb, the outpatient physician, proposed admission to a ward. The patient asked to return home to arrange for the care of her baby. Then, once again, an irate husband appeared.

'I cannot let my wife come in,' he declared. 'The baby is not old enough to be left.'

To Elsie this was monstrous. That difficulties should stand in the way! That one human being should settle for another whether or not she should be cured! Did he realise the pain his wife was suffering? What if he had to bear it himself?

Helen Webb,[7] a kindly woman of excellent judgement, followed this heated outburst with a quiet, rational appeal. The man remained as deaf to her reason as he had been to Elsie's ranting. The two young women told him he was a brute. 'At least get a good doctor to see your wife at home' they begged; and watching him go, knew he would never do so.

Elsie fumed helplessly. He was an obstinate mule, a beast, a selfish cad; but she was as much inclined to blame the woman. Why could she not have stood up for herself? The only way to

* This Bill, defeated in 1892 by a very small majority, was the last occasion when woman's suffrage was defeated in the Commons as a straight issue.

educate such people was to get the franchise!

'Bravo, bravo,' cried Miss Webb enthusiastically.

Elsie was astonished. She had had no idea that here was a fellow traveller. A great friendship was struck up. Miss Webb* it now appeared was a keen worker for the Cause, in trouble with her branch of the Liberal Women's Association for her championship of the suffrage movement. Elsie herself was impatient of the way Liberal women allowed party interests to come before the vote. 'Women are awful fools to truckle to their party instead of putting their foot down about the Franchise', she wrote to her father.[8]

Life at the New Hospital might bring new comradeships. It certainly brought a tremendous amount of work. She wrote to her father 'I will tell you what I think of the Home Rule Bill† tomorrow—that is to say if I have time to read it. It is really a case of officers and men here just now. I can't say "go on" instead of "come on". I cannot order cold spongings and hot fomentations by the dozen and then sit in my room and read the newspapers, can I?'[9]

She found, however, time to make her debut as a speaker. The occasion had its comic side. Mrs Wolstenholme Elmy was another pioneer of the movement: a tiny, sweetly smiling lady who well into the twentieth century wore the fashions of her youth, the Victorian black dress, shawl and bonnet identified equally with Miss Nightingale and Charley's Aunt.[10] Mrs Elmy, belying her aura of lavender and lace, was an indefatigable campaigner on all the most controversial fronts: she had been active in the Married Women's Property Act agitation and had worked alongside Josephine Butler for the repeal of the Contagious Diseases Acts.[11] A great encourager of young blood, Mrs Elmy now asked Dr Inglis to speak on British medical education. Even Elsie's self-confidence boggled ('too great cheek in a house surgeon') so when Mrs Elmy proposed a speech on suffrage instead, Elsie felt unable to refuse.

Arriving at the meeting in a rush (she was seldom early for anything: managing time was never easier for her than managing money) she found an alarmingly fashionable audience being

* At this period and for many years the title Miss or Mrs was used interchangeably with that of Dr for medical women, whether surgeons or not. Dr Inglis used them interchangeably throughout her life.

† Second Home Rule Bill, 1893.

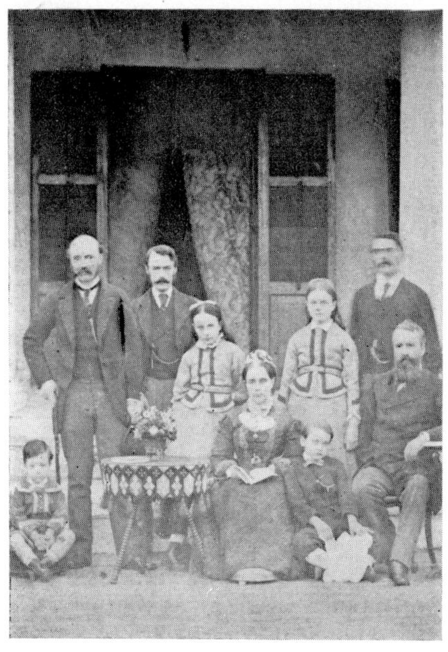

Left Family group, about 1879. *Standing, l. to r.*: Robert Simson, Hugh Inglis, Eva, Elsie, Cecil Inglis. *Seated, l. to r.*: Henry Simson, Harriet Inglis, Horace Inglis, John Inglis.

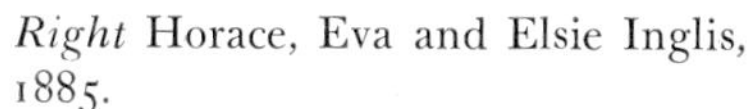

Right Horace, Eva and Elsie Inglis, 1885.

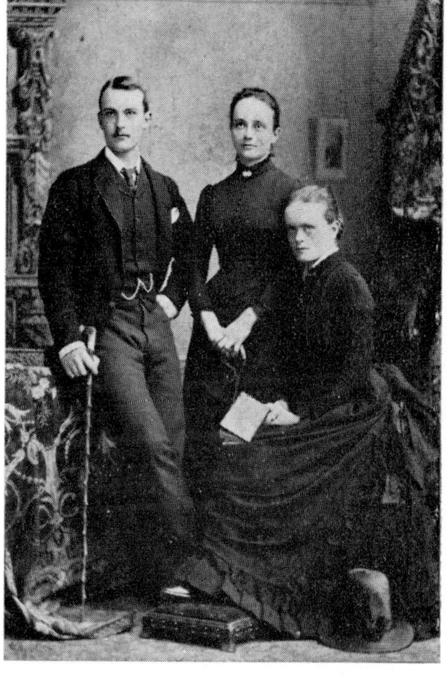

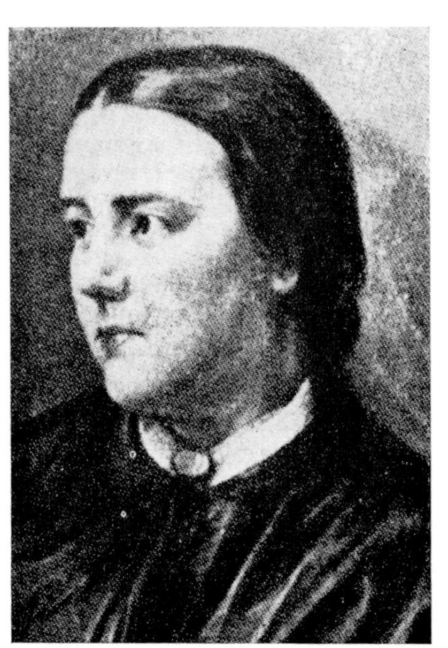

Left Sophia Jex-Blake, from the painting by Samuel Lawrence.

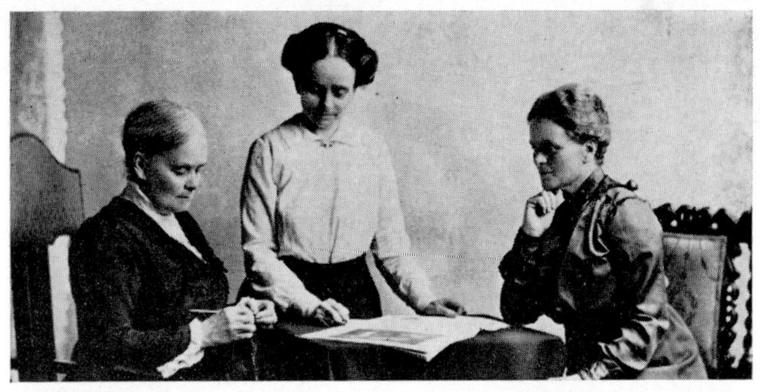

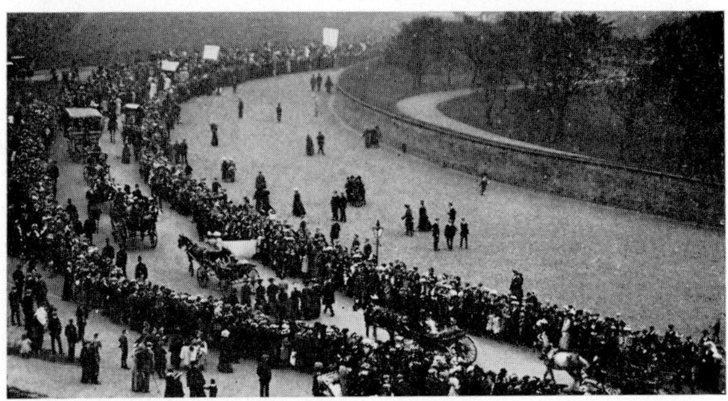

Top Mrs Simson, Mrs McLaren, Elsie Inglis, about 1912. *Above* Suffrage March leaving King's Park, Edinburgh, 1913.

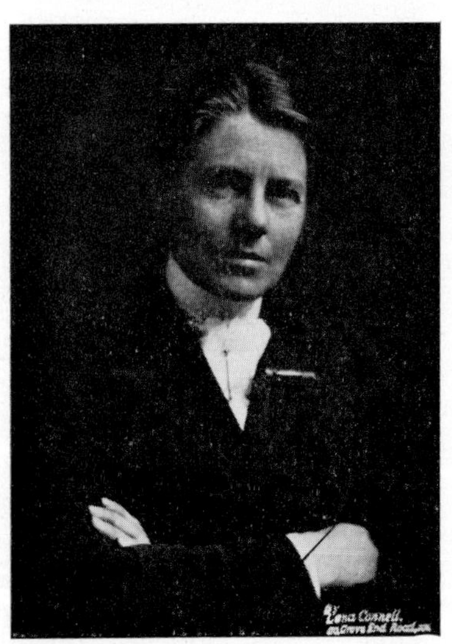

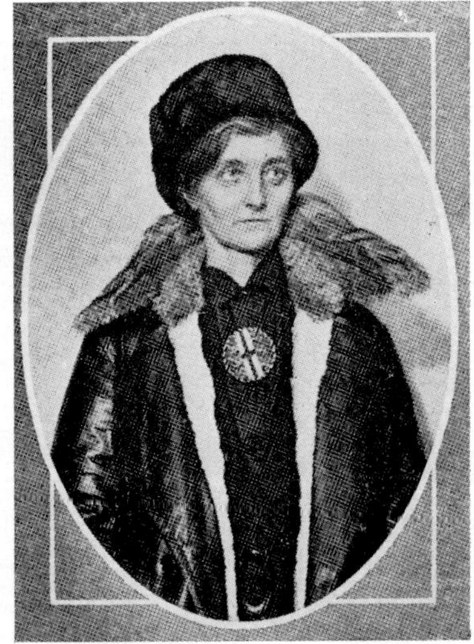

Left Mrs Eveline Haverfield. *Right* Dr Alice Hutchison.

harangued by a clever-looking man—and along the same lines as her own ideas. She congratulated herself: clearly her thinking had been sound.

The speaker finished. Joining in the applause, Elsie noticed Mrs Elmy beaming and nodding to her. Light dawned. The dear old encouraging lady had merely wanted her to second the motion. And the first speaker had just said almost everything that she had thought of saying.

Panic seized her. Then an adaptability which was to serve her in more serious crises came to her aid. 'I was in such an awful funk that I got cool', she wrote to John Inglis, 'and got up and told them that I did not think Mr Wilkins had left any single thing for me to say; however, as things struck people in different ways I should simply tell them how it struck me, and then went ahead with what I meant to say when I got in.'[12]

She was encouragingly received. Mrs Elmy was kind and reassuring; so were others. Soon Elsie was an engaging and fluent speaker both on medical subjects and on politics.

Life was not all work and campaigning. There were family connexions to be visited, among them the Pownalls of Blackheath, for croquet or lawn tennis, then just passing its first vogue. There were long solitary tramps round London's sights; and she managed to hear most of the famous preachers even if she usually hurried late into the church.

There were also theatres. One of her first visits was to *King Lear* at the Lyceum. Her father had imbued her with a love of Shakespeare, but like most of the London theatre public which took its opinions ready-made from the critics,* she was more impressed by Ford Madox Brown's scenery and storm effects than by Irving's Lear, which she found 'not a bit kingly, but just a weak old man', though she thought Ellen Terry, at thirty-six at the height of her powers, 'splendid'.[13]

Her hospital seniors were kindly. Mrs G. Anderson took her to a dance, was a 'capital chaperone' and saw to it that Elsie danced every dance; 'you may make up your mind, papa dear, that I go to all the balls in Edinburgh after this,'[14] she wrote enthusiastically.

The dark-eyed and serious Mrs Scharlieb was also 'awfully nice

* Irving's Lear was a first-night disaster on November 10th, 1892, feeble, inaudible and incoherent. Graham Robertson five nights later found Irving 'magnificent and terrible' but by then damaging notices had done their work and the play was taken off in January.

and kind. She said she hoped I would get on always as well as I had here. Was it not nice of her? I said I hoped I would do much better ... She says everybody has to make mistakes. The worst of being a doctor is that one's mistakes matter so much.'[15]

Elsie watched her own health with a regime of cold baths, long walks, and open windows; and observing that 'a patient with a well-balanced nervous system will get well in just half the time that one of these hysterical women will', she went on 'I agree with Kingsley: one of the necessities of the world is to teach girls to be brave and not whine over everything, and the first step for that is to teach them to play games!'[16]

She took a keen interest in the development of the Medical College for Women in Edinburgh, and conducted her own campaign by sending the New Hospital's annual report to prominent Edinburgh doctors. 'The [out] patients have to pay a small sum, yet they had over 20,000 visits this year ... Who says women doctors are not wanted!'[17] She heard from her father that Sir William Muir, their old family friend from India, who was now Principal of Edinburgh University, had rallied to their support. 'It is splendid having Sir William Muir on our side', she wrote in February 1893, 'and I believe the bulk of the Senators are all right—they only want a little shove.'[18] And when Bailie Walcot of Edinburgh visited London she took him all round the New Hospital as an example of what a women's hospital could be. 'He says our girls are going to Dr Littlejohn's class with Jex's girls at Surgery Hall (sic). It is wonderful how these men who would do nothing at first are beginning to see it pays to be neutral now.'[19] The future Sir Henry Littlejohn, the great public health pioneer and Edinburgh's Medical Officer of Health, was perhaps the most influential convert of all. The college's future was safe.

And always there were the hopes, the ambitions. 'If I don't get into the Infirmary in Edinburgh, I mean to build a hospital for myself, like this one. Indeed I don't know that I should not like the hospital to myself better!' she wrote; and again, '[Mrs Scharlieb] said she expects to be called in as my consultant when I am a surgeon. Won't my patients have to pay fees to get her up from London!'[20]

Before she could confidently set up in Edinburgh—which her London chiefs considered a very lonely place—Elsie needed more midwifery experience. She decided to go to the Rotunda, Dublin, then as now one of the world's leading centres for obstetrics. Apart from its excellence, 'mixed classes' were the accepted thing there, so a principle was involved.

Almost the first thing she saw on landing in Ireland on November 17th, 1893, were the headlines of the *Irish Daily Independent* announcing a defeat of the Government on a woman's franchise question: married women had won the right to vote along with spinsters in parish council elections. Once more suffragist hopes ran high. Elsie was jubilant and eager to make her views known, but after an 'awful argument' with one of the Rotunda's senior surgeons, in which she failed to convert him, she resolved not to re-open the subject.[21]

On other subjects, too, she learned to be wary. Ireland at the peak of the Home Rule agitation showed her a prejudice she had never imagined; for the only time on record, she admitted herself scared into silence. A fervent Home Ruler herself—Irishmen, like Englishwomen, surely deserved to control their own affairs; Home Rule was the one subject on which she disagreed with her father —she was dining with Presbyterian friends before church when a clever young doctor, Miss Emily Dickson,[22] who attended the same church, was mentioned. 'We don't know her,' said the hostess firmly. 'They are Home Rulers, both she and her father; though I for one would not mind that, if they did not obtrude their politics so much.'

Elsie resolved not to obtrude her own politics. But her hostess's next remark was 'You must take a side, you know, and say distinctly what side you are on when you are asked.'

'So I thought', Elsie wrote home in amusement, '"Well, I'll wait till I *am* asked" and I have got through today without being asked. But positively they used the word "boycott" about those Dicksons. They have been boycotted by the congregation.

'It must be rather hard to be a Home Ruler and a Presbyterian just now in Ireland,' she added. 'Positively they frightened me so I nearly squirmed under the table. However, when I looked round the congregation I thought I should not mind being boycotted by them.'

The sermon that evening, she did not fail to note, was on forgiving one's enemies.

Night calls to confinements were frequent, meals irregular, and health must still be watched. 'I am not such an idiot as to miss my meals, Papa dearest. My temper won't stand it!' she wrote. 'I always have a glass of milk and a biscuit when I go out at night.

I am as sensible as I can be. I know you cannot do work with blunt instruments, and this instrument blunts very easily without food and exercise.'[23]

Before long she had a small but sweet triumph. Assisting at an operation the surgeon who had opposed her suffrage arguments, she was concentrating entirely upon the matter in hand when he suddenly, with a casualness which masked a *volte face*, remarked, 'By the way, you are right about the suffrage, Miss Inglis.'

Had her own demeanour convinced him? Had male disbelief been worked away? 'I found', she wrote, 'he had come over about the whole question. As a convert is always the most violent supporter, I hope he'll do some good.'[24]

She wanted to go to Paris for further study. But money was the problem. Moreover, John Inglis was now seventy-five and his health, which had been causing anxiety for months, was failing rapidly, though this he hid from her.

On February 10th, 1894, coming down to breakfast at eleven o'clock after a night interrupted by a confinement, Elsie found a letter from him saying Paris was out of the question.

Any disappointment she felt was instantly put behind her with a joke about the difficulty of settling to punctual habits again when she returned to Edinburgh. Then she turned without repining to consider her next move, and as so often was to happen for her, as one door closed, another opened, and with an extraordinary promptitude.[25]

Jessie MacGregor, with whom she had had 'awful rows' over the Jex-Blake affair, who had stayed with Sophia and in 1893 been appointed as junior medical officer at Sophia's little hospital,[26] had written to Elsie renewing their old acquaintance; the letter arrived by the same post as that from John Inglis. Miss MacGregor proposed that they should become partners in Edinburgh. The suggestion was surprising. Elsie weighed it carefully. They *had* disagreed, bitterly, at the Edinburgh School of Medicine, but as Miss MacGregor was careful to point out, that had not been a personal quarrel.

'We certainly got on very well before that', Elsie wrote to her father. 'I am quite sure Miss MacGregor is Scotch enough not to propose any arrangement which won't be to her advantage ... The question for me is whether it will be for my advantage. I am rather inclined to think it will.'[27] Miss MacGregor had far fewer social connexions than had Elsie, who guessed she would be supplying her partner with patients rather than the other way about. But then, Miss MacGregor was so very clever, and a splendid pathologist; and two women in partnership would be spared the tiresome necessity of calling in a male opinion. And having referred the plan to her family, and heard that Eva, the fey one, had an 'instinct' in favour, she was fully ready to accept it and to build new castles in the Edinburgh air. 'We'll end by having a hospital like the Rotunda, where students shall live on the premises' she prophesied. It was no mere fancy, but a resolve she was to hold to for many years and finally, in a modest way, realise.

John Inglis kept going long enough to see his favourite child and receive her gratitude. 'I do thank you so much for having let me come here ... The money has certainly not been wasted. But it was awfully good of you to let me come. I am sure it will make a difference all my life' she assured him in almost her last letter before her return home early in March.[28]

She arrived just in time to nurse him through a last short painful illness. On March 13th he died. Two days later she wrote to her brother Ernest in India. 'He never once complained. I never saw such a patient' she reported. 'He always said that he did not believe that death was the stopping place, but that one would go on growing and learning through all eternity. God bless him in his onward journey. I simply cannot imagine life without him.'

She remembered the castles in the air, the walks when, half-joking, half-serious, they had forecast her golden future. 'We had made such plans', she wrote to Ernest, 'and now it does not seem worth while to go on working at all.'[29]

CHAPTER 7

It took Elsie years to get over her father's death. Yet though immersed in grief, she was not submerged by it. A woman of deep feeling, she neither paraded nor repressed emotion; instead it became for her a source of driving power.

She flung herself into her work, but with a difference. 'The question for me is, whether it will be for my advantage', she had written of Jessie MacGregor's proposal. No one, from now on, heard her mention her own advantage. The element of personal ambition was henceforth quite absent. No more do we hear a note of glee at the thought of getting expensive consultants up from London. Her character had always been unselfish; it now became selfless.

John Inglis's death posed practical problems. Eva went to relations in India,[1] but for Elsie it was the moment of becoming in fact as well as theory the self-supporting independent 'modern woman'.

She was competent to do so. Besides her professional skills she had optimism, determination, adaptability and the power to infect others with these qualities, attributes even more valuable to a physician then, when medicine was not the science it is today. Normal saline was one of Dr Inglis's most frequently prescribed remedies, a nurse noted:[2] determination had to make good the age's deficiency of knowledge. Anaesthetics even were still in their infancy—Elsie's early student letters make frequent mention of 'chloroform scares' and her belief that only Scottish medical men really understood anaesthesia.

Following the plan already made, she set up with Dr MacGregor in Atholl Place; before long they removed to the fashionable Walker Street. The partnership was happy. Both held decided opinions, and Jessie MacGregor even continued on excellent terms with Sophia Jex-Blake, but each had matured since the days of the awful rows and they could agree to differ. Elsie, even while struggling on behalf of the breakaway medical school in 1892, had been able to write to her father, 'We have a lot to be grateful to J-B for.'[3]

To be a woman's doctor in the eighteen-nineties was to have religious faith and medical theory sternly tested. In this same Victorian Edinburgh, R. L. Stevenson had observed with disgust that respected men of his acquaintance, good citizens, pillars of the church and the law, literally killed their wives through their sexual exploitation.[4] Birth control was held immoral and almost continual pregnancies were the lot of rich and poor alike. These were the women among whom Dr Inglis's work lay, whether in the elegant Georgian streets of the New Town or in the ancient dark evil-smelling wynds and closes where the six-storey tenements with only one water pipe to each building overflowed with pallid children and wives old before their time.

She saw the inroads of unemployment upon the self-respect of the working class; the drunkenness, the squalor, the near-starvation. In 1889 the Borough Engineer of Edinburgh estimated that over 60,000 people were living in families in slum tenement dwellings of one apartment only.[5] Moreover during the twenty years Elsie Inglis was in practice, things got worse; national prosperity increased, the purchasing power of the working man declined.[6]

Responsible people did not condone this. They were distressed, but could not imagine how to alleviate the suffering without incurring what they felt to be worse evils. When Dr Barnardo visited Edinburgh in 1889 the *Scotsman* roundly declared that his work merely encouraged parental neglect;[7] on similar grounds the intelligent and compassionate Mrs Fawcett was to reject, all her life, the argument for family allowances.[8]

For Elsie, medical work offered a constructive approach. It was often enough work without reward. The free dispensary at which doctors worked without fee, and the voluntary hospitals, were all the help available to those who could not pay; even when the National Insurance Act came, in 1911, it covered only wage-earners. Furthermore, before 1902 midwives were mere handy-women, untrained and unsupervised.

Soon Elsie had a substantial practice. Her poorer patients adored her, named their babies after her, relied on her for more than medical care. She paid for treatments from her own pocket, arranged holidays for them often at her own expense, and equipped them with clothes for such occasions.

Like most women doctors she was begged for contraceptive

advice and abortions which the morals of the age compelled her to refuse. It was a relief to dissolve in laughter when one mother of a large family of girls, having sought to avoid bearing another child, produced a longed-for son and said to Dr Inglis with pawky humour, 'Ye canna say I haena likit ye—at the hinder end at onny rate.'[9]

She remembered the smallest details about her patients' families, and greeted the children in the street or waved to them at the windows; invited poor women to tea to unburden their troubles; was fearless in penetrating the dark closes, but accepted with unforced delight a torch patients subscribed to buy her; talked sternly to husbands who thought wives exceeded their prerogative by needing an operation or convalescence; and argued suffrage with politically-minded ones.

She injected them with her own vitality, lectured them up hill and down dale if they ignored her advice, and when they offered payment was likely to reply with a laugh, 'Now, you go and buy a nice chop for yourself instead.'[10]

Rich patients got the same blend of personal friendship and trained skill. To a neurotic woman she could hand a prescription and follow it with a kiss: the kind of thing that awakened more than one patient to a sense that she was of value in the world, and inspired new courage.

Even the written prescriptions were not always strictly pharmaceutical. 'I want you', ran one, 'never to miss or delay meals. I want you to go to bed at a reasonable time and go to sleep early. I want you to do your work regularly and to take an interest in outside things, such as your church, and suffrage.' Another, 'We should not let these Things (with a capital T) affect us so much. Our cause is too righteous for it to be really affected by them—if we don't weaken.' Again: 'My dear, the potter's wheel isn't a pleasant instrument' and, 'Realise what you are, a freeborn child of the Universe. Perfection your Polar Star.'[11]

In 1894 Edinburgh University opened its medical degrees to women, and ambitious students flocked to the city. Remembering her own student days, Dr Inglis knew they mostly had a miserable existence in drab lodgings with little guidance through the moral or social pitfalls of university life. She befriended them, invited them to Sunday tea, encouraged them. She wanted to do more; and in 1898, with the Muirs, she promoted the opening of a Hall of Residence for them in George Square, becoming its secretary and medical officer, an interest which she continued throughout her life.[12]

She herself graduated M.B., C.M., of Edinburgh in 1899 and was appointed lecturer in Gynaecology at the Medical College for Women.[13] Now she took the first practical step towards founding a hospital of her own. She had already taken the lead in forming a Medical Women's Club in the city, of which she was the secretary and which met usually at 8 Walker Street. Many old friends, including Dr Cadell, were members, and one of the avowed aims was to open a small hospital staffed wholly by women and to which any of them could send their patients.

Before any further steps could be taken, Elsie heard through Jessie MacGregor that Dr Jex-Blake was proposing to extend and modernise her own small cottage hospital* and hand the whole concern over to trustees before retiring to Sussex.

Now, apparently in response to a suggestion of Dr MacGregor, Elsie set aside her own ambition and on January 29th, 1899 wrote on behalf of the Club to the committee of Dr Jex-Blake's hospital; she offered to raise half the money for the new extensions, provided the Club was given a fifty per cent representation on the hospital's committees. Jessie MacGregor had already made an informal approach to the formidable J-B and had apparently not been snubbed; and Elsie's letter must have been encouragingly received, for three days later she wrote again specifying £4,000 as the sum she and her friends could raise.[14]

The Bruntsfield committee considered this on March 18th and replied that although it welcomed support, the request to nominate committee members could not be granted; even had the Hospital wished to agree, the proposed new constitution would have prevented it.[15]

Elsie discussed this with her friends and wrote again. 'It was unanimously decided that if the Club was to give the promised aid, their condition must stand in the main ... The Club will not undertake to collect this money for the Hospital unless they are assured by your Committee that the half representation will be conceded to them when the money is collected.

'The Club has the fullest intention of establishing a Woman's Hospital in Edinburgh and feels that it would be much better both for your interests and theirs to form one strong Hospital

*The Edinburgh Hospital for Women and Children, later known as the Bruntsfield Hospital.

than to divide forces.

'If your Committee see their way to considering our proposals favourably, our delegates are authorised to meet your sub-committee at any time or place you name.'

The suggestions are generous; but the tone is hardly conciliatory. It is possible to see from it why enemies called Elsie Inglis domineering and even friends sometimes found her lacking in diplomacy.

She *had* friends on the executive of the Bruntsfield. But J-B still had the last word, for after discussion a snub went to Dr Inglis. 'Dear Madam, Our executive committee have considered your letter ... and can only account for its tenor by a belief that you are labouring under a misapprehension of the wishes and intentions of our Exec. Committee. Under these circumstances they think it best that the present correspondence should cease.' And although the letter added that informal conversations might perhaps be more helpful, at the same meeting the Committee adopted the new Trust Deed and so put a rapprochement beyond the bounds of possibility.[16]

Elsie now returned vigorously to the idea of a hospital of her own. She enlisted the support of medical women; of her sisters (Eva, having returned from India, was at this time preparing for her marriage to the surgeon John Shaw McLaren);[17] and of the friends who would always rally round John Inglis's daughters. She launched an appeal for funds and persuaded Dr Hugh Barbour to put 11 George Square at their disposal rent free.[18] All this had been done when towards the end of June the Bruntsfield committee wrote again, having had second thoughts; they offered two seats on their committee to the Medical Women's Club.

Elsie replied that 'for the next three years all the energies of the Club—both in the way of work and money—must be devoted to making the George Square home a success ... The Club in no way desired to start a rival institution to the Edinburgh Hospital for Women and Children and ... it appears to them quite possible that eventually the two schemes might be worked into one. Even if this were not found feasible the Club might at the end of three years find itself able to take an active part in helping both.'[19]

The small George Square hospital was a modest affair, only seven beds, attended by resident nurse and probationer; but Dr

Inglis was radiant when she attended the opening, in November 1899. It was a beginning, it filled a real need, it was something she had always dreamed of, one more step forward for women. 'The lady medicals are forging ahead' commented the *Caledonian Medical Journal* the following January. 'Is this the nucleus of a new Infirmary?'

During the next few years, all varieties of disease among women and children were treated there; and any medical woman in Edinburgh could send in patients. A bed in one of the three private rooms cost one guinea a week, or in the four-bed ward, half-a-crown. It was, probably, the undertaking closest of all to Dr Inglis's heart. In the next twelve years she missed only three meetings of the medical committee, and wrestled personally with all the tedious minutiae; the nursing sister who scorned the authority of a woman doctor, the details about supplies of carbolic, the releasing of nurses for the Boer War, the arguments about allowing students to witness private operations, and, above all, the never-ending struggle to raise money.

Dr Cadell was on the medical committee; so was Jessie MacGregor, who the previous July had become 'attending medical officer' at the Bruntsfield and so had a foot in either camp. Dr Inglis was unperturbed. The success of the work and the interests of the patients mattered; private feuds did not. 'Elsie', remarked Dr MacGregor to Eva, now Mrs McLaren, about this time, 'is so exceptionally generous in her attitude of mind, it would be difficult not to get on with her.'[20] Dr MacGregor, Mrs McLaren wrote later, was the first to comment upon a quality others were to notice; it was always the work as a whole, not her own importance or recognition, which counted with Elsie.

Her hope of uniting women's medical work in Edinburgh seemed a step nearer realisation when in June 1901 the constitutional arrangements at the Bruntsfield were altered at a special meeting, to the displeasure of J-B who from Sussex still kept a watchful eye upon the hospital she had founded.[21]

The new arrangements gave more control to the lay committee, less to J-B and the doctors. Now Dr Inglis might hope for a consultant post there; and when the lay committee next met to vote new appointments, it was found that the senior post had gone to Dr Mona Chalmers Watson (Elizabeth Garrett Anderson's niece) while the votes for the 'junior assistant physician' were exactly divided between Dr Inglis and a Dr Marion Erskine; and that a re-vote would be necessary.[22]

At this interesting point, several pages of the minute book of the Bruntsfield Hospital have been removed; from subsequent records it seems clear that Dr Inglis was somehow defeated. In the light of later events it would probably not be fanciful to suppose J-B had again been the determining factor. Elsie had to accept the setback for the moment.

Early the next year the future of the little George Square nursing home came under review as the lease was running out. In other circumstances, the two competing hospitals might now have been worked into one. As things were, Dr Inglis determined that her own experiment should not be abandoned. She drafted a minute which is revealing of the determination and optimism with which she approached a problem.

'The Medical Sub-committee', she wrote '... realise to the full the trouble the House Committee must have in carrying on the Home and they regret that these duties must be rendered more difficult owing to the small amount of money with which the Home has to be carried on. They wish to point out, however, that this is a difficulty in the way of most small charities.

'Looking at the question from the point of view of the work done—the statistics show that the Home has been largely and increasingly taken advantage of during the three years of its existence.

'They are aware that several subscriptions were guaranteed for three years until the question of the usefulness of such a Home had been tested by experience. Some of these subscriptions will probably in view of the above fact be continued; and they believe that any that lapse can be made up, for the same reasons.

'In view of all these considerations they see no reason why the Home should be closed.'[23]

'Looking at it from the point of view of the work accomplished'—that was always Elsie's attitude. But new premises must be found. As the work that seemed to her most valuable was the attending of poor women during their confinements, it was decided to take premises in the Royal Mile.

The choice fell on 219 High Street: a house with finely proportioned rooms and Adam fireplaces, which had once been a respectable inn, abutting on Old Stamp Office Close where in Jacobite times had lived the Countess of Eglinton, and where Flora Macdonald went to school. Its attraction for Elsie Inglis was partly historical, but she also knew that in these once noble habitations now become murky slums was the front line of battle against dirt, poverty, ignorance. Outwardly dismal, inconvenient inside with its narrow twisting staircase, the old building had still—in her vision—an exciting future. She renamed it, romantically, The Hospice.

The opening was in January, 1904. The Hospice was to be a surgical and gynaecological centre with its own operating theatre, and was also a centre for district midwifery. It was one of the first hospitals to make anaesthetics in childbirth available to the very poor. There was also a general dispensary and accident department. So successful was the work that in December it was found necessary to appoint a resident medical officer, Dr Alice Hutchison;[24] at about the same time Mrs Simson's daughter Evelyn joined the nursing staff.

Elsie Inglis had been in practice almost ten years. Little girls she had treated for earache or measles were now young mothers who turned to her to deliver their first babies. Women she had known as young wives now boasted six or eight children, many of whom had been slapped into their first cry by the 'wee sandy-heidit doctor'. She was the friend of whole families. Even the husbands did not always disdain her help—who else would fight the War Office for months to get his rights for Private Bell when he returned from the Boer War, and refuse to give up till his request for false teeth was granted?

This Bell family were among the many from whom she took no fee; she visited their children in hospital even when not professionally involved; arranged for the baptism of the baby, named, inevitably, Elsie Maud; and not only accepted with delight a gift of South African ostrich feathers from Private Bell, but called later to show how well they set off the hat she was wearing to a wedding.[25]

Such a well-meant gift was perhaps the only thing that could make Elsie interest herself in dress. Short, and by now turned forty and tending to stoutness, she had neither the makings nor the inclination of a fashion plate; though now the cropped hair had been grown to a decorous length and student sloppiness turned to a disciplined neatness suitable to the dignity of medical women. Ignoring of the allurements of fashion can have unexpected results. A photograph of a large group of founder-members of the Federation of Scottish Suffrage Societies shows serious-minded women who nevertheless in the fashion of 1906 appear to have got themselves up like prize poultry: Elsie almost alone wears simple clothes that to a modern eye seem classically tasteful.

Her methods as a doctor were imaginative. One poor woman, about the time The Hospice was opened, had lost two babies through malnutrition. When a third was born, Dr Inglis arranged for her sister, at that time a nursing mother, to visit the family daily and feed the baby—an unorthodox arrangement, Mrs McLaren's acceptance of which demonstrates that Elsie was not the only unusual woman in the family.[26] Sad to say, the child died notwithstanding; but Elsie succeeded in saving a fourth child, by the determination and regularity with which she herself went to the home daily, no matter what her other arrangements, to sterilise bottle feeds.

Her practical knowledge of the poor led Elsie to undertake research into their nutrition, a quite new field. She persuaded the town council to subsidise this, the first municipal authority to do such a thing. Two medical men collaborated in the scientific tables, but Elsie organised all the field work and wrote most of the report.

It bears the stamp of her dry humour ('We must remember that taxes are paid only once a year and rent only twice, and this being a Canongate house no one would think of preparing to meet them long beforehand'), her ready appreciation of others ('Mrs O. deserves great credit for ... helping so willingly as she did. She does not know what wage her husband gets. During the week of the study she fed a household of six on 9s. 11d.').

The report adduces some startling comparisons—one woman was subsisting on a diet less than the ration allowance at beseiged Ladysmith—and mentions 'the question of how far it is right that the diets of prisons and poorhouses should be better than that of the free labouring classes.'

'Our experience' she ends 'has convinced us that the steady, thrifty poor who feel the difficulty of making both ends meet would appreciate and would benefit by simple instruction on the rules of diet.' It proposed the distribution of simple tables of food values and some instruction in the subject for district visitors and others with an entree to poor homes. Seventy years on, this may no longer sound remarkable. At the time, it was unusually imaginative and practical.[27]

CHAPTER 8

In April 1905, Dr MacGregor made the sudden decision to go to America for family reasons. It was unexpected. A week earlier she had applied for a five-year reappointment to the Bruntsfield.[1] She left at once. Almost exactly a year later, at Denver, Colorado, she died.[2]

Elsie was sufficiently established to keep 8 Walker Street on alone. She was one of the most prominent women in the city. In July, the Bruntsfield Hospital offered her the appointment vacated by Jessie MacGregor, because of 'her ability and outstanding position amongst the women doctors of Edinburgh'.[3]

When Sophia Jex-Blake in Brighton got wind of this she wrote intimating her intention of resigning her own position (she was still a consultant) if Elsie's appointment went through. The committee begged her to reconsider. They invited her to become a Vice-President. They did not, however, offer to drop Elsie Inglis. And when J-B declined their overtures and pressed her resignation, they contented themselves with expressing regret at the severance of her connexion with the hospital she had founded.[4] Sophia's story contains the essence of tragedy, as her biographer Dr Margaret Todd truly observed (while omitting all mention of events involving Dr Inglis). Sophia's own qualities would always, inevitably, defeat her.

Elsie was working harder than ever. Besides her new appointment, her work at The Hospice and the dispensaries, her private practice, she had become, gradually, inevitably, and almost unremarked, a leader of the suffrage movement.

Medical work had, from the outset, strengthened her original conviction that the women's vote must be mobilised. Only women really understood the needs of children, of the sick, of the poor; they *must* have a voice in legislation.

In the new century, she devoted more and more time to this cause. Suffrage was becoming a crucial issue, although the struggle was still peaceful, constitutional, essentially ladylike. The very word 'suffragette' was unknown; suffragists as they called themselves aimed at the conversion, not coercion, of public opinion. Every village in England had its Women's Suffrage Society[5] and in their National Union Mrs Fawcett was developing the strongest, most tightly organised yet most responsive, democratic, and flexible political movement ever known in England. She was helped by having a cause which for its adherents had all the force of a religion. But their task was hard. Apart from theoretical considerations, the creation of millions of unpredictable new voters all thinking for themselves is something few M.P.s would face with equanimity.*

In Scotland the movement had lagged, owing to the more scattered population. From 1900 on, Elsie Inglis threw herself into building it up, inevitably impressing herself on much of its policy. She spoke at sometimes as many as four meetings a week; no open-air meeting on Porthleven Sands was complete without her. She travelled widely, addressing audiences as far away as Shetland and Orkney; making hasty dashes by train or car to arrive at some remote spot, having foregone a meal, after her full day's work; and returning by first light next day to begin her rounds on time.[6]

Meetings in smaller places could be heavy going. Lady Frances Balfour openly declared them 'like speaking into the middle of a pincushion'.[7] In such disheartening conditions Elsie's optimism was a formidable asset. 'My dear', she once consoled a worker who expressed disappointment over a poorly attended meeting, 'I was not counting the people, I was thinking of the efforts which had brought those who *were* there.'[8]

Many of those who *were* there had the dull acceptance of woman's inferior lot that had shocked Elsie years before; even the educated were only too likely to lump suffragists with vegetarians, total abstainers and Christian Scientists as sincere, but cranky.

Hence Elsie Inglis's contribution was novel, and valuable. Many in the movement were still leisured gentlewomen with limited contacts with the seamy side of life. Mrs Fawcett herself managed an afternoon rest beforehand whenever she addressed a meeting. Elsie's experiences were different and she used them astringently. Once she startled a complacent audience by describing an inter-

* At this period only men over thirty had the vote. When in 1918 the vote was granted to men over twenty-one and women over thirty the electorate increased from 8 millions to nearly 16 millions.

view earlier that day with a man who, deaf to persuasion, refused consent for his wife to have a necessary operation. 'Who is to get my porridge?' he had demanded, and condemned the woman to a suffering which death alone would end. Dr Inglis's voice was well-bred, gentle and feminine with a light, bird-like quality;* she never raised it to emphasise her words. But her deep feeling infected her audience; few of them forgot the episode or failed to draw the moral. Educated women must seize the vote, because only so could they effectively help their downtrodden sisters in the slums.

More perhaps than any other woman in the campaign, Elsie Inglis was the apotheosis of 'the modern woman'—emancipated, supporting herself in an exacting profession, high-couraged, yet gentle, well-bred, *womanly*; and personally fulfilled in family links and friendships. The sight of her opened the eyes of many who had previously supposed suffragists were only in it because of their own frustrations; in the words of one nurse who worked for her, 'she couldn't drink her tea for telling you how marvellous life was'.[9]

By 1906 Elsie Inglis was to the Scottish groups what Mrs Fawcett was to the English; when they too formed themselves that year into a Federation, it was Elsie who became its secretary.

She acted as hostess to other distinguished speakers, the Snowdens, the Pethick Lawrences, Maude Royden and many more, putting them up at 8 Walker Street and surrounding them with comforts she hardly had time to enjoy herself.[10]

By 1906 the militants had embarked on the dramatic methods which earned them their colourful niche in history. The evening in October 1905 when Annie Kenney and Christabel Pankhurst interrupted a meeting of Sir Edward Grey's marked the beginning of the change, and the word 'suffragettes' was quickly coined by the *Daily Mail*; although it was another three years before the first stone was thrown, at the windows of 10 Downing Street.

The militant phase coincided with the enlistment to the cause of many working-class women, and with the realisation among suffrage workers that they must pin their hopes on the Labour Party. Dr Inglis had been connected with liberalism since her father's day, but the time had come to end all that; suffrage alone must be her cause. The Liberals, Lady Frances Balfour owned,

* Personal information, Mr Moray McLaren and others.

received her resignation with something like relief; they had never been able to rely on her to truckle to her party instead of putting her foot down about suffrage.[11]

The new Federation of Scottish Suffrage Societies worked under difficulties, and could not at first even get a telephone from the authorities. Then by one of her lucky coincidences, Dr Inglis was approached by the Post Office to surrender some of her 'back green' at Walker Street for a telegraph post. In the words of Miss May Simson, who acted as her secretary, 'my aunt came spanking in, bubbling with amusement, to announce "My dears, we've got our telephone".' Low cunning? Dr Inglis's interpretation would more probably have been in the phrase often on her father's lips, 'All things work together for good to them that trust in Him.' She could seize an opportunity, but devious manoeuvring, however innocent, was beyond her; nor did she believe it brought permanent gains.[12]

The strain of campaigning was great. To the physical effort of travelling were added skimped meals, burning the candle at both ends and (since she was an obstetrician) often in the middle as well. She was human enough privately to feel that bed was always especially comfortable when the night bell rang;[13] but forgotten now was the maxim of student days that women should not make themselves ill by overworking. She did not complain. Indeed, she kept pretty silent about her own concerns. Lady Frances Balfour noticed that when joined by a friend, after church, for a walk, or socially, she more usually waited to hear what was their overriding preoccupation, and into this poured her interest and sympathy.[14]

Her resilience was a byword among those who knew her. It was entirely the product of her determination *never* to be beaten by mere circumstance. There was a night when Elsie was driving with Maude Royden, distinguished already as a writer and lecturer, and later to be famous as a preacher at the City Temple. They were going to a suffrage meeting at a remote village, on an evening of stormy wind and rain. Miles from their destination, their car was halted by a tree across the road. The two women were in the evening gowns and thin shoes still the wear for formal meetings; but they got out and struggled to help their driver move the obstacle.

When it seemed hopeless Miss Royden suggested walking the rest of the way. The look Elsie turned on her she never forgot.

Only later did she remember that she could hardly have managed the walk; she was lame. At the moment, Elsie's own determination infected her to the point of confidently offering the impossible. As it turned out, however, the tree in the road also seems to have felt in the end the force of Elsie's determination. Inanimate things did, from time to time. The walk did not need to be made.[15]

Those who campaigned in these conditions gave the lie to opponents (Beatrice Webb among them) who opposed suffrage because 'the emancipating process has now reached the limits fixed by the physical constitution of women'.[16]

The physical constitution of women occupied the minds of some opponents obsessively in those pre-Freudian days. There is a clear connexion between the entry of women like Elsie Inglis into medicine and a change in the accepted notions about women's constitution during the generation preceding 1914.* Girls in fact, were learning 'to be brave and not whine over everything'; were becoming, gradually, the physically tough and energetic creatures who in the Great War would drive ambulances in hair-raising emergencies, break and school horses at remount depots, or nurse horribly wounded men in primitive conditions.

Even more valuable, perhaps, was the deep comradeship of the suffrage campaigners. Friendship, said the ancients, is only for the good and noble; a modern writer has pointed out that the first condition of having true friends is that one shall care deeply for something else more than for friendship.† Now for the first time in all history, women, *ordinary* women, broke free of the imposed relationships of family and social life to find this condition in themselves.

In the women's campaign every step of the common journey was, in ways humble but never trivial, testing those engaged in it. Duke's daughters stood shoulder to shoulder with mill girls. Class, party, income, status, profession, ceased to count. The suffrage campaign, and later the Great War, gave to women a taste of that special comradeship which had seemed reserved for men and which, once experienced, makes any other relation-

* See Sir Almroth Wright's notorious letter to *The Times*, March 28th, 1912, which was described as 'pornographic' at the time, presumably because it contained the expression 'change of life'; and the subsequent correspondence.

† C. S. Lewis, *The Four Loves*, p. 77.

ship pale into dimness. It was a comradeship for which Elsie Inglis was particularly fitted.

Her enthusiasm, however, compromised her professional future. Hospital boards responsible for senior appointments never favour cranks; and suffragists were seen as cranks.[17] Only the Bruntsfield could consider her, and when the senior consultant there retired, Elsie Inglis succeeded to the post. At her suggestion, and perhaps because she rated suffrage claims on her time above professional ambition, Dr Cadell was brought in not under her (the normal thing) but as co-equal.[18] The following year Dr Inglis became an extramural lecturer in gynaecology to the University; and a lecturer for nurses taking the examinations of the Central Midwives Board set up in 1902. 'As a lecturer', a colleague wrote, 'she proved herself clear and concise and the level of her lectures never fell below that of the best established standards.' In 1908, too, she opened at The Hospice the first infant milk depot in Edinburgh, and began the systematic inspection of babies which laid the foundation of future child welfare services in the city; and also, with Dr Beatrice Russell, began lecturing to the new Voluntary Health Visitors Association.[19]

She was now Edinburgh's foremost woman practitioner; making, outsiders judged, probably between £2000 and £3000 a year, a considerable income for the period. 8 Walker Street, a Georgian house of well-proportioned lofty rooms, with a graceful oval staircase with elaborate cornices and wrought iron-balustrade, was elegant and, Lady Frances Balfour considered, 'well run'[20] by Lizzie the faithful table-maid and a cook, housemaid and charwoman who were less permanent fixtures. At wages of £25-£35 a year for indoor staff this would have been a modest establishment for a professional man, but was handsome for a self-supporting single woman. The staff were trusted to work in their own way. Occasional troubles were briskly dealt with: 'If you can't agree, you'll *all* have to go.' They usually agreed. Dr Inglis did not inquire how. Results alone concerned her.[21] 'Always so bright and cheerful, and kind in her manner, and so frank and easy to do for and told you at once if anything was not right' was the verdict of one domestic, a dispensary caretaker.[22] Only one rigid rule obtained at 8 Walker Street: family prayers before breakfast, for staff and visitors alike.

Promptly at ten the hired victoria, chosen on principle as the vehicle giving the maximum fresh air, would arrive from Scott

Croall's coach yard; keeping her own carriage was one of the purely personal ambitions now quite thrown out. At each stop on her rounds, the coachman was carefully instructed to park end on to the kerb lest the shafts weary the horses. In the mornings there would be dispensaries at St Cuthbert's, St Anne's, Morrison Street or the Little Sisters of the Poor, as well as hospital visits; on most afternoons, attendance at the service at St Giles' would be fitted between lectures, visits, private consultations in the room at 8 Walker Street lined with her father's books. There would be a committee, or a visit to the Y.W.C.A., where she injected some of her own cheerful confidence into the delicately-named 'servant department', the welfare section for unmarried mothers. Finally, in all likelihood, a late visit or two to some grimy slum where the leading woman doctor tucked up her sleeves to show some poor ignorant mother how a baby should be bathed; or made tea and toast for a patient too ill and apathetic to get herself food.

Dinner at Walker Street was nominally at seven, in the dining room dominated by a Raeburn portrait of great-aunt Katherine Inglis; but more often, it was a quarter to eight when Dr Inglis came spanking in; now as in student days, she usually undertook too much for the available time. Lizzie knew she must have her bath before dinner. 'Plenty of hot water day or night' was the only personal amenity she demanded (and the one to be remembered most regretfully in Serbia and Roumania). For others she could be autocratic in tiny things as well as great. Mrs McLaren's daughter Amy, staying at Walker Street, expressed a wish for a certain pudding. The bell was instantly rung and the pudding ordered, although it was little more than an hour before dinner.

The Simson children were now grown up, some of them married, and great-nephews and -nieces were growing up alongside the small McLarens and Inglises. Elsie made garments for each new baby, though she was a careful rather than an enthusiastic needlewoman; and as they grew, managed to make each child feel it had a special niche in her heart. They found her 'a darling', with a soft shoulder, a fund of bedtime stories, and the ability to get as excited as any of them over a close-run race on school sports-day.

Sunday evenings were family occasions in the Simson household and there Elsie would go for supper after the evening service in St Giles'; usually, again, arriving late, for she liked to pace after the service in long and earnest conversation with the Dean, Dr Wallace Williamson, and his wife, who, outside her family, were her closest friends.[23]

Her own hospitality included family and friends, suffrage speakers, colleagues, and patients. A woman doctor arriving on a visit discovered that a party of six had left only the day before: a patient and her five children, the mother having badly needed a rest but having an unsympathetic husband and no relations to help her. Visitors were made free of the house; they might borrow anything and forget to return it—except her father's books.[24]

Elsie was almost at the peak of her success and—ironically—within a few weeks of realising her ambition to unify all women's medical work in Edinburgh, when in October 1909, when she was forty-five, an incident occurred to bring out all of the ardent, uncalculating fighter, youthfully willing to throw away all rather than compromise on a principle, that still remained in her.[25]

The Bruntsfield Hospital had been involved in a lawsuit over alleged negligence by a nurse. In his judgement against the hospital, the judge declared the committee had approved a letter which was 'not fair and honest' and seemed determined to clear itself at all hazards.

Elsie Inglis was not personally involved, but when the final day for appeal had passed with no action from the hospital, she wrote resigning her position. The judgement she considered wrong and insulting. The hospital authorities had failed to back up their own staff and 'from that point of view alone I cannot act any longer with the committee. But apart from that I do not think that anyone, or any body of people like the committee, are doing right when they allow such statements to be made about them without protest. There are some things which if they are not denied, are admitted, and these statements about the methods of the committee were made not by an irresponsible newspaper, but by a judge from the Bench. The only way of contradicting him is by appealing against his judgement. The committee obviously do not agree with me and feeling as strongly as I do on the point, the only course left to me is to resign.'

They could not accept this. A committee member who was a

fellow suffragist, Miss Margaret Houldsworth, suggested a compromise; if details of her protest were placed on record, would Dr Inglis agree to carry on?

Elsie was usually prompt in replying to letters, but she had not answered this one when a few days later Miss Houldsworth died, leaving £3,000 'for the advantage of medical women and in pursuit of gynaecology and midwifery'.

What conversations next took place we do not know, what appeals to 'low cunning', nor whether Dr Inglis was somehow induced to remember that she had once thought the best way to deal with calumny was simply to live it down. But some weeks later she wrote to Miss Houldsworth's successor, saying that as the committee wished it, she would gladly carry on.

The following day, with little discussion—it had obviously been well thrashed out beforehand—the committee placed on record its decision to apply the Houldsworth bequest to bring about what Elsie had always dreamed of, the amalgamation of the Bruntsfield Hospital with The Hospice. The Bruntsfield should be enlarged so that all medical and surgical cases could be treated there, The Hospice continuing with maternity and child welfare work only.

It must have been a bitter pill for Sophia Jex-Blake, who still had three years to live in her Sussex retirement.

For Elsie, however, almost everything she had aimed at had now been achieved. By February 1911 the Bruntsfield Hospital was enlarged and united with The Hospice. Official approval sealed the work when on July 18th Queen Mary, on her coronation-year visit to Edinburgh, visited the hospital and was proudly escorted by the radiant Dr Elsie Inglis round the new surgical unit.[26]

Professionally, she could rest on her laurels.

The suffrage campaign had meanwhile become even more controversial. Since 1905 the forceful methods of the Pankhurst party had attracted attention; papers which ignored the constitutional 'suffragists' fell over themselves to publicise the 'suffragettes'. Yet though the suffragettes' devotion cannot be questioned—many had their health broken by imprisonment—it remains open to doubt, and certainly Elsie doubted, why mature women should expect tactics like the tantrums of a frustrated child to persuade anyone of their fitness to vote. She could not approve their methods. Discussions—and there were plenty: Mrs McLaren was for a time a member of Mrs Pankhurst's organisation—left her unmoved.[27] Herself capable of great sacrifices—including some, such as the sale of the Raeburn great-aunt to swell the coffers of the cause, which were made by stealth[28] and greatly to the irritation of her family when they found out—she never saw sacrifice as valuable in itself. Since the success of a cause was all, the role of the individual (herself or another) nothing, why then, talk of self-sacrifice was simply irrelevant.

The militants were at first content to suffer violence without retaliation. The gentle and sweetly-smiling Mrs Elmy who had given Elsie her first chance as a speaker was, still in her black dress, shawl and bonnet, a speaker at the first meeting of Mrs Pankhurst's W.S.P.U. in Trafalgar Square in 1906. But in June 1908 the militants moved into the aggressive phase which involved breaking windows and throwing stones (often, it must be confessed, with inaccurate aim: Dr Ethel Smyth had to give secret lessons in stone-throwing to Mrs Pankhurst who had never played ball games in her girlhood). It was now their turn to split their own ranks. Mrs McLaren was one of many prepared to suffer but not to exercise aggression, who now left the Pankhursts. The suffragettes' violence antagonised the public; it antagonised the constitutional suffragists, if possible, more. For a time it was an open question whether the two branches of the movement were more concerned to demolish the 'Antis' or one another

Scottish suffragettes slashed and burned golf courses. They tried to tear the clothes off Mr Asquith at Lossiemouth.[29] Was this likely to convince anyone of their fitness for responsibility? Dr Inglis could not think so. Had not one of her own followers been told, when trying to book a village hall for a perfectly peaceful meeting, 'It's suffragettes ye'll be. Are ye not ashamed o' yersels, rantin' and reivin' round the country?'[30] She felt the danger, later to be expressed retrospectively by the *Glasgow Herald* in a leading article on 'Heroines of the War' in December 1917: 'Looking back on those days ... the multitude were dangerously wrong, although perhaps with excuse, in making the excesses of overwrought and hysterical women a pretext for ignoring the solid claims seriously advanced by women of the calibre of Dr Inglis.'[31]

They were difficult and depressing times for those who chose to plod the less exhilarating path of peaceful propaganda. The reactions of one typical new convert were described by Mrs Abbott of Edinburgh. She had gone to the suffrage centre to offer help, but found the committee rooms 'a depressing empty shop' and the job she was asked to do, 'giving out handbills in a rainy street', neither inspiring nor apparently effective. Then Dr Inglis rushed in on a wave of vitality, to arrange speakers for meetings. Mrs Abbott found herself being told firmly 'You will speak ...'

'I must explain,' she interrupted. 'I am quite new. I don't speak at all. I have never spoken.' In fact she had resolved—having presumably listened to some suffrage speakers with more enthusiasm than expertise—that she would never inflict herself upon an audience without proper training.

Her protests were waved aside by Dr Inglis. 'Oh, but you *must* speak.' She spoke; only later realising that it had simply not occurred to her to press her refusal. Soon she was one of a growing band of full-time organisers planted by Elsie all over Scotland.[32] It was one of Elsie's strengths as a leader, to give her followers confidence in themselves and in one another. Even when the human material was unpromising she had an eye for hidden capacities, and a useful knack of inspiration.

By 1910 the movement in Scotland was as tightly organised as in England. There was now enough backing in the country for a Parliamentary Conciliation Committee to be formed to support a Bill to give the vote to women householders. The militants called a truce while it went forward. It looked as if the day were won.[33]

Twenty-five years before, Elsie Inglis had written of 'the habit of dreaming, which must be given up'. Now some at least of the dreams seemed to be coming to fruition.

If her life appeared to those around her happy, fulfilled, extroverted, that was only what everyone who knew her would have expected. She had apparently every cause for satisfaction. It is true that some people found her preoccupied, a little aloof even. But everyone who has left any record seems to have thought of her as a happy woman. Was this the whole story?

It is not easy to find evidence of Elsie Inglis's personal feelings. She kept no diary, lived surrounded by her family and friends and so wrote few personal letters; did not put her feelings easily into words. Even with her father, 'I wish I could have scragged that beast!' or 'I want to pass awfully well' were about the extent of her self-revelation. One must not therefore assume she was uncomplicated. She was a Victorian lady; one trained, in Shaw's words, 'to the utmost attainable degree in the art and habit of concealing her feelings, and maintaining an imperturbable composure under the most trying circumstances'.[34] Nine-tenths of her nature, therefore, lay below the surface. In personal contact she often managed to communicate with few and conventional words, or even without any. From Serbia and Russia, when circumstances were trying enough in all conscience, even her personal letters to sisters and close friends were to make use of the same thoughts often couched in the self-same restrained phrases, as her formal official reports. Her achievements, as Mrs Abbott later wrote, are there for the world to see; 'but the things behind all that, the character that conquered, the spirit that inspired, the incredible courage, optimism, indomitability ... all that, it seems to me, had to be gathered in and understood from the tiny incident, the word, the glance'.[35]

There are, however, some few clues to her inmost thoughts at this time, a few papers discovered locked in her desk after her death, which must have been kept because they held significance for her: that old sheet of resolutions made after her mother's death; one or two letters of her parents'; a copy of a hymn by F. R. Havergal, a writer whose unfashionable mawkishness of expression tends to obscure, today, the sturdiness of much of her religious thought.

> ... I turned aside
> With aching head and heart most sorely bowed,
> Around me cares and griefs in crushing crowd;
> While inly rose the sense, in swelling tide
> Of weakness, insufficiency and sin
> And fear and gloom and doubt in mighty flood rolled in.
>
> ... O Saviour I have proved
> That Thou to help and save art really near.
> ... The cross is not removed
> I must go forth to bear it as before
> But leaning on Thine arm I dread its weight no more.

Weakness, insufficiency, fear and gloom and doubt are not what the world saw in Elsie Inglis. What she felt, she concealed to the utmost degree. The sheet of paper in her desk hints at another story.[36]

There is another clue. About this time she wrote a novel. Mrs McLaren knew of it for the first time after her sister's death, and recognised it as autobiographical.[37] From internal evidence it can be dated at somewhere around 1910. From this manuscript also, it is clear that Elsie was far from immune to depression and self-doubts, although by the time she wrote *The Story of a Modern Woman* she had largely solved them. The interest of the book lies solely in its self-revelation; it has no literary merit.

The novel's heroine is a teacher, a spinster, facing middle age, outwardly cheerful, inwardly oppressed by loneliness, depression, doubts. She is involved in a near-fatal boating accident, an episode Mrs McLaren recognised as taken from life.

> Self-revelation (Elsie wrote now of this) is not usually a pleasant process. Not often do we find ourselves better than we expected ... But very rarely ... the flash may, in a moment, reveal unknown powers or unsuspected strength.
>
> And Hildeguard, sitting back in the boat, suddenly realised she wasn't a coward. She looked back in surprise over her life and remembered that the terror which as a child would seize her in a sudden emergency was the fear of being parted from her mother, not any personal fear for herself, or her own safety.
>
> Such a pleasurable glow swept over her ... 'Why, no,' she thought: 'I wasn't frightened.'

Physical courage was hardly looked for in Victorian or Edwardian ladies. The Glasgow professor had noted with amusement that Elsie was afraid of nothing and would make an excellent surgeon; nor did those who knew the murky wynds and closes underestimate the courage needed to enter them. For the most part, though, it was only in the Great War that even Elsie's close associates realised that, like her grandfather Thompson, she had nerve enough for anything and a heart never seen to fail for an instant. She herself had a reassuring inkling of it years before.

On her personal philosophy of life the novel is also revealing. She had grown up in a family that was God-fearing but not narrow; and her own faith in a divine providence was expressed in her choice of an inscription for John Inglis's tomb: 'Like as a father pitieth his children, so the Lord pitieth them that fear him.' But although, as Lady Frances Balfour observed, Elsie's reserve on these matters was not often broken, she once admitted to her sister that she was passing through a crisis of faith. 'I go to church still because I do not wish to cut myself off from the religious life of my day, but I confess I do not know what they all mean.'[38]

In *The Story of a Modern Woman* it is the remark of a Quaker friend* which shows the heroine the key to her problems.

> 'Christmas' (*says the friend*) 'is a hard time with all its memories. I think I have found out what we lonely women want. It is a future ... You see other women with their families—it is the future to which they look ... their life goes on in other lives.'

When her Quaker friend dies, a sudden intuition strikes the heroine, some words come to her mind: 'The Power of an Endless Life.' She becomes a woman transformed. She involves herself (another autobiographical incident) with the suffrage cause, but that is only part of the story. She looks at some old photographs.

> For long these old photographs had stood to her as symbols of a past glowing with happiness ... But now as she looked her thoughts did not turn to the past. In some unexplained way the loves of long ago seemed to be entwined with a future so wonderful and so enticing that her heart bounded as she thought of it ...
>
> 'The Power of an Endless Life'—the words seemed to hover around her, just eluding her grasp, just beyond her comprehension, yet something of their significance she seemed to catch ... No mystic she, to whom an ineffable union with the Highest was the goal of all. Never even distantly did she reach to that idea. Rather she was one of God's simple-minded soldiers, who took her orders and stood to her post. The words thrilled her, not with the prospect of rest, but with the excitement of advance, 'an Endless Life' with ever new possibilities of growth and of achievement, ever greater battles to be fought for the right, and always new hopes of happiness ... She began dimly to feel the power of the idea, the life of which she was a holder only 'part of a greater whole', Earth itself only a step in a great progression. Ever upward, ever onward, marching

* Marion Holbourn, formerly of Edinburgh Meeting of the Society of Friends, writes: 'Elsie Inglis never attended Edinburgh Friends Meeting and I think I should have known if any of the Friends – very few in those days – had known her personally.'

towards some 'Divine far-off event to which the whole creation moves'.

It had taken Elsie years to resolve her problems of belief. Her father 'said he did not believe death was the stopping place'. But no one takes over ready-made a living faith from another; to quote R.L.S. who (perhaps because he once wrote of God as a surgeon) was among her favourite writers, 'every man is his own doctor of divinity in the last resort'.[39] Death was no more the end in her philosophy than in her father's. But personal immortality? She was after all a 'modern woman', influenced by Darwin, Huxley, Wells. 'The power of an endless life' is an inspired phrase, to be found of course in Hebrews 7, 16 and meaning many different things to different people. For Elsie it had come to be a phrase reconciling traditional beliefs with the new ones expressed in Wells's 'I do not believe I have any personal immortality. I am part of an immortality, perhaps, but that is different.'[40]

She had found her solutions to the universal problem. And the greatest of her achievements lay ahead.

Her private life was indeed happier by 1910 than at any time since John Inglis's death. Her brother Ernest's widow and children came in that year to make their home at 8 Walker Street, and filled it with the lively concerns and laughter of the young. They revelled in Aunt Elsie's company; to a formidably authoritative adult's power to make the rules, she added a childlike delight in living. On holiday in the Highlands, she heard one child remark how much she would love to see the wooded hills by moonlight. 'So would I,' responded Aunt Elsie promptly and the thing was arranged. The children were got up in the middle of the night and the whole party tramped out in outrageous high spirits on a never-to-be-forgotten expedition.[41]

The children had filled the only real gap in her life. For one is bound to ask why a woman so vital, so full of the qualities most men seek in a wife, never had a husband and children of her own. She had an affectionate heart, and 'womanly' is one of the adjectives most often used by men who knew her. Her sisters married happily; did she alone fail to inherit Harriet's quality of being the kind of girl men drive fifty miles to dance with? Did she feel it her duty to stay with her parents? Or was there some might-have-been of which we know nothing?

One possible answer can be ruled out. Marriage and a medical career were not mutually exclusive; of fifty registered women doctors in 1885, just before Elsie began training, eighteen were married.[42] Marriage was, however, a bar to even junior staff posts, and this did weigh with some women doctors.

Another possible explanation is that men of the time fought shy of the 'advanced' woman. Certainly women discovering in the face of age-old tradition that they could stand on their own feet, were understandably unwilling to indulge in that superficial feminine behaviour which even men as able and intelligent as Asquith find so strangely flattering and reassuring. The dilemma of the womanly woman is that the more womanly she is, the more she requires that a husband shall be one she can really look up to, not merely affect to do so. If she is also intelligent, forceful and idealistic, the field is narrowed; if she spends years of her youth studying for an exacting profession in segregated classes, it narrows almost to vanishing.

Elsie had experienced a close relationship with one male paragon, her father. Anyone else would have had much to live up to. However, it is the opinion of men and women who knew her that she would certainly have married had the right man presented himself. People noticed that in her public speeches she did not, like many suffrage campaigners, denigrate the male sex. 'I do not think we are nearly careful enough to make it quite clear that we do not hold that we women alone could have done a bit better—that we are proud of the great work our men have done,' she liked to say, adding that only when men and women worked as partners would the best solutions be reached.[43]

She was lucky, however, in that her instincts were mainly, and strongly, maternal. It is a fallacy that such a woman needs children of her own to fulfil her; it is the unmaternal woman whose instincts need physical motherhood to awaken them. Elsie found fulfilment in her work and in the family circle. 'The babies as they arrived in the families [of her relations] met with her special love,' wrote a niece. 'In her short summer holidays with any of us the children were her great delight.' The women of the slums were her sisters; her medical colleagues, comrades in arms; but to men, even her contemporaries, her attitude was maternal; every one of them was seen as some woman's son.

They felt it themselves. A dour business man met her only once, when his sister, a friend of Elsie, had been staying at 8 Walker Street to be near another brother who was dying. As they finally drove away after saying goodbye, the hardened man of affairs found his eyes filling with tears. 'I should have liked to kiss her like my mother,' he said.[44] The same quality was to be noted later by the Serbs. *Srbska maika iz skotske* they called her, Serbian mother from Scotland. A man such as the young Russian air officer in the Dobruga might escape with a mild and maternal glance at his good intentions after some disregard of instructions that would have brought down torrents of wrath on the head of any of her nurses. But then of *women*, or at any rate of *British* women, higher things were expected.

By 1912, for all her optimism, Elsie was feeling a certain strain. Now in her late forties, for years she had never rested except during her September holidays in the Highlands, which she spent cycling, sketching and walking. She drove herself hard, lived in a perpetual rush, could not always count upon an uninterrupted night's sleep.

Nor did she have the small extra comforts that money could have given. Her income was adequate, her home comfortable, but others had more time to enjoy it than she did. Such spare money as she had, went to innumerable private benefactions ('philanthropist' was the second word chosen for her epitaph by those who knew her) and to the suffrage campaign. She was not hard up, but there were economies. She postponed repairs to the house, saved on clothes, took inexpensive holidays. For years she had rushed and skimped even her meals.[45]

In 1912 there was a suffrage setback. Asquith had promised that his government would not oppose the Conciliation Committee's Bill introduced in that year. But after the first reading had passed comfortably, many Liberals were drawn to oppose it on the grounds that enfranchisement of more householders would only favour the Conservatives. The Bill was thrown out.

The women were led to believe that they could be included in the Manhood Suffrage Bill shortly to be introduced. When the appropriate amendments came up in January 1913, however, they were ruled out of order; the Bill's title referred only to men. The only course for the frankly relieved Asquith, who with the Home Rule controversy and the Marconi Scandal had his hands over-full anyway, was to withdraw the Bill altogether.[46]

The disappointment of the women was intense. Forty years' work, said Mrs Fawcett, was destroyed. The militants broke out with redoubled fury. Now the Rokeby Venus, exquisite portrayal of woman-as-plaything, was slashed by Mary Richardson. Now Emily Davidson threw herself beneath the King's Derby runner and was killed. In Scotland, Asquith himself was ambushed and attacked with dogwhips while motoring to Stirling.[47]

To Elsie, the setback was also the signal for renewed effort; but still on peaceful lines. 'Our secretaries have been most extraordinarily unconcerned over disasters in the House,' she wrote to one local secretary, Mrs Cursiter of Orkney. 'Not one of you has suggested depression, and most of you have promptly proposed new work! That is the sort of spirit that wins.'[48]

To maintain the spirit that wins, however, takes its toll. Soon she was forced to admit that she had been doing too much. She resigned from her dispensary at the Little Sisters of the Poor, giving as reason 'health, and the other demands on her time'.[49] She stayed in Edinburgh until after the big suffrage procession with its banners and flowers organised for Assembly week, then went to America. The sea voyage meant rest, but once there she spent much time visiting hospitals and collecting new ideas to incorporate in a hospital at home.* The return voyage failed to restore her and when she got home she was seriously unwell. In September a colleague urged her to close The Hospice and take things easily.

Her reply was made with concentration and earnestness. 'Give me one more year. I *know* there is a future there, and someone will be found to take it on.'[50]

After one more year, however, the sword was again casting its shadow. It was not the future of The Hospice that lay in the balance, but of the civilised world. History was about to present Elsie Inglis with her last and greatest challenge.

* They were, according to a typewritten note in Minute Book 2 of The Hospice and Bruntsfield Hospitals, incorporated when the Elsie Inglis Memorial Hospital was built five years after her death.

CHAPTER 9

In July 1914 Austria invaded Serbia in hit-or-miss retribution for the murder at Sarajevo of the Austrian Archduke Franz Ferdinand. Within days Russia was giving support to Serbia and France to Russia; Germany aligned herself with Austria and attacked France by way of neutral Belgium, thus bringing England—a guarantor of Belgian neutrality—on August 4th into the struggle that would come to be known for a brief twenty years as the Great War.

Elsie Inglis was at this time close to her fiftieth birthday, ill, and ready, if not actually to give up, at least to consider it. That was now forgotten. The war was to her a challenge to all women to prove themselves worthy of the vote. Service to the country became for her service to the Cause. One of the unanswerable arguments of the anti-suffrage lobby had always been that since authority must ultimately rest on force, women who took no share in fighting for the nation clearly deserved no say in its councils.[1] Elsie saw a chance to refute that. Women could serve the army as doctors and nurses. Although most women, untrained for anything but running their homes, received scant welcome or direction from authority, for a surgeon there would surely be no problem. She had for weeks been organising the training of V.A.D.s for hospital work, and now gave over the main rooms of 8 Walker Street as a hospital depot for the rolling of bandages and packing of dressings, taking her own meals off a tray in a tiny back room till Mrs Simson carried her off to the comfort of her own house in Grosvenor Street. She needed the cossetting. Where more extroverted women found the effort to get into war work exhilarating, Elsie was downcast by the tragedy of it. 'We shall live all our lives under the shadow of this war,' she said.[2]

She heard that Mrs Garrett Anderson's daughter Louisa was forming a field hospital unit and wrote to ask if a surgeon was needed; only to be told regretfully that a full team was already assembled.[3]

She offered her services next to the R.A.M.C. representative at

Edinburgh Castle. Miss May Simson* was alone in the drawing room at Grosvenor Street when her aunt returned more dejected than Miss Simson had ever seen her.

'He said "My good lady, go home and sit still",' she said, in reply to her niece's eager question. She lit a cigarette and smoked in silence for some time. At last Miss Simson asked, 'What are you going to do now?'

Elsie threw the stub into the fire. 'I know what we'll do, May. We'll offer help to the Serbs, and to the French.'

'Go home and sit still' was to become in the Scottish Women's Hospitals the kind of joke that is a watchword. ('What's the next job? My dear girl, go home and sit still!') But that was in the future. In the summer of 1914 it was still merely what military men at every level did say to women who attempted to trespass on the entrenched male preserve of a European war. 'Ye'd be better at hame knitting socks for the lads' was the gibe thrown by a sergeant at another woman doctor as she too, a little later, left Edinburgh Castle after unsuccessfully applying to the R.A.M.C.[4]

Where was the difficulty? Did the War Office take its direction from the Secretary for War, Lord Kitchener of Khartoum, who is generally supposed to have had a monastic distrust of women unless they were very well-connected and influential?[5] It is true that Kitchener experienced during the Boer War such a rush of female amateurs to the hospitals as would scare most professional soldiers for life.[6] It is equally true, however, that Mrs Fawcett got on famously with him when she headed a committee investigating Boer refugee camps. She liked Kitchener better than any politician, found her interview with him the most businesslike she had ever had, and amusedly remarked it was the compliment of her life when he invited her whole committee to dinner and took her in himself.[7]

Mrs Fawcett was the exception which proves a rule. Not rich nor influential, and still at fifty-four a pretty and charming woman, she was also supremely intelligent and in a masculine way.

Kitchener's aversion to women was not *simply* monastic. He disliked them as silly havering creatures who argued emotionally, seldom troubled to inform themselves correctly and when not

* The late Miss Simson kindly furnished me with her first-hand recollection of an incident of which there are various conflicting accounts.

spreading defeatist propaganda were keeping a war going unnecessarily by their fanaticism.[8] And Kitchener was right. Pre-1914 woman *was* like this. It was not her fault; the restricted conditions of her life had moulded her; the very conditions that the suffragists fought to change.

Kitchener's attitude, however, his belief that war was for professional soldiers only, his well-known conviction that medical services merely wasted the taxpayers' money,[9] his equally well-known habit of bowler-hatting subordinates who propounded views contrary to his own, all this in 1914 combined to discourage a subordinate—if indeed any such existed—who might have wished to allow women doctors to serve the country.

'My good lady, sit still' was however precisely the attitude, when struck by an opponent, to ensure that Elsie Inglis did not do so. She smarted under the snub to medical women in general, and was quite incapable of taking no for an answer when she saw a chance to kill three birds with one stone: to serve the nation, demonstrate women's fitness for the vote, *and* advance the claim of medical women to do general work and not only gynaecology and paediatrics.

On August 12th, at the first meeting of the federated Scottish suffrage societies after the outbreak of war, she proposed that they should offer a fully equipped hospital unit staffed by women, to the Red Cross for use at home or abroad.[10] With Mrs Laurie, a supporter from Greenock, she went to see Sir George Beatson, head of the Scottish Red Cross.

The Red Cross, Sir George told them, was in the hands of the War Office and could have nothing to say to a hospital staffed by women. (Three years later, had they but known it, both War Office and Red Cross would be trying to coax Dr Inglis into a prudent course of action and would be made regretfully aware that they had got no jurisdiction whatever over the infuriating woman.)

Sir George, however, knew Elsie of old; she had studied under him in Glasgow in the Nineties. He understood, too, the disappointment of having one's inspirations rejected: his own successful treatment of cancer was not followed up until after his death. 'There is no knowing what they may do before the end of the war,' he added, to mitigate his refusal.[11]

The hint was enough for Elsie. She went on planning, and wrote to the ambassadors of Belgium, France and Russia asking if their countries could use her women's unit. She opened a fund with £100 of her own money.[12] Subscriptions followed slowly, but volunteers came flocking, and soon her imagination, flying ahead of mere account books, envisaged several units. Each of them, she told her committee early in October, should be responsible for 100 beds and consist of two senior and two junior doctors, ten trained nurses* with ten auxiliary staff; to equip and run such a hospital for six months would cost £1000.† At this point one of the committee interrupted with a groan, 'We might as well ask for a million at once.' Ignoring this, Dr Inglis went on to propose a national appeal with a target of £50,000. It seemed an impossible sum for a women's movement accustomed to thinking in terms of needlework sales and homemade jam.[13]

Dr Inglis, however, *knew* she was right. And when she *knew* she was right, experience had taught her, to yield to the pressure of others was merely to invite unfortunate results; she had once said as much, perfectly matter-of-factly to her friend Miss Sarah Mair.[14] Now she stood firm. Ten thousand copies of an appeal went out over Scotland. Within two days the funds had doubled. A fortnight later *The Common Cause*, weekly paper of the women's movement, headlined its main news story 'Dr Inglis has her first £1000'. One hospital at least was secure.[15]

There was debate over the organisation's name. The Committee had proposed Scottish Women's Hospitals. Dr Inglis, already planning a wider appeal, had wanted it called the British Women's Hospitals, and demolished as too limiting Mrs Fawcett's idea that 'suffrage' should be somewhere in the name. 'If the hospitals were called by a non-committal name it would be much easier to get all men and women to help' she wrote to Mrs Fawcett on October 9th.[16] It was perhaps one of her few concessions to low cunning; in the event the name was never changed and though the hospitals drew support from England, the Dominions, India, the colonies, and neutral America, it was

* Prior to the Nurses Registration Act, 1919, there was no legal definition of a trained nurse. Two years was normally recognised and the Army required nursing recruits to have had three years; but many women styled themselves trained after six months. Three years was the period stipulated by the Scottish Women's Hospitals.

† In fact £1000 was a low estimate, based on the assumption that some doctors and all untrained staff would give their services. Senior doctors were to have an 'honorarium' of £200 a year, juniors nothing, nurses the standard rate of £50 a year.

as the Scottish Women's Hospitals that they won imperishable renown.

Mrs Fawcett however (unlike the Pankhursts) had organised her supporters on sound democratic principles and though the leaders had given Elsie Inglis ready support she had now to carry the rank and file.

At a mass meeting at Kingsway Hall on October 20th, she faced the biggest task of persuasion of her life. She was billed to speak on 'What Women Can Do to Help the War'. Many of those present were unconvinced that women *should* help the war. Some were strongly pacifist; others influenced by the idea that 'it will be over by Christmas' which accompanies the start of every war. They pleaded that suffrage energies, and suffrage funds, should be salted away till propaganda could recommence. Those who were present on that night still recall impassioned pleas for and against.[17]

Finally Dr Inglis stood up to speak. She began and continued simply, with no histrionics. Her theme was that 'something very big' lay before the Hospitals. She had taken the precaution of getting first-hand and horrifying details[18] about some of Serbia's front-line hospitals from Mme Grouitch, the American wife of a Serbian minister, who was then in London trying to collect a few nurses for that primitive and unhappy country. She described her own vision of the Scottish Women's Hospitals, much as she had described it to Mrs Fawcett in a letter of October 9th:

'We get these expert women doctors, nurses and ambulance workers organised. We send our units wherever they are wanted. Once these units are out, the work is bound to grow. The need is there, and too terrible to allow any haggling about who does the work. If we have a thoroughly good organisation we can send out more and more units to strengthen those already out. We can add motor ambulances,* organise rest stations on the lines of communication, and so on. It will all depend on how well we are supplied with funds and brains at our base. Each unit ought to be very carefully chosen and the very best women doctors must go ...

'From the very beginning we must make it clear that our

* Motor ambulances had hardly been envisaged by the authorities. The B.E.F. of 1914 had none. The official plan was that wounded should come back from the line in the empty horse wagons which had gone up with the daily meat supplies.

hospitals are as well-equipped and well-manned as any in the field, more economical (easy!) and thoroughly efficient.

'I cannot think of anything more calculated to bring home to men the fact that women *can help* intelligently in any kind of work. So much of our work is done where they can not see it. They'll see every bit of this ...

'The money is the thing now. It must not be wasted, but we must have lots. And as the work grows, do let's keep it together, so that however many hospitals we send out, they all shall be run on the same lines, and wherever people see the Union Jack with the red, white and green flag* below it, they'll know it means efficiency and kindness and intelligence ...

'I can think of nothing except these Units just now! And when one hears of the awful need, one can hardly sit still till they are ready.'[19]

She swept the audience off its feet. The rank and file voted overwhelmingly to back Elsie Inglis and the Scottish Women's Hospitals. The money which began to roll in that night did not stop until four years and £450,000 later.

The need was indeed awful. So awful that the authorities dared not fully disclose it. The B.E.F. lost 50,000 men in the first battle of Ypres, the French 300,000 in the first month of the war, a rate of loss never later equalled. Belgium was being overrun. In Serbia the Austrians had destroyed the only military hospital. Official preparation for the flood of casualties was lamentable.

The response of the women was immediate and generous. Money arrived by every post now, and as Elsie had foreseen, not from suffrage supporters only. 'I am so glad you are doing something useful at last' wrote one of her personal friends tartly, enclosing a generous cheque.[20] Women up and down the country organised flag days, collections of waste paper, sales of home produce. The Cambridge women's colleges promised to support one unit for six months. Suffrage groups from Ascot to Orkney, from East Grinstead to Bridge of Weir, opened subscription lists. Glasgow suffragists put on a 'Dickens entertainment', Edinburgh women students organised a collection, Gilbert Murray endowed four beds, Glasgow Tramways staff had a whip-round, children in Crieff organised a sale of their handwork.[21]

Volunteers also came flocking. Elsie had, while in London, also addressed the Medical Women's Federation. Miss Frances

* Colours of the National Union of Women's Suffrage Societies.

Ivens, a leading Liverpool surgeon, and Dr Eleanor Soltau, a capable woman with a talent for organisation, enrolled. Dr Katharine MacPhail turned her pretty young face to the path that was to lead to a lifetime of work in the Balkans. Dr Isobel Emslie, having been warned by male colleagues that 'It won't last, these shows run by women never do', and 'You'll be quarrelling with each other the whole time', bought a pink ostrich-feather hat to give herself enough confidence to hand in her hospital notice: she never wore it again for two days later she was in the hodden grey of the Scottish Women's Hospitals and on her way to France.[22]

Women with no qualifications became orderlies: Cicely Hamilton, the writer; Mrs Harley, the dashing widow of a Colonel of The Buffs and one of the two embarrassingly independent-minded sisters of the C.-in-C., Sir John French; Madge Neil Fraser, the Scottish Ladies golf captain, who had prepared herself by taking First Aid and Home Nursing classes; Olive Kelso King, the daughter of an Australian millionaire, who enrolled as a chauffeuse. Edith Stoney, physicist and Cambridge wrangler, was probably the most brilliant of those who joined and certainly one of the most outstandingly useful.

These were the comparatively privileged. From the big city infirmaries and tiny cottage hospitals all over Scotland came also a stream of trained nurses: the Jessies and Margarets, Floras and Christinas who had mostly never been outside Scotland or even far from their homes, but who blithely assured well-wishers that they would 'soon be learning the French tongue, for it iss ferry like the Gaelic'.[23]

A vast amount of detail had to be settled. Uniform—its bonnet strings of Gordon tartan caused the nurses to be dubbed with Tommy Atkins's usual affectionate irreverence 'Skittish Widows';[24] money—it was to be taken abroad in sovereigns, acceptable anywhere, money belts being advised for safety, preferably of 'an admirable pattern with compartmented pockets as gold is so remarkably heavy';[25] equipment—a sign on all crates would simplify recognition at crowded stations, and it sounds strangely to the generation of fifty years later to learn that the sign chosen was the swastika.

There was only one difficulty. Where could the units work?

Dr Inglis's letters had drawn no useful response. True, the Belgian consul in Edinburgh had grasped at her offer, but his small country had virtually ceased to exist, being occupied already by the enemy. R. Seton Watson, the Edinburgh scholar and Balkans expert, agreed to contact the Serbian government in Belgrade, but there was again delay.[26]

The French offered the best hope, the more so as Louisa Garrett Anderson's hospital was by now actually in Paris. Rendered independent by Garrett Anderson money; accepted by the French apparently under the impression that stores only, not women doctors, were being offered; installed in the newly completed Hotel Claridge not altogether with its directors' approval; Louisa Garrett Anderson, a chip off the old block, had charmed and bluffed her triumphant way through.[27]

Financial problems, and a certain finicking regard for truth and protocol, had slowed Elsie Inglis, but on November 5th she again approached the French. The reply was positive. Two days later the first emissary of the Scottish Women's Hospitals crossed the Channel.

Alice Hutchison, M.D.,[28] former medical officer of The Hospice, was remarkable even among the remarkable women of the S.W.H. Her tiny stature, rose-petal complexion, and masses of soft red hair would have suited a women's magazine heroine; they never completely concealed the ox-like constitution, the matter-of-fact courage and the gift for disciplined organisation which caused subordinates to dub her, only half-jokingly, 'the little General'. A medical missionary's daughter, who had worked in the Canongate slums, served through an Indian cholera epidemic and in a convoy corps during the First Balkan War, she was one of the very few women doctors with experience of war and of primitive countries; an invaluable asset this, for not only had few British doctors ever seen a case of typhus or cholera, but often enough the professors who lectured on these diseases had not seen a case either.[29]

Dr Hutchison was to negotiate the establishment of a Scottish Women's Hospital in France, but when she arrived in Calais, Belgian wounded were pouring in and Depage, the Belgian surgeon whose Brussels clinic was staffed by nurses from the Cavell school, and who knew what English standards meant,[30] had already telegraphed to the S.W.H. Now Dr Hutchison agreed to supply two doctors and ten nurses to work under him. She hurried to Paris to see the French authorities, returned to Edinburgh to report, and by November 19th, with one nursing sister, was back in Calais to begin work.

Still there were curious delays. Only when, a few days later, typhoid fever broke out in Calais, where sanitary services were inadequate for the rush, could Depage get the Scottish Women accepted by the military. Then he installed Dr Hutchison in a special typhoid annexe in the Rue Archimède.

'I quite realised that the Generals were not dying to have us,' she wrote. 'But I determined that they should arrive at the stage of being loath to lose us, before long.'[31] Ward after ward filled rapidly. The epidemic was severe and prolonged. Until ten more nurses and one other doctor arrived, even Alice Hutchison found herself doing many things she had never dreamed of doing. When the epidemic ended, three months later, and statistics became available, it was seen that the lowest mortality rate in Calais had been in the Scottish Women's Hospital in the Rue Archimède.[32]

Elsewhere things had been moving. On November 8th Seton Watson telegraphed that the Serbian Government accepted the offer of a Unit with gratitude.[33] On December 6th another Unit took possession of the disused Cistercian Abbey of St Louis at Royaumont, twenty-five miles from Paris, allocated to them by the French Red Cross.

The Abbey, romantically beautiful and in a state of preservation surprising considering its age and that it had stood empty for years, was to become perhaps the finest of the Scottish Women's Hospitals. For five years the work of healing would go on there under Miss Frances Ivens. The first penny notebooks of records would grow to a complex filing system. To Royaumont would come pathetic wounded *poilus,* enormous bewildered Senegalese, gaunt Arabs and tough outcast legionnaires. Somehow the spirit of the place would take possession of them, so that with little external discipline the devotion and service of the women drew from the patients a response which was to make 'the Royaumont spirit' an almost tangible influence in all their lives.[34]

But now, in early December 1914, the Abbey was empty, neglected, full of grime of years, without light, heat or water. Nurses, orderlies and junior doctors all turned to and swept and scrubbed for a fortnight; cleaned floors, washed walls, opened packing cases, carried heavy equipment upstairs 'as if they were born housemaids' wrote Dr Inglis. 'Really I am proud of them! They stick at absolutely nothing.'[35]

By Christmas everything was ready. 'What it is', commented Mme Goüin, wife of Royaumont's owner, with a feline touch in her admiration, 'to belong to a practical nation.'[36]

Before patients arrived, Dr Inglis had to inspect. She was unusually optimistic, having come direct from seeing off the Unit which was going to Serbia under Dr Soltau and Dr Edith Hollway; it had as administrator Mr William Smith of Aberdeen, one of only two or three men ever to serve in the organisation. The Admiralty, approached for transport to Salonika, had been more co-operative[37] than the War Office; Churchill, who had once declared he would never be henpecked into giving women the vote was, as ever, ready to try *anything* that might help win a war.

'Everything is splendid here now', she wrote from Royaumont on December 22nd to Mrs Simson, 'and if the General from headquarters would only come and inspect us we could begin. The wards are perfect. I only wish you could see them with their red bedcovers and little tables ... The Abbaye itself is a wonderful place. It has beautiful architecture and is placed in delightful woods. One wants to spend hours exploring it, instead of which we have all been working like galley slaves getting the hospital in order. The equipment has come out practically all right. There are no thermometers and no sandbags. I feel they'll turn up. Yesterday I was told there were no toothbrushes and no nail-brushes, but they appeared. After all the rush, you can imagine our feelings when the "Director", an official of the French Red Cross, who has to live here with us, told us French soldiers don't want toothbrushes.

'We have had to get a new boiler in the kitchen, new taps and lavatories, and electric light, an absolute necessity in this huge place, and all the theatre sinks. We certainly are no longer a mobile hospital, but as we are twelve miles from the point from which the wounded are distributed ... we shall probably be as useful here as anywhere. They even think we may get English Tommies.'[38]

The French authorities, like the Belgians and the British, had not been dying to have the Scottish Women. The military of all nations doubted, not so much the medical and surgical work of women, but their disciplinary powers. The French began by treating Royaumont with caution, sending the simpler cases and carrying out frequent inspections at which the good behaviour of patients came in for comment revealingly emphatic. Within four months they were asking for the accommodation to be doubled and for another Scottish Women's Hospital to be opened.

On the way home from Royaumont, Dr Inglis passed through Paris, where she had an extraordinary experience.

Elsie Inglis had never, to outward appearance, been one for the supernatural. Eva was the fey member of the family, the intuitive one who had 'feelings' about things and whose photograph as a grown woman shows the same dreamy sensitivity she had had as a child. Elsie was in everything the practical one. She expressed interest in the supernatural only once, when in 1883 she asked her father's opinion and was told that he believed in uncanny communications but believed too that 'all these things are hidden from us'. Nor is there any record of Elsie's ever having had a 'call' such as Florence Nightingale and Elizabeth Fry had received. In adult life, she simply responded unquestioningly to the claims of duty and religion as understood by the world in which she moved, but they had been part of her life from childhood. The only remarkable thing was the vigour and enthusiasm with which, as an adult, she embraced their claims. There had been no one dramatic moment, no turning-point in her life.

Now in Paris,[39] wanting peace for reflection and prayer, she went, as perhaps few other good protestant Scots would have done, into Notre Dame. She searched for an isolated corner where she would be undisturbed and alone, and settled to her devotions caught up, deeply absorbed, she sat there while the minutes passed timelessly. How long she had been there she did not know, when she was aware of something obtruding upon her self-imposed solitude. Gradually the feeling grew that she was not, after all, alone. No one had passed her. Yet someone was behind her, someone who must have been there unnoticed all along.

She felt a strong impulse to turn, but resisted it, unwilling to disturb another's devotions. The impulse grew, strengthened. At last it was so insistent that almost without her own volition, she turned around.

No one was there. Now, however, she saw what she had not perceived before in the dimness: a statue of Joan of Arc, a statue which seemed imbued with life, which seemed indeed to have some message to impart to her.

That was all. Statues do not speak; not in the twentieth century, not to a Modern Woman, not to the scientifically trained, not to a middle-aged Protestant doctor so devoid of any sense of self-importance that one of her favourite sayings was Celsus's 'I bound up their wounds, God healed them.'[40] Nothing more happened and Elsie left the cathedral.

Back in Edinburgh, she, who seldom spoke of her personal experiences, confided in Mrs McLaren. 'Wasn't it curious?' she ended her tale. 'I would like to know what Joan was wanting to say to me!' She remained convinced that some message had been in the air, unspoken, unapprehended.

What is to be understood from this? Simple, trivial even, as it sounds in the telling, there is no doubt that the episode made a deep impression on her. Was she deluding herself? Or did something happen, unaccountable by the normal standards of the physical world?

It would be easy to write off the story as an affair of auto-suggestion. Dr Inglis was at that age when women are said to be liable to strange ideas; she was in an exalted state, imbued with a sense of mission. What more likely than to take up, unconsciously perhaps, a position near the statue of an admired figure and then imagine a 'supernatural' message? So the argument would run.

The rational argument, however, runs counter to all that is known of Dr Inglis's own character; and it is worth remarking that Lady Frances Balfour, who knew her well and who had a brisk no-humbug mentality, was not prepared to write the story off as nonsense.[41]

Elsie had been given to 'making up stories' when young; but there is no evidence that she thought of them as anything but irrelevant daydreams, an evil to avoid, not to be confused with reality. She seems to have been certain that the Joan of Arc episode was an objective event, not a self-induced fancy.

Here it may also be remarked that Joan of Arc was not, in 1914, the dramatic saint of modern thought. Ten years earlier she had been raised from plain Joan the Maid to become the Venerable Joan of Arc and in 1908 the Blessed Joan of Arc. Canonisation was yet six years off and so was the flood of literature which that event released. The figure familiar to English people in 1914 was the Maid of France of Andrew Lang's biography with its rational, non-committal verdict that 'in some sense not easily defined, Joan was inspired'; by no means an obvious choice for a middle-aged Protestant doctor seeking an anchor for self-deluding visions.

Elsie Inglis was a medical woman, trained in sifting fact from fancy; although it is clear from her prescriptions quoted earlier that she knew the effect of mind upon matter it is also clear that she knew the separate sphere of each. Medical men and women are usually the last people to suspend scepticism in such an affair.

Lastly, all who knew Elsie Inglis testify to her lack of any sense of her own importance. To her the cause was everything, her own activity in it, nothing; a quality, it may be remarked, which she certainly shared with the Maid of Orleans. It is not to those with this degree of reckless humility that self-fabricated visions come.

The key to the episode lies perhaps, in the phrase seized upon by Elsie earlier, 'The power of an endless life.'

Many who are not orthodox believers would agree that there is a reality behind this phrase. A later agnostic biographer of Joan of Arc, V. Sackville-West, wrote of 'one comprehensive, stupendous unity of which we apprehend but the smallest segment', and of certain persons who 'are in touch with or shall we say receptive to, the influences of a unity for which we have no adequate name'.[42]

Joan, Socrates, Teresa, Buddha, are all widely accepted as having been such persons. But there have probably always existed thousands of more obscure souls as receptive in their less dramatic way as these great saints, to the influences of that unity for which we have no name: people who do not ordinarily speak of their experiences, but are content to act upon them in the spirit of soldiers taking orders and standing to their posts. Of these, it seems clear that Elsie Inglis was one, and it is to be believed that the power of that life which she and Joan both served, brought together the spirits of the two women in some timeless and space-defying communion of a kind which, after all, modern physical science itself makes to seem not impossible.

Those who are indeed subject to auto-suggestion in visions and messages (and let us admit that they too abound) are seldom in doubt as to what message is intended. To dig the whole thing out of one's own unconscious is at least to be clear what it is all about. Elsie Inglis's uncertainty over the incident also argues the case for the supernatural. Something unaccountable happened, there was a message, it was to come through Joan of Arc ... but the reception was imperfect. She did not know what it was.

Speculation here carries us into mere hypothesis. Was the message to do with her mission to help France, or Serbia? A prediction that that mission would cost Elsie her life, as Joan's mission had cost hers? An admonition that she must nevertheless go forward without fear, as Joan's own voices had admonished her?

Elsie Inglis did not know and no one else ever will. But inspiration and the giving of courage are not less potent, and can be more so, when not expressed in words or apprehendable thought. To the end of her life, Elsie Inglis held that Joan of Arc had had some message. It may be that she drew strength, in her own ultimate trials, from whatever it was that happened on that winter day in the Cathedral of Notre Dame.

Back in England she plunged again into organisation. She travelled all over the kingdom appealing for funds, writing innumerable reports and letters, harrying officials, attending committees. She still hoped to win authority's agreement to her Units working for Britain. Not only did Tommy Atkins have first claim on her loyalties, but also the secondary object, the suffrage cause, could best be advanced through work for Englishmen.

Her main preoccupation was to build an organisation that could function in her absence. At one of the earliest meetings for the S.W.H. she had spoken of her own wish to work in the field.[43] That meant ensuring continuity of organisation at home. By early 1915 this was well advanced; besides the original Edinburgh committee, a London Committee was formed with Miss Edith Palliser, an elderly Irish lady who had devoted her whole life to the suffrage cause, as Chairman; Mrs Flinders Petrie, wife of the archaeologist, as Secretary; and as Treasurer Viscountess Cowdray, whose husband was one of the country's richest men; and local committees had been formed in various provincial centres.[44]

All these workers felt the impact of her forceful character. Her method was simple; she convinced by the force of her own conviction. She was helped by the conditions forged in the suffrage campaign in which she had built up over many years personal friendships which could bridge great gaps in time and distance. One incident may be quoted as typical. The organiser of the

Glasgow Suffrage Society met Dr Inglis by chance in Sauchiehall Street soon after the Kingsway Hall meeting of October 20th, and was drawn in to take tea under Copland and Lye's Rotunda dome. In this incongruous setting Dr Inglis expounded her ideas, spoke of her determination to go abroad herself and concluded, 'We shall need you behind us at home.' Thrilled, Mrs Cochrane-Shanks pledged her efforts and those of her group, and was rewarded with Dr Inglis's spirited and sunny smile, a smile never forgotten by those who saw it.[45]

Simple? Schoolgirlish, even? It sounds so ... until one understands that from then on the Glasgow Suffrage Society sent a sum, never less than £1,000 each month, to the Scottish Women's Hospitals. That, and at 1914 monetary values, is neither simple nor schoolgirlish.

This, however, was the response Dr Inglis expected and this was the response she got. Of her descents upon 2 St Andrew's Square, her Edinburgh headquarters, Miss Mair wrote of 'a certain stir of feeling ... Had the impossible been accomplished? If not, why? Who had failed in performance? Take the task from her, give it to another. No excuses in war-time, no weakness to be tolerated —onward, ever onward ... No one must pause, no one must waver; things must simply be done, whether possible or not, and somehow by her inspiration they generally were done ... she appeared as in herself the very embodiment of wireless telegraphy, aeronautic locomotion, with telepathy and divination thrown in.'[46]

In mid-January came news which made Dr Inglis more determined than ever to press on with the work. Dr Hollway's Unit had arrived in Kragujevatz, Serbia, on January 5th, where they were the nearest foreign hospital to the front. It was the physician of the Unit, Dr Eleanor Soltau, who telegraphed home within a few days of their arrival:

> Dire necessity for fever nurses. Can you send me ten or more overland? [Also] equipment, mattresses, covers, blankets, linen, milk, typhol, carbolic, tow, castor-oil.[47]

Unable, for censorship reasons, to be specific about the emergency confronting them, Dr Soltau had worded her telegram with care, hoping those in Edinburgh would interpret correctly its dreadful meaning.

CHAPTER 10

Serbia, as English-speaking people by the end of 1914 had learned to call that tiny inland kingdom which now forms north-eastern Yugoslavia, was to most of them just a name; and that a variable one. When in July she had been accused by Austria of instigating the Sarajevo assassinations, and invaded by an Austrian punitive force, English people still knew her as Servia.[1]

The first of Turkey's European provinces to revolt, Servia had won some independence in 1804, led by a pig-farmer named Karageorge; and had become a kingdom in 1882. Scholars knew her heroic pre-Turkish past—that same Lord Lytton whose arrival in India had signalled John Inglis's retirement had once enlivened a junior diplomatic appointment in Vienna by making the first collection of heroic Servian ballads; but the public image of her as a modern kingdom was unappealing.

The squalid wranglings of her first modern king and queen, the sordid assassination in 1902 of their son and his queen, the accession of a rival dynasty believed (probably wrongly) to have been implicated in the murder,[2] all left insular Englishmen with the impression that Servian affairs were conducted in a way more appropriate to an Anthony Hope novel; while 'Brigandage in Servia' was the kind of useful headline newspapers of the day kept in standing type.

Probably Queen Mary summed up the feelings of the man-in-the-street when she wrote on July 28th, 1914, 'God grant we may not have a European War thrust upon us & for such a stupid reason too, no I don't mean stupid, but to have to go to war on account of tiresome Servia beggars belief!'[3]

Tiresome Servia that autumn made Europe change its mind about her. Austria and Austria's ally, Germany, had written her off in advance; so scornful was Austria that though the Servian commander, Vojvode (Marshal) Putnik, was in Vienna at the outbreak of war, he was, with imprudent chivalry, allowed to return home.[4]

Twice in the early weeks he repulsed Austrian invasions;

rugged soldiers of a rugged land, his men were the only Allied troops to win a victory. Then Austria invaded a third time. She could not be made a laughing stock by this tiny nation with its eleven divisions of infantry, one of cavalry, armed off the scrap heap.[5]

Both sides had fought almost to a standstill when in December the ageing and crippled King Peter addressed his men.

'Heroes,' he said, 'you have taken two oaths. One to me as your king, and one to your country. I am an old and broken man and from your oath to me I release you. From your oath to your country no man can release you. However, if you wish to leave the trenches you may go. For me and my sons, we remain. If you decide to return to your homes, and if we should be victorious, you shall not be made to suffer.'[6]

They did not return to their homes. They flung themselves upon the invader. The Battle of the Ridges, December 3rd-6th, was a classic victory. The Austrian rout was complete, and nine days later the last fugitive was back across the Danube.[7]

Tiresome Servia had become heroic Serbia.

The Austrians had left, however, a deadly fifth column behind: forty thousand prisoners of war, many of whom had surrendered without firing a shot rather than fight their brother Slavs* but of whom many came from Galicia where typhus was endemic.

Serbia anyway faced appalling conditions that winter. G. M. Trevelyan and R. Seton Watson went in December to report for the Serbian Relief Fund, of which Seton Watson was Hon. Treasurer. They telegraphed on December 30th reporting many hideous cases of gangrene and frostbite with a high percentage of amputations; and three weeks later wrote that every extra blanket might mean an illness averted, that there was a great shortage of disinfectants, dressings and surgical instruments; that many hospitals were without even sterilisers; and that the Austrian prisoners, working on roads and railways everywhere, were mostly verminous and had no spare clothing.[8]

The Relief Fund's chairman appealed in *The Times* on January 14th, 1915, for help, but held, probably rightly, that to ask Britons to provide a change of underwear for enemy prisoners would make his fund a laughing stock.[9] So *p. vestimenti*, which knows no

* Of every one hundred soldiers of Austria-Hungary in 1914, nine were of Serbo-Croat origin, two Slovenians, thirteen Czechs and four Slovaks.

distinction of friend or enemy, was left to spread the germs of typhus from one end of Serbia to the other.

The Second Scottish Women's Hospital Unit had arrived, before Seton Watson's report was published at Kragujevatz, Serbia's great arsenal town and military key point. To deal with the hundreds of wounded, every sizeable building in Kragujevatz had been turned into an emergency hospital, where a few doctors and unskilled orderlies were doing what they could; almost no Serbian girls had nursing training. When the Scottish Women arrived they were directed to a school building, full of wounded; typhus was not yet known in the town.

Bullock wagons trundled over the town's cobbled streets, laden with injured whose wounds had had no attention for a week or more. Those who survived to the hospital doors had often to lie for hours on the pavements before being admitted. Inside, conditions were equally pitiful. Miss Nightingale's reforms had never reached the Balkans. Patients worn to skeletons by suffering and hunger lay two or three to a bed, or on the bare floor. Soldiers in their early twenties looked like old men through privation. Men who had just endured the amputation of a limb—with a folded bandage to bite on, for anaesthetics had given out early—were huddled beside those in acute stages of typhoid and dysentery. Sheer neglect often cost a man a limb, or even his life, for of nursing in the Western sense there was none. 'They are splendid men, magnificent even when they are dying of fever, but it is a most dreadful waste of human beings' wrote one of the women.

The Scottish Women set to, scrubbed and whitewashed, unpacked heavy equipment, broke the windows to get ventilation, set up beds, started sterilisers, opened an operating theatre. They did it under the hardest conditions, but within a week the place was transformed: neat wards; patients, washed and tidy, in clean beds.[10]

The women, having gone to nurse a hospital of 100, unexpectedly found themselves able to take on 250, for Austrian prisoners were given them as orderlies. They took over four small inns to which the less seriously ill could be moved, to give more room in the wards; they increased as much as they dared the numbers in the wards themselves; but the flood of suffering rolled on. On January 23rd, to add the last note of horror, came the news that typhus had broken out.[11]

The people of Serbia succumbed in thousands. Whole villages

died without a visit from any doctor. Indeed, one third of the country's 450 doctors themselves died. The incidence was in three months equal to that in one year in the great Irish epidemic of the potato famine years; and one tenth of all the cases in the country were at Kragujevatz.[12]

Dr Soltau sent off the telegram already quoted. It had to be cryptic but Dr Inglis understood. Her immediate response was to send five extra doctors and on February 9th twelve fever nurses and £600 of equipment.[13] Without waiting for these, Dr Soltau had taken over a typhus hospital and called for volunteers from the existing Unit to staff it. As Elsie Inglis had forecast, once the Units were in the field, the work was bound to grow.

A former barracks was made over to the Unit and they found that, again by overcrowding it by British standards, they could get in two hundred typhus patients, to be looked after by three doctors and fourteen sisters with the prisoner-orderlies. Later a third hospital, a dilapidated two-storey building, once a palace, was taken over, and a department opened for women and children. By the end of March the Scottish Women were responsible for 550 beds, more than five times their original estimate of work.

'You are perfectly right', wrote Elsie. 'I knew when you went out that we could trust you to take the best line under the circumstances and not to be bound by red tape or any conventions whatsoever.' She added, 'I very much hope I shall be able to come myself with the next Unit if we send one.'[14]

The Scottish Women's Hospital in Serbia was certainly not conventional. Its kitchen, laundry, and bath-room were improvised in sheds in which the orderlies also slept; water was fetched from a well in a central courtyard; oil lamps provided the only light. Wood for the stoves came by ox-cart from the surrounding Shumadija or forest region, but as the nearer plantations were soon demolished and oxen killed off for food, on many of the bitterest days the Hospital had only one fire.[15] Even so the Scottish Women's Hospital seemed like 'selfish luxury' to Madge Neil Fraser when she visited another in the town. She wrote home:

'The most terrible sight I have seen here is the big fever hospital ... There were only a few doctors for their hundreds of cases, otherwise only orderlies terrified for their own safety, crowding in corners doing nothing unless driven to it. All the windows were shut and the place smelt like a sewer ... Clothing and bedding were filthy and verminous and the helpless cases are simply left to become filthier and filthier.'[16]

It was the last letter she wrote. She caught typhus and died on March 8th. Her funeral, outside the cathedral as no indoor services were held for fear of infection, was with military honours. Under the grey sky, with snow on the ground, Orthodox priests in robes brilliant with gold and silver embroidery and carrying great flaming candles, led the chanting, attended by red-and-gold-robed acolytes bearing aloft huge gold stars and a cross with the name of the dead woman. The royal band played a march as the hearse plunged and swayed through mud inches deep on the long road to the cemetery. And if the Scottish Women kept a stiff upper lip amid the uninhibited wailing of the crowd, many of them found it an unforgettably moving experience; though not a few of the good Presbyterians expressed themselves appalled at 'all this popery'.[17]

Miss Fraser's death received wide publicity at home, and golfers subscribed for a complete new Unit for Serbia in her memory. Other help, too, was coming to Serbia now. Early in March an R.A.M.C. advisory mission under Colonel William Hunter arrived; they surveyed the country, insisted upon notification of typhus, stopped all army leave and other traffic for one month, disinfested units coming from the battle areas, inoculated the whole army against cholera. Besides the wounded they found 37,000 sick in the Serbian army, nearly half of whom had typhus, typhoid or relapsing fever. In Kragujevatz the mortality was fifty per cent, and unburied bodies lay about in heaps of up to two hundred. It was almost more than he could bear, Hunter later wrote, not to give immediate help to the sufferers; but his orders were to concentrate on a programme to reduce the disease; in ten days after his arrival, its incidence had fallen by half.[18]

It was found that even a moderate amount of good nursing for patients who lay helpless for days could make the difference between life and death. The Scottish Women's Hospital, with its trained staff, scored heavily, and learned never to give up hope.[19]

As the details filtered through to Edinburgh, Elsie Inglis became more and more restless. Seton Watson was urging her to send out more Units, and she longed to be in the fight herself. So far as her own patients were concerned, she felt free to go. Someone, as she had predicted, *had* been found to take on The

Hospice: Dr Grace Cadell, the stormy petrel of the Edinburgh School of Medicine all those years before.[20]

But if she went abroad, who would take charge of the all-important fund-raising? 'We need huge reserves in hand, in case e.g. Royaumont wanted more beds or the Servian unit a cholera camp' she had written to her Edinburgh organiser on December 11th. 'Therefore the scheme depends on two things:

Good work by women at the front

Plenty of money raised by women at home.

'I told Miss Leaf we must have £30,000 and she said we should have it.'[21]

But could those at home be trusted not to flag? Were their ideas on a large enough scale? She was still uncertain, when things once again worked together for her.

The London Committee, shortly after its setting up early in 1915, had needed a secretary. An inexperienced, pretty, shy girl had taken on the job. She had been in the office a month, when Dr Inglis bustled in, radiating enthusiasm. The French had just asked for a second Unit. The money promised by Girton and Newnham would finance it, the staff were ready. Elsie turned to the new secretary. 'Do you speak French?'

'Yes.'

'Very well. Go and write me a letter to General de Torcy, telling him we accept the building he has offered at Troyes.'

Some cautious soul suggested that so important a task should be given to a more experienced hand.

'Nonsense,' Elsie retorted. 'I know the type. That girl probably speaks six languages. If she says she speaks French, she does.' When the resulting letter was finished, she hardly glanced at it before signing it.[22]

She was right. That girl had in fact been brought up in France. She had ability, but she had something more valuable to Elsie Inglis. Of Irish parentage, someone in her ancestry had undoubtedly kissed the Blarney stone. For a month Elsie had her under scrutiny. Did she know for sure that she had found the answer to her problem? At any rate, when in April the news came that Dr Soltau, weakened by anxiety and overwork, was ill, Dr Inglis announced that she would go in person to take over. The typhus was still at its height—April 3rd was the worst day of all—and since all previous epidemics had lasted several years, no one could say when the Serbian disaster would be overcome.[23]

A meeting of university women had been arranged at Oxford which Dr Inglis could not now address. 'That girl' had better go instead. For young as she was, and whether or not she spoke six languages, Dr Inglis now knew that she certainly spoke the one language needed above all, the language of heartfelt appeal which could coax hard cash out of pockets and purses, out of private bank accounts, out of the funds of clubs and societies, out of the profits of business firms, and into the coffers of the Scottish Women's Hospitals. Elsie Inglis's capacity for bringing out in others hidden qualities which matched the moment had achieved, perhaps, its most striking result.

So Miss Kathleen Burke assumed the role of fund-raiser in chief. 'The thousand dollar a day girl', as she became known, made tours in America and Canada, addressing meetings of up to five thousand people and raising, herself, well over one quarter of all the money spent by the organisation. In 1916 she was allowed by Pétain—who called her 'knight of tenderness and pity across the world'—to visit the fortress of Verdun,[24] the only woman to do so. When her account of this was read to his congregation by the Rev. S. Baring-Gould, author of 'Onward Christian Soldiers' and himself no mean organiser of emotion, he several times found his delivery impeded by tears.[25]

In the S.W.H. offices Miss Burke's talent was treated less reverently. When funds were low because a new Unit was being equipped, 'Miss Burke had better write a letter to the papers at once in her most heart-wringing style' was the proposal. It usually worked well.[26]

Elsie remained only to complete the arrangements for the Troyes Unit and to arrange that Alice Hutchison, no longer needed in Calais, should take one further Unit to Serbia. Then, on April 24th, she set off.

In London she met—whether by arrangement or one of her fruitful accidents, is not clear—the Hon. Mrs Haverfield, a woman three years younger than herself and widely known among suffragists as one of their more intrepid supporters. An enthusiast of the hunting field and a brilliant horsewoman, she had acted as a mounted marshal, riding unconventionally astride, in suffrage processions, and had been in the middle of a horse-caravan propaganda tour when in June 1909 she was called upon to stand trial at the Old Bailey, with the Pethick-Lawrences, for her involvement in suffrage agitation. Tall and beautiful, impetuous, dashing, warm-hearted, Eveline Haverfield was to work with Elsie in the next two difficult years and to devote the remainder of her life to the Serbian nation, until dying at Bajni Bashta in 1919 she was buried as she had asked to be 'in a field where horses can walk over me'.[27]

'Mrs Haverfield is delightful ... She may make an administrator,' wrote Elsie to Mrs McLaren now. 'She left the W.S.P.U. when you did, and for the same reason.'[28]

Together the two women travelled overland to Brindisi, calling at Royaumont on the way. 'It is a *huge* success', Elsie wrote to her sister, 'and I do think Dr Ivens deserves a lot of credit. The wards and the theatre, and the X-ray department, and the rooms for mending and cleaning the men's clothes, were all perfect.'[29]

They arrived at Brindisi on April 27th. Looking from the window, the insular and single-minded Elsie wrote that it was 'queer to see the red, white and green flags and to think they mean Italy and not the N.U.W.S.S.'.[30]

There were frustrating delays at Brindisi and Athens; although it was a public holiday she stormed the shipping office at Athens to claim a refund on their tickets for no details escaped her and 'the Scottish Hospitals have plenty to do with their funds besides paying unnecessary hotel bills' she wrote to Mrs McLaren who was working with the committee. 'Do make them look into the route Cook sends us ... there is absolutely no necessity whatsoever to stop anywhere between London and Brindisi especially as the Committee gives us sleepers.'[31]

Arrived at Kragujevatz on May 5th, almost her first action was to telegraph home for six motor transport vehicles, in view of the difficulties of travel in Serbia. On May 11th she made her first report.[32]

'Both the operating theatre and the room for the dressings [in the surgical hospital] are beautifully arranged and managed by Sister Boykett, and are very creditable to an improvised hospital ...' she wrote. 'The Hospital is at present under Dr Chesney, who is doing excellent work. It is understaffed as regards Sisters, most of them having been drafted over to the Typhus Hospital ...

'The Typhus Hospital ... holds 200 patients, is overcrowded, from our standard, but is clean and fresh and well arranged. It is comparatively well staffed, fourteen Sisters, and when the new ones arrive, sixteen. But its equipment might be immensely improved. The doctors who are working there are, Dr M'Vea, Dr Corbett and Dr Laird.

'The Relapsing Fever Hospital ... was empty when it was turned into a hospital. It is in two storeys. A long corridor runs the whole length of the building, both upstairs and down. Off them open the rooms, downstairs the patients are received, upstairs are the wards, comparatively small square rooms, all overcrowded. The place will hold 200 beds and has now 170 patients. The kitchen and laundry are outside.

'It has no equipment to speak of, and is being worked by Dr Brook and one Sister, namely Sister Hollway!* This, of course, sounds ridiculous, and it is so in a sense. There is very little nursing or doctoring. But there is no denying that those two women have worked wonders in the place. The Austrian orderlies are kept up to their duties. The patients, at any rate, get the medicines which are ordered for them, and the place is fairly clean ...

'This is the work the Unit has undertaken. It means that they made themselves responsible for something like 570 beds! One can quite understand how they were almost driven into it, in the face of the awful need of the country, and there is no doubt at all that they have done it excellently and with a wonderful self-devotion. The standard in all three hospitals is distinctly higher than that of the ordinary hospital here, and the Surgical Hospital is really well equipped and well arranged.'

The women had in fact been trying to cope with modern artillery warfare casualties in almost medieval conditions. Praise came from all sides. General Subotic, the Chief Medical Officer of the army, described their hospital as the best in Serbia. Major Protitch the hospital Director (liaison officer) said the same. 'They are very good at saying pleasant things here,' Elsie commented drily. The praise of fellow countrymen was the most acceptable: the British Minister at Nish, wartime seat of government, 'could not speak too highly' of the Scottish Women, and Lady Paget, wife of the previous British Minister, wrote a little later, 'The Scottish Women's Units are doing splendid work ... their courage and the way they overcome almost insurmountable difficulties is extraordinary ... of all the Units out here the S.W.H. have done the best work.'[33]

* Not to be confused with Dr Hollway. I have been unable to discover, however, if they were related.

Elsie Inglis's original idea was bearing abundant fruit. She had at the outset planned one unit. Now four were in the field. As well as Royaumont and Kragujevatz, the Troyes Unit was now installed in a tented hospital, the first experiment in nursing *poilus* under canvas[34] though this was customary in the British army. The fourth Unit, under Dr Hutchison, destined for work in Serbia, had sailed at the end of April in S.S. *Ceramic*, a White Star liner carrying ammunition to the Dardanelles.[35]

In the first week of May, *Ceramic* arrived in Malta. Summoned unexpectedly into the presence of the Governor, Lord Methuen, the women were told that a sudden unforeseen strain was to be put on the island's medical services. Methuen proposed to detain the women for two weeks until reinforcements arrived from home.[36]

On May 4th an avalanche of casualties arrived: New Zealanders, Australians, and 'just plain British' from the Dardanelles. They came from the boats, many of them, in as shocking a state as had been the Serbs at Kragujevatz; still in their filthy uniforms, many of them totally helpless, their wounds untouched since they left field dressing stations ten days before when the Gallipoli landings began. The War Office, so confident that it needed no interfering women around, had once again utterly failed to make suitable provision for the wounded.

'It is lovely to have the chance of looking after our own men,' wrote Dr Hutchison, 'and I have been thrilled and appalled at the account they give us of the landing of our troops ... The Australians arrived here first and are very interesting as a character study.' They were 'delightfully frank and easy to get on with', and 'always ready to jeer at the sentimental effusion of the *Malta Chronicle* over "our wounded heroes".' 'It will cost us a big pang to say goodbye to our British Tommies,' she wrote on May 15th. 'I'm so glad, *ever* so glad to have had this little chance of serving them ... and it's a great joy to us that they should so quickly be enthusiastic about their women doctors.'[37]

When the Unit sailed for Serbia, they had converted more than the Tommy to the notion of women as doctors. Lord Methuen, who at the start of the Boer War had been the senior British general in the field and who in its course had won 'that special place in English minds reserved for men who did not give way to adversity',* was perhaps the one soldier free to speak his mind

* Rayne Kruger, *Goodbye Dolly Gray.*

despite Lord Kitchener. He wrote, 'It is not in my power to express my gratitude sufficiently for the help given me by the Serbian Unit ... They leave here blessed by myself, surgeons, nurses and patients alike.'[38]

The idea underlying Dr Inglis's scheme had been sufficiently proved. Besides the work of her own Units, medical women were now replacing in general hospitals at home men going into the R.A.M.C. In many other forms of war work, the women were converting public opinion. If the Prime Minister could still hold out against the notion that women deserved equal citizenship, the average Englishman at least had been convinced.

On August 4th, the first anniversary of Britain's entry into the war, *Punch* spoke, as so often, for the collective unconscious of the nation. A Wallis Mills drawing showed an irrepressible wounded Tommy grinning at a severe-but-kindly woman doctor. The caption read:

> Eminent Woman Surgeon, who is also an ardent Suffragist, (to wounded Guardsman): 'Do you know, your face is singularly familiar to me. I've been trying to remember where we've met before.'
> Guardsman: 'Well, Mum, bygones be bygones. I *was* a police constable.'

The women, it was already clear, had worked their passage. The pay-off date, however, was still uncertain.

CHAPTER 11

When Dr Inglis arrived in Serbia in early May, the typhus figures remained as high as in February. The trains reeked of formalin, the Scottish nurses of camphor and naphthalene; the black flag denoting a typhus death was still seen on houses in Kragujevatz. Two more Scottish women had died of it; others had had it and recovered. The cafés still closed for the daily cleansing prescribed by emergency law. The hospital Director still burned methylated spirit on his plate before all meals. In the mess, the Scottish Women's light-hearted chatter was still largely on the entrancing subject of lice.[1]

The bell of the fourteenth-century cathedral still tolled for the morning funerals of important civilians; in the afternoons the Crown Prince's* band lent military honours to soldiers' burials; at night dead carts rattled over the cobbles taking the humble to a common grave.[2]

People, however, were beginning to hope. Many convalescents had gone home, or expected to. The sun shone, spring cast its spell over the country. Primroses, cowslips and violets starred the fields, fruit blossom and lilacs frothed overhead. To a Scottish eye the hills and valleys, woods and streams recalled those of home, only with a heightened colour, a larger scale, that transformed Serbia into the fairyland of childhood imagining.[3]

Help was now coming in many forms. Large sums had been raised for relief, a Board of Health set up. Food was more plentiful; earlier, the Scottish nurses had to be prevented by threat of instant dismissal from supplementing the patients' scanty rations from their own hardly more luxurious ones. Now the authorities made hospitals an allowance of meat, eggs, milk, and sugar in old-fashioned huge cones which needed pounding up. Patients supplemented their rations in strange ways. One man produced a fresh

* Alexander, Crown Prince and Regent of Serbia, the second son of King Peter, was at this time twenty-seven. As Alexander III of Yugoslavia he was assassinated in Marseilles in 1934.

egg each day; only later was it discovered he somehow kept hidden in his bed a live hen.[4]

This was one comical aspect of the serious overcrowding so shocking to Dr Inglis. But she too fell under the spell of Serbia. 'This is a lovely place, and the Serbians are delightful,' she wrote to Mrs Simson on May 20th.[5] At the age of fifty, she had fallen romantically in love at last; not with a single man, but with a nation.

The Serbian soldier—contemporary observers are surprisingly unanimous in saying—was a simple, open soul, brave, uncomplaining, with the natural and dignified manner of an old-fashioned Highlander. 'My word, Clarke, but I tell you these men are great,' an American doctor had earlier told the *Daily Mail* correspondent. 'I feel so small beside them that I could hide myself. Pain! Suffering! You've not seen bravery until you've seen these men suffer. I'd take off a hand, an arm, or a leg—without anaesthetics, mind you—and will the fellow budge?—no, not an eyelid. And if you hear them say *Kuku lebe* (oh dear) that's as much as you hear, and not often that much. And die! They'll die without a sound—unless it is to thank you, if they can, before they go. Where this race of soldiers sprang from I don't pretend to know, but I tell you right now they are God's own men.'[6]

God's own men inevitably appealed to all the deepest qualities in Elsie Inglis. Her love for them was strong; it was also, characteristically, maternal. They were magnificent; but magnificent children, who, like children, could sometimes be infuriating.

Apart from a few who had studied in Austria or France, the whole nation, right up to its generals, retained the sturdy slow outlook of the yeoman farmers they were. Her Unit had worked magnificently; but their praised adaptability had led them to put up with conditions that could, that *must*, be improved. She lost no time, for instance, in bullying Major Protitch into promising that cement floors should be laid in theatre and dressing-room over the old wood boards that were impossible to sterilise; it was however mid-July before she could thankfully report that the work had actually been done. She had already requested six motor cars from Edinburgh. She got them in June;[7] not before a determined effort had been made to hijack them for use elsewhere in Serbia. Cars were a rarity; ox-carts were the normal form of transport, the roads being ill-adapted for anything heavier;

the motors arriving in 1915 were the first seen in many villages and subject to attack by the long-horned traction oxen.[8]

The language was another problem. 'Sometimes', she wrote, 'you have to get an orderly to translate Serbian into German, and another to translate the German into French, before you can get at what is wanted.' The nurses managed well and held long conversations with patients despite knowing almost no Serbian; they spoke English and the Serbs, observant of tone and expression, managed to follow; when the patients spoke, the doctors noticed that these simple men, who mostly could neither read nor write, talked so expressively and mimed so well that the sisters soon knew their life history.[9] Dr Inglis, aware of her limitations—after all she was half English, she liked to say, so could not be so linguistic as the Scots—did not waste time trying to acquire Serbian. She had other fish to fry.

Typhus had diminished under Colonel Hunter's measures. The figures, however, shot up again after the resumption of railway travel (against his advice) on April 15th and by May were almost back to the February figures.[10] As late as May 18th, 100 new cases arrived in the Scottish Women's Hospital. The surgical hospital was also busy: Dr Inglis herself performed twenty-three operations in the last week of May.

Throughout May and into June she was occupied on an important scheme. The main railway junction used by troops on leave was Mladanovatz, where they often hung about for days in conditions ideal for the spread of infection. It was the key spot in Serbia for the control of typhus, typhoid and cholera. Hunter approached Dr Inglis to establish a quarantine and disinfesting station with a tented hospital to nurse cases appearing there. She agreed. There were, however, curious delays. Hunter approached the Serbs at intervals throughout May, but she did not get her orders until the 28th. The Serbs also were, some of them, not dying to have either Dr Inglis or Colonel Hunter's plan.[11]

The plan itself developed: Mladanovatz would be supported by two other Scottish Women's Hospitals, 'blocking hospitals', one near the Roumanian frontier to be run by Dr Hutchison, another east of Belgrade staffed by new recruits from home.

As soon as Dr Inglis had her orders she went to choose a site and establish the key hospital at Mladanovatz, taking with her Colonel Lazar Gentitch, medical chief at the Serb G.H.Q. and Dr Milan Curcin, head of the department dealing with foreign personnel. Curcin, young, energetic, painstaking, cosmopolitan, of partly Austrian descent,[12] was of all the Serbs the one who best understood Dr Inglis and whom she found most congenial. They also had with them Mrs Haverfield and the young Dr Janet Laird who had been in Serbia since February.

It was Dr Inglis's first experience of road travel in Serbia. 'The wildest drive I ever had in my life,' she wrote. 'We skidded at least fifty times in the course of the day, but we never upset. We bumped all the day and at one time charged a string of boulders, which had been used to mend the road, and *got over them*; but it was the most glorious run as regards scenery. For a long way the road ran along the top of hills and valleys, and the lights and shadows were magnificent. I don't know when I enjoyed anything so much.'[13]

Arrived at Mladanovatz, there was the old difficulty.

Colonel Nicolayevitch, the commanding officer, was a giant of a man who could put his fist through a door or break a horseshoe in his bare hands; a member of a cavalry family, one of whom later commanded Serbia's Third Army, and himself a superb horseman, he was said to be the most popular soldier in Serbia. He had the cavalry officer's distrust of innovation, and that attitude to women perhaps best described as chivalrous contempt. Towards them his voice and manner were surprisingly gentle for so huge a man.[14]

Dr Inglis spent a weary hour discussing plans with him. At the end of it, nothing was settled. Suddenly, Curcin said in English, 'Don't lose heart, Madame; things go slower in Serbia than in England.' Her laugh broke the tension. Then, providentially, Captain Clements, one of Hunter's men, arrived. Nicolayevitch would accept him. 'So we got a very good site, gently sloping ground with a good water supply and an iron shed at the back where we can put stores.'[15]

Before the other two blocking hospitals could be established, there was more characteristic Balkan muddle to contend with. The venue of Alice Hutchison's projected hospital was changed, and the reason given to Dr Inglis was that a railway bridge had been washed away by floods and would take time to rebuild. She was puzzled and annoyed. It 'knocked the scheme on the head'. Her puzzlement increased when, en route for Nish to collect equipment for the two hospitals, she met Mrs Haverfield and learned that the destroyed bridge was in fact a myth. So why was

Dr Hutchison being sent elsewhere? Was it, Dr Inglis wondered, because the original town was too near the frontier? The Serbian Government was worried about security and in May had formally requested a stricter control upon British personnel going out. Or was it just typical muddle? She concluded irritatedly that in this strange country one seldom got the real reason for anything.[16]

The real reason may have been simpler than she supposed. She was still waiting at the junction three hours later when a train from Nish actually brought up Dr Hutchison and her Unit, accompanied by Hunter who now learned for the first time of the changed plan for his blocking hospitals. But their trains moved on before he could tell her that (as he wrote to Mrs McLaren after a rather different account had appeared in *The History of the Scottish Women's Hospitals*) he himself had been pleased about the change of plan when Dr Inglis told him. Valjevo, the new location, was in his view a more important centre of possible trouble than the original town. It was as simple as that, though why the tale of the railway bridge was put about remained a mystery.[17]

At Nish, Dr Inglis learned from Sir Ralph Paget, head of the civilian health commission, of Lord Methuen's eulogies of the Scottish Women. 'I wonder', she wrote home at once, 'if the War Office would let us send a real Unit for our own men there?' It was no good; she was too far from the centre of things to press the idea.

At Nish, though, she got enough equipment to get the Mladanovatz blocking hospital opened almost at once. Dr Beatrice MacGregor, another of the Bruntsfield Hospital stalwarts, was in charge of it; and Mrs Haverfield went as administrator, which solved—temporarily—a nagging problem.

The Hon. Eveline Haverfield, like so many people who are at their best with horses, had so personal and passionate an attitude to everything that she was prone to sudden and violent antipathies. Dr Lilian Chesney, one of the five reinforcements sent out in February, and one of the steadiest workers the S.W.H. ever had, was everything people meant who spoke of the 'new woman': determinedly un-feminine, a lone wolf, with a dry humour liable to be misunderstood and the uncertain temper which goes with extreme conscientiousness.[18] By now she and Mrs Haverfield were misunderstanding one another with determination and persistence.

Dr Inglis now tactfully sent Mrs Haverfield to Mladanovatz. She was exactly the woman to hit it off with Nicolayevitch; and Dr MacGregor, having been assistant to J-B for years, could surely get on with anyone.

Dr Inglis went herself to help open the new hospital. The site was well drained and timber expensive. She decided not to put down the wooden floors brought from home anywhere but in the operating tent, but instead to use them for partitioning stores. That saved £40 and she had always a Scottish sense of economy. Other tents were set up on ground stamped down hard; it was the floor of most houses, schools and even barracks in Serbia.

She entered enthusiastically into this first experience of starting a war hospital from scratch. 'I wish you could see our kitchen—the quaintest little place, in a shed which was here when we came, and to which we have added another shed, the whole open all round. And our incinerator—which I built. It burns up everything so beautifully,' she wrote on June 16th.[19]

She was full of a youthful zest all through the summer. Indeed it was the grand climax of her life, the fulfilment of her achievement, and was to be the last period of unalloyed happiness she knew. She was doing the work she had always been ambitious for, general surgery, and had won the respect of Serbian medical men for it. She and her colleagues were accepted as competent to treat grown men, something hitherto unimagined. She was consulted, deferred to even, by men like Hunter and Paget, men of position and influence. Her administrative talents had for the first time something approaching full scope. She was even devising radical improvements for the country.

To Anny Christitch, the Serbian writer and feminist who was reporting for the *Daily Express*, she confided one such scheme. 'When the war is over,' Miss Christitch reported her as saying, 'I want to do something lasting for your country. I want to help the women and children; so little has been done for them and they need so much. I should like to see Serbian qualified nurses and up-to-date women's and children's hospitals.'[20]

To a Serbian officer she outlined an even more radical scheme. 'You suffer in Serbia, and are often subject to epidemics, through nothing else but bad water,' he described her as saying. 'I have been thinking it over and would like to ameliorate as much as possible this deplorable state of affairs.' She went on to speak of

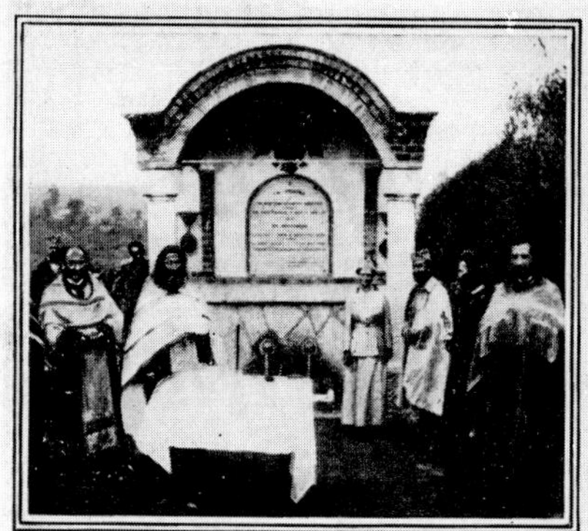

A Tribute to British Nurses by Serbia

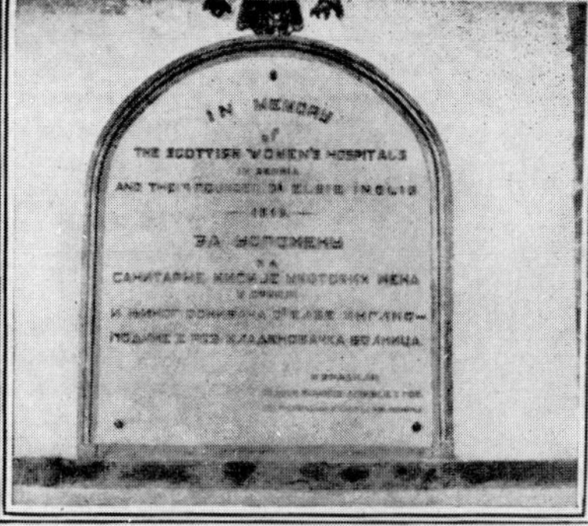

The Inscription on the Memorial Fountain at Meladenovatz

Meladenovatz was recently the scene of a high tribute paid by the Serbians to the good work done by the members of the Scottish Women's Hospitals in Serbia and their director, Dr. Elsie Inglis. A beautiful fountain was built quite close to the camp hospital there, and on October 7 there was a formal opening ceremony, at which a religious service was conducted according to the rites of the Greek Church. Afterwards Colonel Nikoliavitch made a speech in which he expressed his admiration of the good work done by the Scottish Women's Hospitals. Dr. Inglis then turned on the water in the fountain, and the ceremony was concluded by the playing of "God Save the King" and the Serbian National Anthem

The fountain built as a tribute to Dr Elsie Inglis and the Scottish Women's Hospitals in Serbia. *Left* Elsie Inglis at the opening ceremony; *right* the inscription.

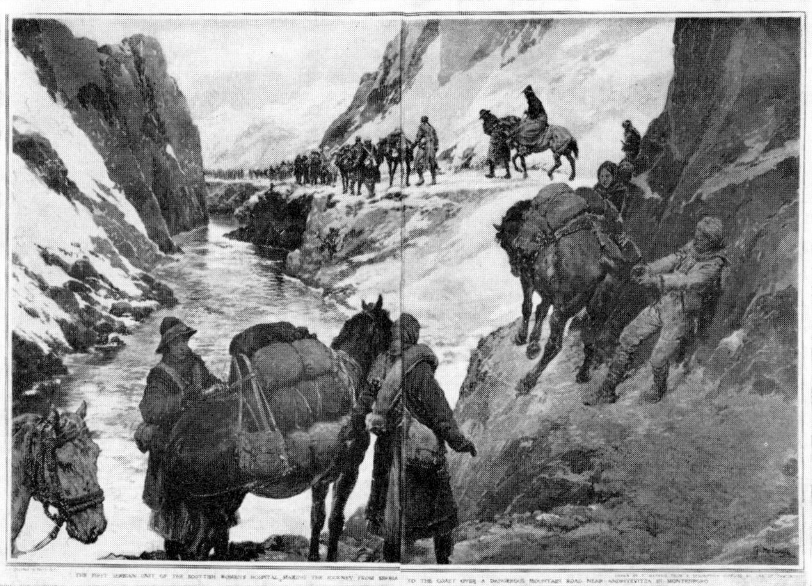

THE FIRST SERBIAN UNIT OF THE SCOTTISH WOMEN'S HOSPITAL MAKING THE JOURNEY FROM SERBIA TO THE COAST OVER A DANGEROUS MOUNTAIN ROAD NEAR ANDRIYEVITZA IN MONTENEGRO

Nurses making the retreat from Serbia through the mountains in Montenegro to the coast. Drawn by F. Matania after personal consultations with the women concerned.

No. 10 + 4. März
+ Jahrgang 1916 +
Erscheint Samstags

Schweizer

Illustrierte Zeitung

Einzelpreis 20 Cts.
Abonnementspreis
Halbjährlich Fr. 4.-

Verlagsanstalt Ringier & Cie., Zofingen

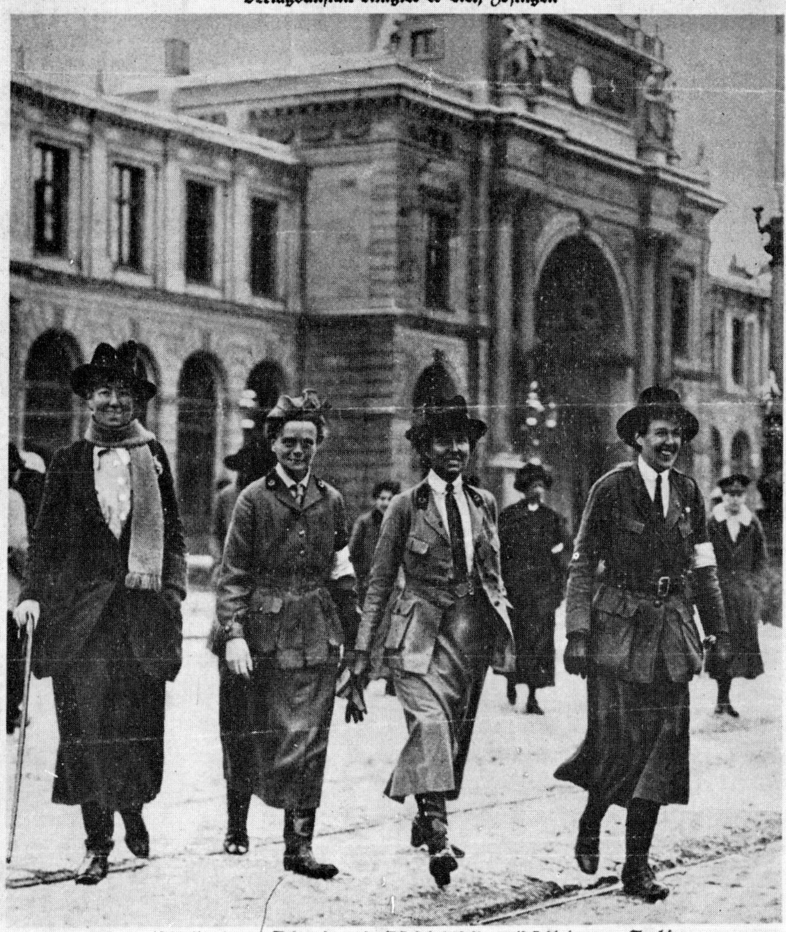

Schottische Rotkreuz-Schwestern in Zürich bei ihrer Rückkehr aus Serbien.

Englische Ärzte und Krankenschwestern hatten fast seit dem Ausbruch des Krieges einen wichtigen Teil des Sanitätspersonals der serbischen Armee gebildet. Bei der Eroberung Serbiens durch die Zentralmächte fielen viele dieser Briten in die Hände der Deutschen und Österreicher. Als ihnen die Rückkehr in die Heimat gestattet wurde, wählten sie zum größten Teile die Reise durch unser Land.

Elsie Inglis and three other members of the Scottish Women's Hospitals in Zurich after their release as prisoners of war during the German occupation of Serbia.

'constructing in each Serbian village a fountain of good drinking water ... It will be, after the war, my unique and greatest desire to do this for Serbs.'[21]

On Hunter her hospitals had made an outstanding impression. Later he was to write to *The Times*, 'I have never met with anyone who gave me so deep an impression of single-mindedness, gentle-heartedness, clear and purposeful vision, wise judgement, and absolutely fearless disposition ... No more lovable personality than hers, or more devoted and courageous body of women, ever set out to help effectively a people in dire distress, than the Scottish Women's Hospital.'[22]

Hunter, however, was ordered to Malta to deal with Dardanelles casualties. His departure on June 10th[23] left her without much-needed backing. In Serbia, Curcin told her, it was not the custom for women to do such work. 'At the bottom of his heart, Colonel Nicolayevitch can never believe that a woman can do a thing as well as a man. And most of the men in Serbia are like that.

'Now I know that that is absurd, and, Madame, I want you to realise that I, and the men who think like me, the advanced party, we are almost more grateful to you for coming out and showing what women can do, than for the hospitals you have given us.'[24] Curcin, like all his countrymen, was good at saying pleasant things, but perhaps a more discreet judge than most of the type of flattery acceptable. Elsie, anyhow, was delighted, and saw to it that his remarks received wide publicity in England.

Even the cavalry colonel however was shortly to be converted and in a way no one could have foreseen. Mrs Haverfield had begged the loan of a few spare horses so that she and the girls might ride occasionally. It would be surprising if he had sent her the pick of his stables.

Mrs Haverfield had learned horsemanship in a school conceded even by continental cavalry officers as among the world's best: the English hunting field. She was moreover a skilful horsemaster; she had, after all, grown up in an England where the hunters of the rich were more pampered than their tenants.

Soon, Nicolayevitch observed that she cared for his animals better than his own men knew how to. The brutes went better for her too. The Gospodja Haverfield was indeed a splendid woman. Perhaps he should admit it—*all* the Scottish Women were splendid people. Since their ideas on horses were so sound, perhaps their notions about hospitals might also have something in them.[25]

As Elsie had always said, a convert is the most violent supporter. Nicolayevitch was influential, and the path of the Scottish Women's Hospitals in all its dealings with the Serbs was to be smoothed in many ways, from now on.

CHAPTER 12

Valjevo, where Dr Hutchison's hospital was about to open, had been the worst-hit town in Serbia during the winter. Dr Inglis visited it in mid-June to find the reek of death still in the air. In the little field graveyards full of wooden monuments with their painted likenesses of proud young warriors, the peasants piously deposited coins, food, even books, and lit small fires on the graves. But the whole district was so full of hastily buried dead that to dig anywhere deeper than an inch or two was to court disaster, and skeletons turned up by animals were a common sight.[1]

The hospital tents were on a hillside looking towards a great range of hills, and down the valley to the little white houses of the town. Dr Inglis reported it well arranged, with six marquees for wards, a large mess tent, kitchens for staff and patients, and bath tents with curtained cubicles. Though baths were appreciated, the nurses noted that soap was a novelty to most patients.[2]

It was so hot that the tents became uncomfortable and *ladnjaks* were built for the women by their orderlies: a kind of willow cabin (for Serbia was of course the Illyria of the ancients and of *Twelfth Night*) made of slender tree trunks bent into an arbour of interlaced branches; a delightfully cool retreat which according to size could be a sentry-box, veranda, improvised stable or field bivouac, and which impressed some British Army observers as better than tents.[3]

The Little General ran her hospital to a series of bugle calls on an instrument she had picked up in Malta, and liked to prowl at 5.30 a.m. because that was the best time to uncover anything amiss. Not, said Dr Inglis, that anything much *would* be wrong with any hospital whose head gave so determined a lead.

Valjevo had a splendid laboratory which became of use far beyond its original terms of reference; and its sanitary officer was a London health visitor whose arrangements achieved such renown that 'May we see your famous latrines?' was the first question of official visitors, who included Marshal Putnik in person. For their water supply this Unit had taken their own pump from Cardiff; but thirty feet of Serbian clay made installation impossible and they fell back on the normal local solution, water carts drawn by oxen.[4]

It was plain to Dr Inglis that an Austrian onslaught was expected. At Valjevo the camp rang from dawn to dusk with clattering musketry. At Mladanovatz, twenty miles from the front, the guns could be clearly heard and files of men daily streamed past in their homespun uniforms. They were in fine fettle, proclaiming, 'We are the only ones who have so far defeated our enemy.'[5] Troop trains were garlanded with flowers and at each halt men jumped out to dance the national *kolo* to the fiddling of the gipsy musician who was normally included in each detachment.[6]

Allied reinforcements were confidently expected, for by the summer of 1915 it had become clear that the Western Front had settled to a static war of attrition and an 'eastern party' in the British Cabinet was urging, principally through Churchill and Lloyd George, that a decision be sought in the Balkans and the Dardanelles.

The summer, however, continued peaceful. Work was slack, and this set Dr Inglis a problem; inexperienced workers dealing with horrors are better without too much time to think. At Valjevo surplus energy was mopped up with improvised entertainments: most of the Scottish Women ended the war much better reel-dancers than they had been at the start, but the Serbs, with their own complex folk music, disdained British singing. They loved to take some simple tune and improvise variations with Slav rhythms and harmonies; what they made of 'Tipperary' had to be heard to be believed.[7]

At Kragujevatz surplus energy was diverted to a sports day for staff and patients, so successful that someone said it was a pity the Crown Prince had not been invited. 'I only wish he had,' retorted Dr Inglis. 'The Crown Prince would have noticed the awful smells in the yard, and something would have been done.'[8]

The more reliable nurses, like the admirable theatre sister, Boykett, could be given leave in small parties; while exploring the country they also ministered to the sores and fevers of ignorant peasants in remote Turkish-style villages.[9]

Still, it was a problem. A bunch of high-spirited women, considering themselves highly emancipated, abroad in a strange country; free for the first time of the regulating influences of Victorian breeding and convention. And the Serbs were striking: bronzed, clear-eyed, tall, with the swinging gait of kilted highlanders; their brown homespun clothes braided with black silk, for only officers wore uniform; camel-skin sandals on their feet over bright socks knitted by some illiterate *maika* or *sestra* in traditional patterns of unimaginable complexity. With a flower stuck in his sheepskin *kappa*, a rifle on his shoulder and a ballad on his lips, the Serbian soldier must have been one of the most romantic-looking men in the world.

Flirting. It was a great worry to Dr Inglis. It seems probable that only fairly harmless exchanges took place. The women were Victorians born, with hair that came down during a struggle with tents in a high wind, skirts to their ankles, language instinctively moderate even in trying circumstances. But they were a new generation of fillies feeling their oats.

'Our naughtiest girls', Dr Inglis wrote later, 'were some of those who had worked right through the typhus without funking or grumbling, grinding on day after day, with an average of twenty funerals a day—& 3 deaths and 9 cases among the Unit themselves—consisting of 30 people.'[10]

She was, nevertheless, down on them with a heavy hand. Strict anyway to the point of prudery, she had the reputation of her Hospitals to consider as well as her responsibility for the girls. The Great War was to kill the age of chaperones in the end but it was not yet dead. One girl was sent home, dismissed: her crime was to have 'been most decidedly frivolous ever since she came' and to have been out in the evening without permission.[11] In mid-July a request reached the home committee that no new recruits should be sent who had not reached an age of discretion: it was put at twenty-seven for nurses, twenty-three for orderlies, who were of higher social standing.[12]

All in all, however, the S.W.H. had fewer difficulties than other units; the head of one poured out his woes to Dr Inglis, ending 'I suppose you never have these troubles. You seem such a happy family.'

She looked hard at him. 'Shows run by women' were more commonly charged with spite and intrigue. And there *had* been that business of Dr Chesney and Mrs Haverfield. Could he be laughing at her? No, he was in earnest. Suppressing a twinkle, she murmured, 'Well, perhaps a woman *can* manage other women better than men can.'[13]

On July 10th, the heads of British units* in Serbia met to confer at Kragujevatz. The country was now healthy and peaceful. Ought they all to turn their attentions elsewhere? Or would they be needed again?

Dr Inglis's view was forcefully put and carried the day. 'My own feeling strongly is that we should wait here in readiness for emergencies *which must come*' she wrote home, reporting the meeting. 'And when they come there will be no country in more need than Serbia—with under 300 doctors and no nurses whatsoever. In the meantime it seems to me there is a good deal we can do here.'[14]

The best way to help the country, she told the conference, was to try to raise overall medical standards. To this end she opened at Valjevo two dispensaries for civilians, and a training school giving four-week courses to Serbian medical orderlies, by which it was hoped to improve standards progressively throughout the army.

Since Hunter's departure nothing had been done about the third hospital of his blocking scheme. Now, in accordance with her own desire to help the country as a whole, Dr Inglis pushed through the idea that she should run this in Lazaravatz, and according to local methods, using equipment made on the spot by local craftsmen, rather than with elaborate devices from Britain. It would then form a demonstration centre to teach the Serbs, using and improving their own methods, and would also show up clearly where the local methods were inadequate.[15]

She had already experimented in this in her own hospital at Kragujevatz. She found a local carpenter to make her an instrument cupboard instead of accepting one offered by Hunter when he left; and arranged with Ristitch, the energetic and progressive arsenal director, for other equipment to be made there on the spot. The resulting X-ray room could, she said, have held its own with any in Europe.

Buying locally was not always easy. One day she set out with Miss Vera Holme, who had arrived at the end of June with a large staff car and a motor ambulance donated by Welsh

* The Serbian Relief Fund had sent two, the Quakers one, and there were other smaller groups.

suffragists. They hoped to acquire a pair of local-style scales for drugs.

In the apothecary's she saw some, but learned that they were used for the business and could not be spared. She bought some drugs, then some more; altogether staying an hour and spending £10, constantly reverting between her purchases to the scales.

'You know,' she said firmly at last, as if it clinched the matter, 'it is for *your* men we want them.'

The apothecary could hold out no longer. He took down the scales and presented them to her. No, there was no price. It would—he bowed—be a pleasure to give them to her.[16]

She was beginning to understand how to deal with these strange people.

Her main problem was that of every hospital in Serbia: sanitation. Sewage normally passed through holes in the floor to an open ditch under each ward, thence to a pool in the central yard, covered with a wooden lid, usually ill-fitting;[17] the method Miss Nightingale had found at Scutari. Dr Inglis estimated that the pit at Kragujevatz had not been cleaned for ten years. It took her five weeks to get it emptied, first with the use of pumps and when they broke, with the local ox-cart method.

Haphazard local ways aroused her fury. Ten Austrians were sent to fill the pit, 'but they sent no picks or shovels! There were exactly two shovels and one pick in Hospital and when I went down, eight Austrians were lying under the trees smoking—two were leisurely throwing loose earth into the pit. When they got to the end, another man dragged himself to his feet, and broke up some more ground with the pick, while the two over-worked shovellers smoked.'

She watched for ten minutes, then descended on them and asked for the officer in charge. There was none.

'Ten Austrian prisoners and nobody in charge, you know!! Eventually we found the Serbian non-commissioned officer *asleep* at the back of the bathroom. I stood over them for two hours and I don't think those Austrians have worked so hard since they came to Serbia ... In two hours we had made the slope where the cart is to stand which is to carry away our dirty water, and thrown all the earth into the pit. Then I went up to Colonel Gentitch's office and said that if they wanted me to spend my time standing over Austrian orderlies I was quite willing to do it, but I thought it was a job for their officers. They were horrified. So all yesterday and today there has been feverish energy and the place is tidied out of knowledge. We have half (!) emptied the cesspool. We have built an incinerator for all the dressings (which before went into the pond!) and solid refuse from the kitchen. We have made a "tamp"; namely, a slope in which a cart for two barrels will stand, and all dirty water will be emptied into them and carted to the fields. We are to have two carts and a yoke of oxen [from the army] but don't be surprised if you find I have bought a yoke of oxen for you, for we shall find it much easier to keep our carts circulating if we control them entirely. And we have filled in the awful pit or pond—*and* the Serbians have tidied up the grass, which is so like them, the dear things. While we struggle with the cesspool they make the grass nice.

'Well,' she concluded with satisfaction, 'that hospital will be a demonstration in Kragujevatz of what they can do or ought to do on their own system with their own implements.'[18]

The struggle dragged on, however. In mid-August she was writing, 'By the way, I bought that yoke of oxen for Kragujevatz. It was quite necessary',[19] and by the end of September she had got the cesspool closed altogether and was using the cart-and-bucket system entirely, with the two oxen—which, inevitably, received pet nicknames from the Scottish Women.

Then she received a surprise; and it is certainly indicative of the tension she was under by this time that it made her laugh until she cried. In this strange, seemingly haphazard country, traction oxen were actually *registered*, by name, for wartime inventories.[20] The Unit had broken the law by re-naming them Huz and Buz.

When she had finished wiping her eyes, Dr Inglis signed the appropriate registration forms and all was well. But when, weeks later, she at last received the oxen promised by authority ('*so* like them') the irrepressible Scottish girls promptly named them Gog and Magog. 'But I have said those must be strictly pet names for I am not going to sign Acts for altering the names of Government oxen.'[21]

There was endless travelling: to Skoplje in August to do emergency operations at the hospital run by Lady Paget; on to Nish to meet new recruits coming out; then to Valjevo where despite the famous latrines typhoid had broken out infecting six of the staff and killing one, a reminder that in this primitive country one must not for a moment relax attention to hygiene; and on to

Mladanovatz, where Dr MacGregor had opened a civilian dispensary and was trying to give local people some health education.

By mid-August she was back at Kragujevatz. The atmosphere was threatening. The Dardanelles campaign was failing, no Allied forces appeared in Serbia. Months previously, England and France had moreover unintentionally placed a time bomb beneath their ally Serbia. It was now ready to explode.

The Secret Treaty of London signed the previous April[22] had the intention of bringing Italy into the war on the Allied side. The flags at Brindisi which Dr Inglis amusedly compared with the suffragist colours, had almost certainly been celebrating the Treaty's signing on the previous day, for it was secret only in the sense that its precise provisions were not publicised; its existence was openly talked of, as was Italy's bargaining for a strip of Adriatic coast to which Serbia also laid claim. Italy entered the war on May 23rd. This, with the non-arrival in Serbia of confidently expected Allied contingents (Tommy's phrase books had been widely distributed)[23], made the Serbs believe they were to be thrown to the wolves.

'What does it matter what a little nation like us feel?' Dr Inglis was asked bitterly by one Serb woman. 'You Great Powers are settling it over our heads.'[24]

There seems no reason to suppose that Allied policy was the result of anything but muddle. For the Serbs it was tragic. On September 6th Bulgaria signed a military agreement with the Central Powers, who now needed only the Serbian section of the Orient Railway to send supplies to their hard-pressed Turkish allies in the Dardanelles. Germans and Austrians were massing on Serbia's frontier.

Whatever Serbs felt about their allies, they had no doubts about the Scottish Women. One woman asked Dr Inglis her opinion of the outcome of the war. Her sturdy reply was, 'We are already victors if we have done our utmost.'[25]

On September 7th, a morning of dazzling sunshine, an unusual ceremony took place at Mladanovatz, the unveiling and benediction of a stone fountain bringing pure water to the village and built by the Serbs to commemorate Dr Inglis's achievement.

She arrived at eleven with Colonel Gentitch and Colonel Mihailovitz; they had started from Kragujevatz only one hour late, she commented, 'quite good for this dear unpunctual country. It is curious how one gets used to things.' The road which had once seemed so awful, seemed this time 'positively quite good'.

The ceremony, attended by men of all branches of the army, many Scottish Women, and a motley group of local people, had the unrehearsed impressiveness of Orthodox ceremonial. On an improvised altar stood a silver crucifix, a bowl of holy water, a burning candle, a bunch of green basil and one of dry. Five priests in flowing robes chanted the service, at the first note of which the soldiers, as one man, swept off their caps and crossed themselves. Blessings were invoked upon the monarchs of Serbia, Russia, and England. The basil, dipped in holy water, was sprinkled over the fountain and the soldiers. A priest spoke, in the dramatic Serbian style of unrehearsed oratory, of his country's gratitude to Dr Inglis. Elsie could not understand a word; but when she got a translation into French, later, she thought it a 'very pretty little speech'.

'I felt as a Suffragist I ought to make a speech in reply,' she added. 'But in the first case I should have had to speak in French, and in the second, I knew they weren't used to women speaking. So I just said I thanked them a thousand times and they did not seem to expect anything more.' She turned on the flow of the fountain and was presented with the basil sprigs. They were, she wrote, certainly among the few things she would always keep.[26]

Then the whole group adjourned to lunch in the hospital's mess tent, beautified with flowers and berries stuck in vases (made from shell cases found on last year's battlefield); there were more speeches, and healths, ballads sung by one of the priests, and haunting violin music from a regimental fiddler. One thing struck the doctors as odd. 'Ladies are never produced,' observed Dr MacGregor quietly to Dr Inglis. 'Not one Serbian lady came to witness the religious ceremony. At lunch the same —all these Serbian men, and not a woman here besides ourselves.'[27]

Later, Dr Inglis was driven on to Lazaravatz where the local-style demonstration hospital was ready. This, Curcin declared, was her favourite hospital—because it had been accomplished in the face of most difficulties. It was scattered, Serbian style, through the village in *gast häuser* and requisitioned houses. The Scottish Women were responsible for 200 patients, plus all the laundry, this last without wringing machines, drying sheds or even water laid on.[28]

She found Lazaravatz busy. A division had passed through to the front, leaving a hundred sick behind, more than filling every bed that was ready. While she was there a message arrived that fifty casualties were coming back down the line.

Here at last was war work as she had always imagined it:[29] exciting, exhilarating, a challenge. Never mind if the rush resulted in overcrowding such as she would have condemned roundly if one of her subordinates had allowed it.

'We went and turned out a gast house, people who had been sitting there in the café helping to clear out the tables and chairs, the proprietors helping too and showing us where extra wood was to be had, and so on. We swept the whole place out to the light of storm lanterns, made a roaring fire, got on some boiling water in the little kitchen place, and then down on us came the patients, beds, bedding, all together. Some of the men were really ill and all of them were dead tired. Fortunately [the wooden] Serbian beds are more quickly made than our iron ones ... We packed that house as no English Hospital would ever dare to pack. But we got a bed for each man. There was no question of bathing, of course! We just tore off their uniforms and their heavy muddy boots ... and it was good to see them sink back on their pillows saying "Leppo, sestra, leppo" which means "It is beautiful, Sister, beautiful".'[30]

It was obvious to Dr Inglis that her three hospitals, strung along a branch railway skirting the foothills to the south of the Danube basin, would be inundated if fighting broke out. On September 15th Miss Pares, the Mladanovatz hospital administrator, wrote home that guns had been heard all day from the frontier twenty miles away; that flour was scarce in the town and meat had doubled in price.[31] In the same week warnings were received of Austrian air raids and the Kragujevatz arsenal, Serbia's principal one, emptied of workmen; 'and they don't stop work willingly just now' wrote Dr Inglis.[32]

Seeing the indecisiveness of the Allies, Bulgaria finally decided to join the Central Powers and ordered general mobilisation on September 22nd; Serbia sent a last appeal for help to her allies. 'What is coming to Serbia we cannot think,' an officer told Dr Inglis. She saw despair all around her; strong men, she wrote, could hardly speak of the coming disaster without breaking down.[33]

Travelling up from Nish on the main Orient line on September 25th, a journey of ninety miles to Kragujevatz took her twenty-one hours, so blocked were the lines with troops and munitions. 'Serbia is exactly where she was a year ago,' an officer met on the journey said to her.

'If only', she wrote to her committee next day in an uncensored letter being carried home by one of the sisters, 'they could have sent a British Expeditionary Force up here this summer, it would have made absolutely all the difference—all the Balkan States would have declared on our side, Germany could not have got ammunition through to the Turks, and probably things would have been easier for Russia. I suppose one ought not to criticise—but to lengthen our line in France and have muddling diplomacy out here! Of course I believe we have poured in money and munitions and stores—but an Army Corps would have simply solved the situation.'[34]

The muddle was one more nail in the coffin of Asquith's shaky coalition government. Lloyd George made capital out of it, and Carson, the Attorney General, resigned because of the failure to help Serbia. One British and one French division were indeed transferred from the Dardanelles, arriving at Salonika on October 3rd (with, for the British, only thin summer uniforms to face the Balkan winter). Along the railways, peasants tied bunches of box to station lamps in traditional welcome. At Skoplje the buildings were beflagged.[35] The help, however, was too little, too late, too ill thought out. Nothing was known about the roads, or lack of them, from Salonika north, or that Serbian mud was so holding that it could take five oxen to pull a car clear even with the engine running.[36] In Salonika, a neutral Greek port, enemy observers were watching openly as the Allies disembarked.

Air raids were by now frequent. On September 30th a German flying machine was shot down in flames in the centre of Kragujevatz and the town went wild; next day the Arsenal was bombed and several people killed.[37]

That day Paget wrote reminding Dr Inglis of points to consider in planning her actions. Firstly, he said, if captured, her Units might be employed in ministering to the enemy; secondly, even if this did not happen, their services would be lost to the Allies; thirdly, the equipment and stores would be of use to the enemy unless removed or destroyed; finally, that according to the usages of war the care of unevacuable wounded should be left to the enemy: 'the wounded, therefore, may reasonably be left without scruple on that score'.

The chance of helping the Serbian Army should, he concluded, decide whether Units should stay or leave; individual personal bravery did not come into the matter.[38]

Dr Inglis had already decided what to do. 'As long as the Serbians fight, we'll stick to them,' she had said in her uncensored letter home five days before; in which may be detected a note of almost pleasurable excitement. Life was still an adventure, not a tragedy. 'Retreat, if necessary, burning all our stores. If they are overwhelmed, we must escape—probably via Montenegro. Don't worry about us. We won't do anything rash or foolish; and if you will trust us to decide, as we must know most about the situation out here, we'll act rationally.'[39]

On October 6th she left Kragujevatz, driven by Vera Holme, to visit Lazaravatz.

Hill and valley stood out in the brilliant sunshine, shadows chased one another across the landscape. Never had that beautiful country looked so beautiful to Elsie. Woods and hedges glowed with autumn colours, the tang of the air was refreshing after the long heat of summer. But on the horizon hung heavy clouds. The contrasted sunshine and shadow were, she reflected, symbolic of her months in Serbia.[40]

The clouds continued to mass as they came down through the poplar lanes to Topola, home and shrine of the Serbian liberator Karageorge. Soon after, the storm broke. The road, from being thick with dust, became a slithery mass of mud. More than once the ambulance skidded right across it. When darkness fell they had a little over ten miles to go, but ahead lay one of the worst descending roads in the country, and they decided to spend the night in the car.

As the hours wore on, the thunder and lightning became less frequent. The beating of rain on the roof lessened. Then in the growing light of morning another sound could be heard: the boom of distant cannon.

A more dreadful storm was breaking over Serbia. The guns they could hear were from beyond the Danube, and they were bombarding Belgrade.

CHAPTER 13

That same day, Thursday, October 7th, the forces of Germany and Austria-Hungary under Mackensen crossed the Danube.[1] Belgrade, virtually indefensible, fell next day, though a three-day suicidal delaying action was fought, street by street, by the *chichas* ('uncles') of the Serbian Army, the over-forty third-line troops commanded by General Mihailo Jivkovitch, the Iron General as he was called.[2]

Everyone knew Belgrade could not last long. On the first day, Dr Inglis, with Alice Hutchison and Beatrice MacGregor, sat in the latter's little office at Mladanovatz, discussing with Paget and Curcin what they should do. The hospital had already been bombed by a solitary Taube, sending patients, nurses and orderlies to hide in ditches or among standing maize. Paget and Curcin felt responsibility for the women, but knew how important the hospitals were to the fighting men.

As they talked, enemy aeroplanes were heard again, probing the Morava Valley. Dr Inglis refused to move: to interrupt their discussion for such a reason seemed to her surrender.

Beatrice MacGregor wanted to fall back with the army and form dressing stations in the rear; the other women felt it their duty to remain where they were.

'We felt as if a heavy burden had been lifted from all our hearts,' Curcin later described this moment. He had become devoted to Dr Inglis. It was hardly possible to imagine, he reflected now, that one man—and that a *woman*—had done so much for the country in so short a time; and with no help other than her own ideals and driving force. But how long, he wondered, could this extraordinary driving force continue to exert itself?[3]

Mladanovatz was, in fact, the first Scottish Women's Hospital to be evacuated. On the main Orient line, once Belgrade had fallen, the town could not be held. Capture of the railway was the German objective; it was only the entry of Italy into the war which decided them to occupy the whole of 'this cold and inhospitable country'.

Dr MacGregor's hospital retreated on October 12th to Kragujevatz, earning Dr Inglis's approval by getting all the precious equipment away at only two days' notice. Within a day or two they were handling nearly 400 cases a day at an emergency dressing station at Kragujevatz.[4]

Alice Hutchison also retreated from Valjevo, on October 29th, to the rural spa of Vrinjatcha Banja where she established a new hospital and dressing station for the wounded, brought down from the hills on pack mules with pannier seats and stretchers,[5] or in ox-wagons, precisely as in Miss Nightingale's day the English wounded had been brought down from Balaclava.

The hopes of the women remained high. Allied help was still expected, and in fact the French General Sarrail landed at Salonika on October 12th and sent his forces up the Vardar valley. They were too late. The Bulgarians launched an attack to block his advance. In mid-December he retreated to Salonika. The best the Serbs could hope for after mid-October was to avoid encirclement and keep their army intact.

Nothing of this was known to the women in the Western Morava Valley. Rumour was rife and as Dr Hollway and Mrs Haverfield at Lazaravatz had still no orders to move, they all felt there was still hope. On October 19th, however, Dr Hollway was given eight hours to evacuate her patients and leave. Somehow the equipment was packed and in pouring rain in open cattle trucks these women too got back to the Western Morava Valley which experienced soldiers believed might still be held. After a three-day journey of 100 miles Dr Hollway's party reached Krushevatz where they were given a single room in which to sleep, at the Czar Lazar barracks which had been turned into a hospital.[6]

They found Krushevatz chaotic, full of refugees, its cobbled streets blocked with bullock carts. Several days of heavy rain added to the misery. Unable to contact Dr Inglis who was still at Kragujevatz, the women busied themselves establishing a canteen for soldiers near the station. Wounded were pouring into this town also, and Dr Hollway was given a barracks outbuilding in which to open a hospital. A former ammunition magazine, it was two storeys high, with wooden racks round the walls on which they could place mattresses. Some of the equipment had vanished during their moves and the rest was soaking wet. Before they could even prepare the place, the wounded began pouring in.

Elsie, all this time, was still at Kragujevatz. She too was working at full stretch for the wounded from the Belgrade battle. She enlarged her hospital, put beds in the corridors; and took over two *gast häuser* with seventy beds in each, noting wryly that men who had been the spoiled-children convalescents of her hospital for weeks during the lull did not take kindly to being pushed out to make way for more urgent cases.

Protitch, the Director, begged her to put three men in two beds, Balkan fashion, but she was resolved to maintain proper standards. The wounded came in batches from the train, sometimes seventy in a day. Among the most common injuries were compound thigh fractures and perforating wounds of the brain,[7] for the steel helmet, only developed that summer, was unheard of in Serbia. All wounds were at least two days old and most were septic.

Looking back each evening, however, Dr Inglis felt she had reason for modest satisfaction. She never refused a case and still had not got unmanageably overcrowded nor dirty. So far as possible, the less serious cases were kept for twenty-four hours' rest before being moved down the line.[8] One who was kept in the hospital was Danials, an English sailor wounded at Belgrade.*

She had to make a stand against Protitch and Curcin over the beds. Dr Curcin had, indeed, become quite excited. 'That is the difference between the Serbian and the English point of view,' he cried. 'The Serbs take in every case that comes. The hospitals, it is true, will get dirty and overcrowded, but all the men will be in. But the English will only take in as many as they can properly manage and they will be beautifully nursed and cared for, and the rest will remain in the street.'

Dr Inglis retorted, 'But that is exactly what would not happen. Nobody lies in the street, under English management.'

'What would you do, then?'

Never had she felt so tongue-tied, so British and insular and muddle-headed. What exactly the English would do in Kragujevatz, where 3,000 wounded lay at that moment, she found impossible to put into words. Impossible, too, to solve the problem

* For the exploits of the small British naval unit which became 'The Terror of the Danube' see *The Times*, July 7 and 15, 1915.

when neither the full facts nor the full responsibility had been given her. She reflected, sadly, how difficult it is for one nation to understand another, and consoled herself that the Scottish Women had at least solved the problem in their own corner of Kragujevatz.[9]

She hoped to remain here—after all, this was where the Serbian stand of 1914 had halted the enemy. The Allies would *surely* arrive soon.

At the start of the third week of October, however, Dr MacGregor's group was ordered to leave Kragujevatz for Kraljevo, where the Ibar Valley runs south from the Western Morava Valley; they opened a new dressing station there. On October 21st the Germans got two bridges across the Danube. Nothing could stop them now and Kragujevatz was their first objective. On October 23rd Dr Inglis too received her orders to retreat.

She was in the theatre when the order came. Wounded men needing major surgery were arriving all the time. As soon as she could she hurried to Curcin. She was pale and wretched; almost desperately she tried to persuade him that he was asking the impossible, that the Unit could not leave.

Curcin had already been through this argument with other doctors. What he had to say to Dr Inglis was the most painful task of all, he wrote later. He had become deeply devoted to her, and hated the thought that by carrying out his own duty he would earn her hostility. 'I knew well with whom I had to deal,' he wrote, 'and I was less willing to depress her than anybody else.'[10]

After some argument, he prevailed, and Dr Inglis ordered the clearing of the hospital. Every man who could so much as walk was sent off by train, by bullock wagon or, in some cases, on foot. The Serbs had given orders that all who could, were to get away, and it was by no means unknown for men on crutches to set off on a thirty-mile walk to the next town.[11] As wards cleared, equipment was packed under the supervision of William Smith, the administrator.

Outside, the town was in an uproar. Kragujevatz was the H.Q. of the army staff. When it became known that they were leaving, with the Crown Prince, a wild scramble to get away ensued.[12] The Austro-Hungarians had massacred civilians at Shabatz the previous year. Now there was the added fear that the first enemy arrivals might be Bulgarian *comitadji*, against whom many Serbs had been engaged in irregular forays for years and who would have old scores to settle. 'You don't really believe that Bulgarians commit these atrocities on prisoners?' a Scottish Woman doctor once asked a Serb boy. His eyes flashed. 'Of course we believe it. You see, we do it too. We like it,' he replied, and explained with gruesome detail the precise attraction of atrocities.[13]

The sound of guns grew nearer almost hourly. The railway was threatened. Bullock wagons, many full of patients in brightly-coloured hospital clothes, crowded the wide cobbled streets. One incongruous sight was plodding oxen harnessed to two smart painted vans bearing the name of Derry and Toms, the Kensington drapers, who had donated them to the Serbian Relief Fund.[14]

White flags hung from houses, shops were barricaded; outside the town, dumps of stores, ammunition, food, even haystacks, were being set alight; it was noticed that though many haystacks, owing to the recent rains, took fire slowly, others burned with a peculiar brilliance and a rattle like musketry.[15]

By the afternoon of the 25th, Dr Inglis's hospital was cleared; but twenty cases were too serious to move. While staff went to the station, two Sisters volunteered to do final dressings. Dr Inglis remained with them, and William Smith refused to leave until every woman was out. Normal British practice is to leave an R.A.M.C. corporal with unevacuable wounded;[16] in the Scottish Women's Hospital at Kragujevatz six untrained Serb orderlies remained; Protitch and three Serb doctors were staying in charge of all the town's hospitals.

At the last moment one man had a severe haemorrhage. Not an instrument was unpacked. Dr Inglis put on a tourniquet and sent him to a Serb doctor. When the stretcher party returned she said goodbye to the hospital she had made the best in Serbia.

They were to travel on the last train before the line was dynamited; but at the station there was delay. She found a few cigarettes from somewhere and ran back to the hospital with them for the men.

The sight that met her eyes was a shock. The windows were shut, offending her British instincts to the core. The beds were awry, the place already looked chaotic. But that was not the worst.

The patients too ill to be moved were out of bed. One man with a fractured femur and an extension apparatus was sitting up with his splint off, winding up his bandages; another, with

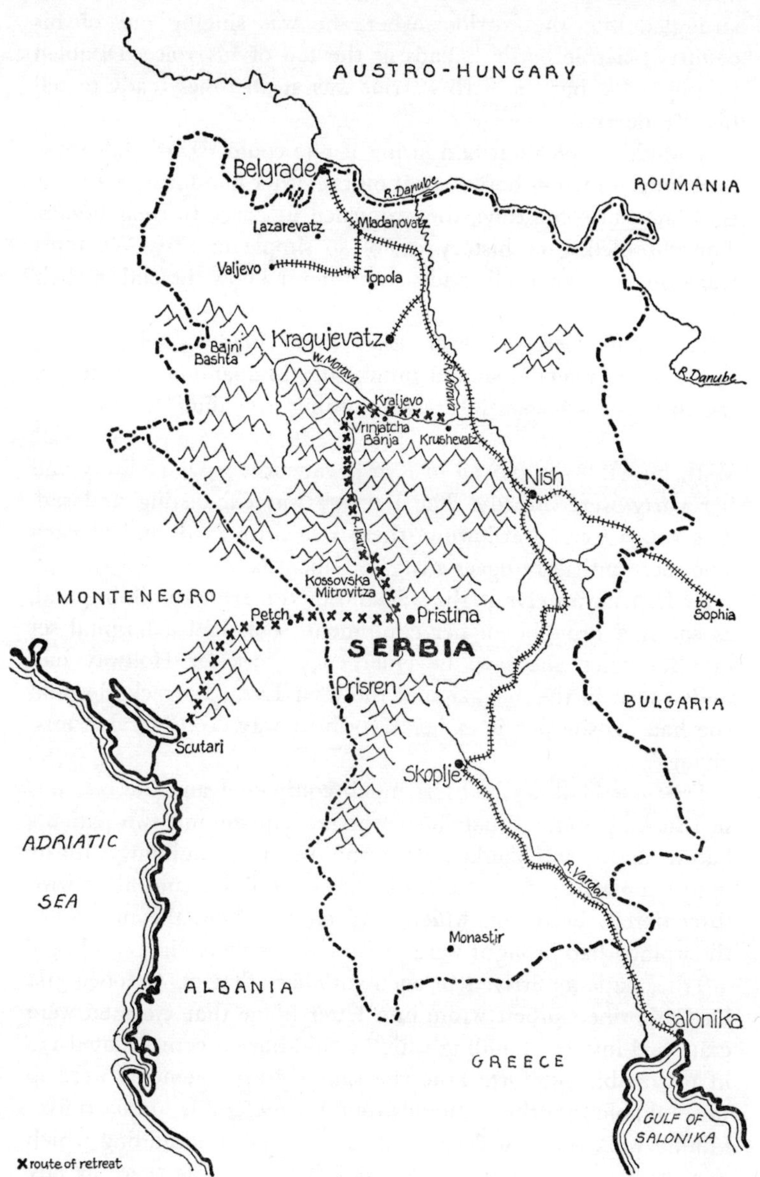

Serbia 1914–15

both feet amputated and paralysed on one side, had somehow struggled into the corridor where he was singing one of his country's heroic battle ballads at the top of his voice. Disabled he might be, but the Serb warrior was at all times ready to sell his life dearly.

It would be pleasant and fitting if one could record that these men indeed died as heroes; or if on the other hand it were known that later, at some time, they returned in peace to their homes. The chronicling of history is not so simple or tidy. We must leave them, as Dr Inglis had to, and never know the end of their story.

Then and there, however, Elsie Inglis made a solemn vow. Nothing, ever again, should induce her to abandon patients for whom she was responsible. And nothing ever did.[17]

With her staff she moved to Krushevatz where Dr Hollway and her party were already. The journey was exhausting and sad. The trains were overflowing, there was little food, and at each stop more pitiful refugees struggled aboard.

At Krushevatz, Dr Inglis was allocated a school building and, as she had brought all her equipment, soon had a hospital set up. But when she saw the emergency work Dr Hollway had undertaken in the magazine at the Czar Lazar Barrack Hospital she had, as she put it in her restrained way, 'considerable misgivings'.

True, Dr Hollway had lost much equipment and the rest was still soaking wet, so that linen was inadequate and two patients had to share each blanket. True, the two-storey building with its mud floor was dark and dirty below, cold above, and filled with three-tiered shelves on which, and on the floor, the mattresses the women had brought were packed as closely as they would go.

True, patients arrived in such numbers that on October 31st Dr Catherine Corbett wrote in a letter home that 570 men were crammed into the building which would have accommodated 150 in reasonable comfort. True the sanitary arrangements were so unspeakable that the fastidious found it preferable to take a five-minute walk through deep mud to the small outbuilding which was the barrack's own original sick bay; nor was there at any time hot water. True, it was so cold and wet that to take uniforms, even verminous ones, off wounded men who had only half a blanket each would have seemed inhuman.[18]

To Dr Inglis, difficulties such as these were there to be overcome. No excuses should be tolerated. 'The organisation of this work was not good,' she wrote censoriously to Miss Mair on November 5th. 'They got the buildings overcrowded, had no way of bathing the patients, and I confess I was horribly worried lest we should have typhus breaking out. However, that won't happen again ...'[19]

The one bright spot was the way the tempers of the women were standing the strain not only of work in these conditions but of living twenty-four in a room which served for sleeping, cooking, eating, sorting and salvaging equipment, sewing and writing by the light of one dim lamp, or trying to rid themselves of vermin picked up from the patients. One or two, Catherine Corbett noted, were not standing it very well, but even they worked hard. Others came out in shining colours.[20]

Dr Inglis set the tone. One night soon after their arrival at Krushevatz, when her Unit had settled for the night, a message came that enemy aircraft were near. Would the Sisters not take refuge? For a moment, panic seemed likely. Then, not raising her head, Elsie murmured 'Everyone will do as they like, of course; I shall not go anywhere. I am very tired; and bed is a comfortable place to die in.' The panic subsided. They all feared Dr Inglis's scorn more than the enemy's bombs.[21]

A day or two later she secured a second magazine building, identical with the first, to be used partly as a store and partly as an operating theatre. It eased the pressure a good deal. By November, however, it was clear that the Western Morava Valley could not be defended; the Serbs were moving men and stores out, and civilians were leaving Krushevatz. The guns sounded nearer each day. The wounded came through endlessly; the sight of them, wrote an American relief worker, was the kind of picture which, once seen, changes for ever the aspect of life.[22]

The only question for the Scottish Women was, who should leave, and when?

Dr Inglis offered everyone the chance to get away. Some had served in arduous conditions for nearly a year and were in no state to face the enemy. Others believed they could help more by retreating with the army. On November 5th a party of twenty women, including Dr Chesney and Dr Laird, was assembled at Krushevatz ready to trek through the Ibar Valley and Montenegro to the Adriatic.[23] Mr Smith, it was agreed, should go in charge, and Danials, the English sailor, would go at the same time.

Although many refugees succeeded in getting south to Salonika it seems that by November 5th this route was thought impracticable. At any rate, the women did not consider it.

During the preceding days Dr Inglis had tried to contact Dr MacGregor at Kraljevo, thirty miles to the west, to settle her plans before the home party left. Getting no reply to telegrams and as there were no trains, she had herself driven, on November 5th, up the valley in the Welsh ambulance, to the undisguised distress of the Serb H.Q. staff. 'We did not see the shadow of a German,' she noted contemptuously.[24] In villages, however, flour had been scattered along the roads in sign of surrender. The tracks were crowded; refugees, army stragglers, peasant women carrying babies and dragging toddlers by the hand, shaky bullock carts piled with household goods, all formed an endless stream. It was a procession by now stretching from one end of Serbia to the other.

At Kraljevo she found Beatrice MacGregor and her staff had already left to trek through the Ibar Valley hoping to open a hospital farther south. In Kraljevo were 700 seriously wounded men left with one officer, Colonel Antitch, and three orderlies to await the enemy. Dr Hutchison was there too; she had come from her own hospital to discover what was happening. The two women again met Sir Ralph Paget and Dr Curcin, and reaffirmed that they both intended staying with their hospitals at all cost. Curcin wrote later that he was intensely relieved, 'because not only did we not know whom to leave with our wounded, but also we had no means of transporting the mission'.[25]

Sadly, Dr Inglis returned to Krushevatz. 'Just now', she wrote to Miss Mair on her return, 'one can think of nothing but these poor little people in this awful hole—with the country they have fought so hard for, overrun from end to end. They can hardly speak to one without breaking down—even strong men among them. They look at one so eagerly and say "When will your men be up?" *When?* ... It is as bad as Belgium ... but Belgium we could not have foreseen. This we could and *ought to* have foreseen. Lots of people did foresee it, but the people in the Government at home were so wise and diplomatic.'[26]

She had, she wrote, decided that if the Scottish Women were really to help Serbia, they must stick to their posts. Sir Ralph had not at first agreed. But events had convinced him that the equipment would anyhow be impossible to save. He had lost the whole of his, when Nish had fallen to the Bulgars. Furthermore, the responsibility for the hospitals in retreat was an extra worry to the Serbs. 'Instead of helping, we were adding to the difficulties', wrote Dr Inglis, 'and if the Committee could have seen Colonel Gentitch's face when I said to him that we were not going to move again but that they could count on us just where we stood, I think they would have been touched.'[27]

This was her last letter to her home committee. Smith was standing by to take it with him. His party left that day, walking or riding in six bullock wagons which Mrs Haverfield had secured for them and piled with tents, bedding and food. Smith was delayed until the following day and Elsie seized the chance to write to Mrs Simson. Shells were falling near the town as she wrote.

'We are in the very centre of the storm and it just feels exactly like having the rain pouring down, and the wind beating in gusts, and not being able to see for the water in one's eyes and just holding on and saying "It cannot last, it is so bad". These poor little people, you cannot imagine anything more miserable than they are ... The hospitals are packed with wounded. We decided we must stand by our hospitals; it was too awful leaving badly wounded men with no proper care ... We all managed wonderfully in our first "evacuations" and saved practically everything, but now it is hopeless. The bridges are down, and the trucks standing anyhow on sidings, and worst of all, the people have begun looting. I don't wonder. There'll be famine, as well as cold, in this corner of the world soon, and then the distant prospect of 150,000 British troops at Salonika won't help much.

'The beloved British troops—the thought of them always cheers. But not the thought of the idiots at the top who had not enough gumption to *know* this must happen. Anybody, even us women, could have told them that the Germans must try and break through to the help of the Turks.

'We have got a nice building here for a hospital, and Dr Hollway is helping in the military hospital. I believe there are about 1,000 wounded in the place. I can't write a very interesting letter, Amy dear, because at the bottom of my heart I don't believe it will ever reach you. I don't see them managing the Montenegrin passes at this time of year! There is a persistent rumour that the

French have retaken Skoplje, and if that is true perhaps the Salonika route will be open soon …

'I wonder', she ended, 'if Serbia is a particularly beautiful country, or whether it looks so lovely because of the tragedy of this war, just as bed seems particularly delightful when the night bell goes!'[28]

By now there was panic in the town. The army, still eluding encirclement, had left the Morava Valley on November 1st. The food shops had been besieged by crowds for days and now everyone was looting. A day or two later Mrs Haverfield was, single-handed, to prevent the theft of the total Serbian Red Cross stores.[29] The Scottish Women had been without bread for ten days, without meat for four.[30]

By the afternoon of November 6th, the last of the escaping party had got away. The women who remained, filled with a sense of anti-climax, were tidying up and preparing for any wounded who might arrive when, in the late afternoon, an enormous explosion blew out most of the windows in the Czar Lazar Hospital and of the house where Dr Inglis's unit were quartered, injuring a nurse and shattering doors and furniture. An ammunition train had been exploded by the Serbs to destroy the railway bridge over the Morava.[31]

The explosion attracted enemy fire and a bombardment followed. It lasted half an hour, with some bombs being dropped from enemy flying machines. Between explosions, the women hurried back through the mud to their patients, uneasily aware of an ammunition dump a few yards from the hospital door. Halfway across the yard, Dr Inglis met Mrs Haverfield and glanced up at her with a quizzical look. 'Eve, we are having some experiences now, aren't we?' she said. How often they had longed to be in the thick of things, really put to the test.[32] Now that had come. They both knew that no scheme existed for exchanging prisoners of war; this was something else to which Kitchener was implacably opposed. Both women were without fear for themselves. But for their sorrow for the Serbs, they could even have felt a sense of pleasurable adventure.

Dr Inglis's party slept that night on the floor of their damaged hospital and moved into new quarters next day. Dr Corbett, taking them a new Red Cross flag from the main stores at the Czar Lazar Hospital, saw that each cottage had some pathetic white rag hanging from the windows and that bodies, victims of last evening's bombardment, lay by the road and in the fields.[33]

The arrival of the Germans that Sunday morning seemed, Dr Inglis said, almost an anti-climax. First, in the square, a handful of Germans appeared and the Serbian mayor read a proclamation telling the inhabitants not to resist. Then, turning a corner into the principal street, she came upon a German regiment drawn up, whose officers saluted her Red Cross badge and let her pass. The discipline and courtesy of the enemy was unexpected; soldiers stepped aside for the women and did not attempt to terrorise the Serbs. At the Czar Lazar Hospital she found German sentries posted, but they let her pass. And when it appeared that the first result of the Germans' arrival was that they had ordered all the hospital's latrines to be cleaned, it even seemed as though there might be something to be said for them.[34]

The following day, the Germans approached Dr Inglis to ask if she would nurse German wounded. Her hospital was now half empty, her staff underworked, and she was, after all, under Red Cross rules; she replied that she would. Over thirty German soldiers were sent to her.[35]

She had been naïve. The Germans now saw what a well-found place she had. Another order came next day: she must remove her Serb patients to the prefecture. She was not allowed to move any equipment, and they simply lay about on the floor until the following day, when she had to move them again, this time into the Czar Lazar Barrack Hospital.

Her colleagues had never seen her look so miserable.[36] 'The double move was quite unnecessary,' she protested. 'One might forgive the Austrians to a certain extent; but in the case of the Germans, with their wonderfully efficient organisation, such ill-treatment must have been deliberate.'[37] The following day she and her nurses were also ordered into the Czar Lazar and she had bitterly to recognise she had been edged out of her own hospital. She protested to the Serbian hospital director, Major Nicolitch. He looked at her strangely. 'But of course they took it,' he said. 'You had made it so beautiful.'[38]

Now both units of women worked at the Czar Lazar, which became an official prisoner-of-war hospital. Dr Inglis was in the main building, by November 11th overflowing with wounded Serbs taken in battles away to the south; and Dr Hollway's party was in the Magazine. The Magazine held three hundred patients, the hospital proper six hundred; often the total numbers in the two establishments rose to twelve hundred. The buildings had been designed to hold four hundred fit soldiers in fair comfort.[39]

The ruthlessness of war was something new to Elsie Inglis, as it was to almost all her fellow countrymen of her generation. The suffrage struggle had seemed, and been, bitter, but was waged against a background of stability, of premises accepted by both sides even when they hardly realised it themselves. With pain and suffering she had for years been familiar, but always they had seemed the result of blindness or ignorance; more education, more effort, and they could be overcome.

Now, a prisoner in a primitive country overrun by a powerful and ruthless enemy, she came, as did so many of those who faced the Great War, for the first time against the fact that the human condition is tragic and man not merely stupid but sometimes evil.

CHAPTER 14

Her earlier months in Serbia had been the fruition of Elsie Inglis's work in medicine. Now began months of imprisonment that tested her spirit.

'The Units left at Krushevatz', she wrote later, 'were the fortunate Units. To them fell the honour of caring for the Serbian wounded through the first three tragic months of the foreign occupation.' She found an exhilaration in working for the grateful, patient men and in helping Nicolitch, so loyal to his country, so conscientious and humane, to bring order from chaos. The unhappiness in the Serbian homes and the physical wretchedness all around, however, were a dead weight on her spirits.[1]

Besides the hundreds crowded into the hospital, from the second day of enemy occupation prisoners, sometimes three thousand in a day, passed through on their way to Hungary.

Each night the new arrivals were turned into the hospital compound to camp. No homely ladnjaks now sheltered them from the biting wind; within the first few days every scrap of wood, branches of trees, packing cases, bits of fencing, all were hacked down for camp fires whose lights flickered fitfully and whose acrid smoke drifted through the unmended windows of the wards.[2]

From the prisoners moving north, squads remained to repair roads and railways: among them Russians who could nightly be heard in the compound singing their traditional evening hymn.[3] From the prisoners, too, came the hospital's sanitary orderlies.

Because of the reputation of the S.W.H., Nicolitch almost at once arranged with Dr Inglis that she should be responsible for the sanitation. 'An Englishman's job all over the world,' she commented drily, 'and our three untrained English girl orderlies took to it like ducks to water. It was not the pleasantest or easiest work in the world; but they did it, and did it magnificently.'[4]

The compound was 'a truly terrible place—the sights and smells beyond description'. The Scottish Women and their squad of

Serbs now dug the rubbish into the ground, emptied the overflowing cesspools, built incinerators and cleaned and cleaned and cleaned. 'Miss Wardle especially developed wonderful powers of command,' wrote Dr Inglis later. 'Managed her men, fed them, clothed them, and left that hospital compound not, it is true, exactly like an English park, but at least clean.'[5]

Dr Inglis considered this as the Scottish Women's most important achievement while they were prisoners. At the same time they were caring for the seriously wounded men at the Czar Lazar. It was the only hospital for Serbs left in the town, and she was running more than half of it. She had to forget her prejudices about overcrowding. She had no choice.

Patients were put three men to two beds. Then there were no more beds; mattresses were placed on the floors, in the corridors, in the outhouses. The Magazine was a sight never to be forgotten. The ground floor had an uneven earth floor, with mattresses upon it; 'not', said Dr Inglis, 'the place one would choose to nurse surgical patients',[6] especially as the grounds were in such a state that everyone crossing them invariably got their feet wet and had to walk on the mud floor.

Upstairs the patients lay on the shelves which ran in three tiers the length of the building; the slightly wounded clambered up and down like monkeys, their incomprehensible chatter heightening the comparison and earning the place the nickname 'the Zoo' from the nurses.

The whole of November was bitterly cold throughout the Balkans. On the 17th the Scottish Women awoke to see two inches of snow, the first of the winter.[7] On the 26th occurred that freak blizzard which clinched the evacuation of Gallipoli. Even before the blizzard, Dr Inglis was worried, for the windows were still unmended and although the wards were tolerably warmed, the corridors and Magazine were so cold that even she saw it was impossible to take away the patients' clothes for stoving or laundering. That her own winter uniform had never arrived from Salonika was a detail compared with the sufferings of the patients. She appealed in vain for blankets; the Germans had confiscated hers and refused to release any.

Cold, overcrowding, fatigue and starvation made typhus a real risk. Dysentery had already broken out among the women. An appeal to the authorities for more premises met with blank refusals. She discussed the situation with Nicolitch and opened a small building at the far end of the grounds as a fever annexe.[8]

The next requirement was bathing arrangements for the patients. Mrs Haverfield, charged with this, could discover no corner for a bathroom, no cans for carrying water from the broken pump a hundred and fifty yards away, no wood to heat the water nor any vessel in which to put it. Under the little doctor, however, bricks must be made, and without straw if none existed. After waiting just one day, Dr Inglis took the matter into her own hands, enlisted a Miss Whitehead* and within hours had a bathroom corner in the Magazine, screened with sheets, with a disinfector machine adapted to heat water which Whitehead carried in buckets from the pump.

With hot water assured, the Scottish Women next took over the laundry. They worked round the hospital, bathing, disinfecting and supplying clean linen every five days. 'In this connexion we must always remember Sister Strange's name,' Dr Inglis wrote later, 'who took over this very necessary if uninteresting work from the point of view of a fully trained nurse, and carried it through triumphantly. We had not a single case of typhus.'[10] Since typhus was rampant in the occupying army, this was an achievement. But Dr Inglis had another she valued even more.

When wounded among the new prisoners were put into the wards there was an outcry from other patients: '*Doktoritza*, if you put these dirty men in among us, we shall all get typhus.' If she had done nothing else in her life, she decided, she had convinced the Balkan mind that dirt and typhus go together. This was more remarkable than it sounds today; the lice-borne nature of typhus was conclusively established only in 1911, and by 1915 there was still in ordinary speech no verbal distinction between typhus and typhoid, in Balkan countries, where indeed, typhus was still commonly presumed to be spread by inhalation.[11]

The food shortage was acute. For a month shops remained barricaded, but a flourishing back-door trade developed and those who had gold still in their money belts could supplement with occasional bits of chocolate, with milk and sometimes an egg, their own and their patients' rations of soup, beans and

* A Canadian of twenty-two who had volunteered for the Serbian Army and was using her leave to work with the Scottish Women when the Germans arrived. Cheerful, energetic, ready to tackle anything from cleaning lamps to chasing looters, she was a tower of strength. I have been unable to discover her later history.[9]

black bread twice a day.[12]

Hardest of all to bear was the isolation. The last letters from home had been three full weeks before the Germans' arrival. Now under the Germans rumour was rife: from Serbian sources came wild tales that the British had forced the Dardanelles, that Constantinople had fallen, that the Russians were at Nish and the English at Skoplje. That Kitchener had been made Viceroy of India and Lloyd George become Prime Minister they read in a German paper. Of truthful news there was none.[13]

On November 24th a curious episode occurred. Accounts vary in detail: Dr Inglis herself wrote of it in *Englishwoman* for June 1916, and a more detailed version exists in Mrs McLaren's handwriting, presumably as her sister told it to her.[14]

The Germans were preparing to leave Krushevatz. Having secured the railway, they were leaving occupation duties to Austria and Bulgaria. Before they went, a German Army doctor called and requested, almost casually, that Dr Inglis should sign a certificate to the good behaviour of the German Army. It was a simple thing, he assured her; a mere formality, to satisfy the officers.

This extraordinary good behaviour, with men getting off pavements and saluting the nurses, had puzzled her. It was so much at variance with what had happened in Belgium. Light had dawned a little when her Unit was ordered to leave their quarters in the girls' school and sent to a villa, part of which was already occupied by Germans; after argument, the women moved back to the school for one more night. Dr Inglis then noticed that the courtesy of the German soldier had not extended to helping the women carry back their heavy baggage. 'In unexpected situations', she had reflected, 'ordinary manners prevail.' The earlier politeness was clearly that of men under orders.

Now, asked to testify to the behaviour of the troops, she hesitated, asked for time to consider, discussed it with her colleagues; and decided to refuse.[15]

'The only absolutely true certificate that could have been given,' she declared, 'was one stating that the German Army had been so well in hand in Krushevatz that it could have been, and probably was, equally well in hand in Belgium and elsewhere.' She would not sign. If she did, 'a statement of the bare fact, taken from its setting that it was signed by a woman shut up in a small Serbian village and cut off from news of everything that was going on in the rest of Serbia—and the rest of the world—might give an absolutely false impression.'

She sent word of her decision. An angry message came back. The High Command was indignant. An order would be promulgated. The certificate must be signed. This vehemence strengthened her conviction that the question, despite the apparent innocence of its original presentation, was important.

What that importance might be, she did not know. But she replied, 'You may send what orders you please; but if I won't sign, I won't.' To angry German protests, which included threats to remove the whole party to Germany, she replied calmly that they could not have it both ways; could not say in one breath that it was of no importance, and with the next that the High Command proposed to issue an order. 'If it is a matter of no importance, I fail to understand why the High Command should know anything about the matter or why it should make them angry. But if it is an affair of sufficient importance to interest the High Command, I wish to know just why it is important, before I sign.'

Twice more she was asked to sign. The last time she was taken into a room full of German officers and given a chair opposite the Commanding Officer. He pushed a paper before her. 'I wish you to sign that.'

When she protested that she must first read it—and it was in German, in which she was far from fluent—he brusquely said, 'It is nothing; just to say you have been well treated and that you have nothing to complain of.'

Then, as she still demurred, 'I tell you to sign it. *I insist.*'

She continued to refuse. Finally the C.O. rose and leaned menacingly across the table. 'Sign at once. I will make you,' he threatened.

Dr Inglis looked at him. 'Make me,' she said.

Then she leaned back with folded hands, closed her eyes and awaited the event. What went on in her mind there is no knowing; but in speaking of it later to intimate friends she would say, 'Afraid? How could I be, with the whole weight of the British Empire behind me?' or 'It was a great day in my life when I discovered that I did not know what fear was.'[16]

The silence lengthened. Seconds, minutes, ticked by.

At last she opened her eyes. The Commanding Officer was looking at her intently. Not a word more was spoken. He signalled to an aide and she was conducted from the room, and allowed to return to her hospital.

Elsie Inglis had only her intuition to guide her, only her own unsupported courage to rely upon. She had been cut off from the world for weeks. She understood that at home there would be anxiety about her Units, but she could not know of any cause for special concern, or that her friend Mrs Laurie had just written to the S.W.H. office, 'I am feeling very anxious about developments in Serbia. After the terrible treatment of Miss Cavell at the hands of those dreadful Germans one feels alarmed for our brave women so far away.'[17]

The news of the shooting of Edith Cavell had burst upon Great Britain on October 22nd with a shock that swept her at once for all time into the ranks of national heroines. 'She has,' said Mr Asquith, 'taught the bravest man among us a supreme lesson in courage. Yes, and in this United Kingdom and throughout the Dominions of the Crown, there are thousands of such women, but a year ago we did not know it.'

The nation might be shocked at Edith Cavell's fate, but *Common Cause* was still capable of a tart rejoinder: 'The war in indeed teaching many things to many people. Is it too much to hope that it may be teaching the Prime Minister something of the value to the nation of the citizenship of women?'[18]

Germany had largely failed to realise the propaganda aspect of the Cavell case.* When they did they were quick with self-justification. The demand, four weeks later, that Dr Inglis testify to their consideration, was one result. Miss Cavell had, until her death, been almost unknown in Britain; Dr Inglis was widely known and respected, a national figure in the women's movement, one of Scotland's leading women doctors, and having friends in uncommitted America. As propaganda, a testimony from her might have gone far to offset Germany's maladroit handling of the Cavell affair.

Her intuition had been correct, her stand effective. Most of the Germans left Krushevatz, and no more was heard of the matter.

The women's isolation was indeed complete. Vrinjatcha Banja

* For an assessment of the similar methods—varying from blandishment to deception and intimidation—by which Edith Cavell in a similar isolated situation was induced to sign a document she did not understand, see *Edith Cavell, Pioneer and Patriot* by A. E. Clark Kennedy, pp. 158-62.

is only about fifty miles from Krushevatz, but Dr Inglis had all this time no word of Alice Hutchison and her staff of thirty-five there. They had in fact been taken prisoner on November 10th when the Germans took the town. Dr Hutchison was allowed to write home: they were all comfortable, she said, in no danger, and had not suffered hunger as she knew others must be doing. She had nothing to complain of. The thing they found hardest was the lack of letters and news. Alice Hutchison was still determinedly avoiding any risk of her Unit's being labelled as a heroic band of women.[19]

Of this Dr Inglis knew nothing. Nor had she any inkling of the fate of the women retreating with the Serbian Army. Clues were sometimes picked up from German bulletins. On November 24th a notice was posted that their armies were approaching Pristina near the head of the Ibar Valley. It was joyful news for Dr Inglis and her colleagues for they had believed the Germans already in Pristina long since, and now they could hope that their refugee sisters who had set off nineteen days earlier might have kept ahead of the enemy.[20]

In actual fact, the fleeing party had taken seven days to reach Pristina, something over one hundred miles, alternately riding and walking, stopping sometimes to have the bullocks shod, sleeping in the open or in tiny mountain huts. From Pristina they trekked on to Prisren close to the Albanian frontier, which when they arrived was the H.Q. of the Government and the army, full of foreign diplomats, medical missions, refugees.[21] A terrible decision had been taken. To save itself intact for the day when it could renew the fight, the army, the Government and all the manhood of Serbia was to cross the mountain passes to the Adriatic, taking with them all boys approaching military age. Serbia was to become a land of women, old men, children, and the enemy.

At Prisren, everyone was preparing for the journey and food had reached famine prices. Only after they had set out again did William Smith discover that the oxen were literally starving; he had been cheated by those paid to stable them in Prisren.[22]

While there, his party had met that of Dr MacGregor who had come by a slightly different route. But Dr MacGregor's party was one short. On November 10th a nurse, Caroline Toughill, had been driving a car in which were several others along a rough mountain track, when it overturned at a corner and bounced down the rocks. The others were only bruised, but Mrs Toughill died a day or two later. They buried her near Kossovska Mitrovitza, beneath a cairn of stones in a tiny village churchyard. Then they trekked on.[23]

On the day when the news of the German approach to Pristina gave Elsie Inglis the first inkling that they might have got clear away, the two parties were in fact struggling northwards again along the rough mountain track between Prisren and Petch. Ahead lay the towering peaks of Montenegro. They were part of an endless stream: foot soldiers, cavalry, boys, refugee women and children, the royal coaches each drawn by four oxen, Austrian prisoners, foreign missions. They crossed rushing rivers on precarious plank bridges. Sometimes they spent the night in tents or round a fire in the snow. The food of the British was scanty and some days they had none, but many of the Serbs were starving. The plight of the Austrian prisoners was worst of all.

Some sights had to be hurried past with averted eyes; the ponies which had slipped over the precipice because their overloaded packs pushed against the rocky walls, and which could be neither rescued nor shot; the oxen which had fallen from starvation and whose skins were quickly taken for footwear, their flesh for food, by those passing; the dying who had fallen out and whom nobody could help; the corpses which there had been no means of burying but which had sometimes been left with a coin, ill spared, on their mouths; the hand of a very small child emerging from a shroud of snow.[24]

Although the number can never be known, it has been estimated that one hundred thousand soldiers perished on the march, and half that number of civilians, mostly boys and prisoners of war. One hundred and fifty thousand soldiers survived. Many English, besides the members of Dr Inglis's Units, made the Great Retreat. One of them, Mrs Stobart, who administered a hospital for the Serbian Relief Fund, was the only commander to bring an entire party through without a casualty. Many of the women were no longer young: Dr Beatrice MacGregor, for example, had been R.M.O. to the Bruntsfield Hospital as long before as 1899.[25]

The bearing of the British women was beyond all praise, Dr Curcin wrote later. Equalling the soldiers in endurance they outdid them in morale, giving to others most of the little they had, putting their last wraps on exhausted soldiers, giving their last small money to Austrian prisoners. Among all the sorrows of the Great Retreat, the women had one overwhelming regret. They had not been of use to the army as they had hoped; and now they felt they had done wrong in leaving their patients. 'I shall never forgive myself for this, as long as I live,' one was overheard to mutter.[26]

So far as was known to those in the Retreat, or to Dr Inglis in her imprisonment, they were the only Scottish Women's Hospitals in Serbia. There was however one other Unit actually working on Serbian soil.

The Troyes party, which Dr Inglis had despatched just before leaving England herself, had been transferred by the French to the force they were sending to Salonika to help the Serbs. This Unit arrived in the extreme south of Serbia and set up its quarters in a disused factory, on the same day, November 7th, that Dr Inglis became a prisoner of war. For one month they remained doing good work before the Allied troops were forced to retreat to Salonika. Among these units were some British soldiers, part of a brigade of the 22nd Division which had been sent north, 'artillery without guns', and caught up in the Serbian retreat near Lake Doiran.[27] One officer, ill and exhausted so that he hardly hoped ever to reach Salonika, fell in with a straggling party of Scottish Women who nursed and helped him back. More than fifty years later he still remembered the pride he had felt in 'the splendid bearing and magnificent endurance of my feminine compatriots'.[28]

Truly these women had learned 'to be brave, and not whine over every little thing'.

CHAPTER 15

The last weeks of 1915 were for Elsie Inglis all gloom, isolation and sorrow; but a sorrow in her own words 'shot through with a strange happiness'.[1] She was sharing the sufferings of people she had grown to love.

If the Austrians of the new garrison were less well-organised, they were, equally, more bitter than Germans against the Serbs. 'Yes, they do die by the roadside like that. So do our men,' said one when charged by a nurse with inhumanity to his work squad of prisoners.[2] The food shortage intensified and the struggle was never-ending to get the routine work done in the face of the apathy of malnutrition.

Dr Inglis came upon a sanitary squad digging rubbish into the ground. She watched, scornful of their lethargy. Then—officers and men again—she seized a spade and began to dig.

When she handed the spade back she said, 'Even the *gospoditza* can dig better than you.'

'The *gospoditza* has more bread,' came the reply. It was true. What could she say?

She remonstrated with the man who carted away sewage. Three journeys a day were insufficient. He *must* make more. '*Doktoritza,* it is impossible. My oxen are unable to do more. They are not fit.'

She looked at the beasts. Their bones were sticking through their hides. 'Why don't you feed them better?' she asked.

'*Doktoritza,* I have no money. Before the Austrians came I got five dinars* for every pool I emptied. But now I must go where I am sent and I am paid nothing. My family are living on the little money we had saved. When the oxen die I don't know what we shall do.'

They were speaking Serbian and Elsie did not trust herself; she believed she must have misunderstood, and checked with the

* Ten dinars was the daily wage of a master carpenter, three or four that of his assistants. It would seem, therefore, that to clear one pit was approximately a day's work.[3]

interpreter. It was true; the man was getting only receipts for his work. She pestered the authorities, unsuccessfully. From then on, she paid him out of her own funds for his work at the hospital; it was the only money he received.[4]

She scoured the countryside, with Mrs Haverfield and a few others, for food for the patients. They had to do it secretly after Nicolitch brought in a quantity of eggs only to have them seized by the sentries. The women had passes to move freely during the day. Their foraging was combined with treating civilian sick, Mrs Haverfield in particular maintaining an aristocratic disregard of the six o'clock curfew if she could help anyone in pain or short of food. Outlying farms had hidden stores, so that they could sometimes get a few eggs, a little milk, or some onions to eke out the official rations.[5]

The prisoners and sanitary workers were on the same meagre rations as the nurses: beans, a little dubious meat, half a loaf of black bread a day. The women supplemented their own *sanitärs'* meals out of their stores, they gave away some of their own rations, but they could not feed the entire enclosure of hungry men.

On the day of the first snow, Dr Corbett noted in her diary that the prisoners had stood crowded in the sleet all night and had no bread. The afternoon before, a mass of prisoners was seen hacking at one another with sticks, to get at a bag of crusts one had found.[6] The Serb orderlies were discovered to have organised a black market in bread. When caught by Dr Inglis or Mrs Haverfield they were forced to give the food away, but the black market persisted. Clearing a drain under supervision, some orderlies found a few beans someone had thrown away. In a moment they were a struggling mass trying to seize them.[7] Crusts found on the ground were seized and eaten, covered in grime as they were.

The readiness of some peasants to profit from their fellow countrymen's need was disillusioning, but Dr Inglis stoutly declared it was explicable in terms of the situation in the country. When the stored food on farms was gone there would be nothing. There was no seed, all animals and poultry had been requisitioned, and only women and old men remained to cultivate the farms.

Something of these conditions was known to the world. Herbert Hoover tried as a neutral to get permission for a visit of enquiry, without success. In London, Seton Watson was urging the government to apply the same principle as for Belgium and send food; but was told that ensuring supplies was the duty of the occupying power.[8]

On November 30th, Dr Inglis was allowed to write to her committee. Her letter was weary, strained and formal. She sent lists of those who were with her, adding, 'I am sure the Committee would approve of our work here. We have charge of the Magazine where the overflow patients from the Hospital are taken ... We are working in the dressing rooms and certain wards in the Hospital—and the Director has put all the sanitation and laundry work in our hands. We live in the Hospital. There are two rooms given to us. On the whole we have been extraordinarily well ... the Committee must not worry about us. We are well and very busy and doing the work they sent us out to do.'[9]

Elsie herself, in fact, was far from well. The illness from which she had suffered two years before was again showing itself. Overcrowding, privation, sickness of heart, all took their toll.

On December 1st there was an encounter which cheered her. Dr Hutchison's Unit had been moved to Krushevatz and in the town came face to face with Dr Inglis, whom they had no idea was still there.[10]

'If', Alice Hutchison wrote later, 'I had up till then felt that we in no way merited the title of "the heroic band of women" I came away from Dr Inglis's Hospital feeling that they *had* earned it. Picture over twenty people—including the head of the hospital—dining and sleeping and eating and washing in one room; picture all their equipment gone and them looking after Serbs in the best way they could in hospital corridors. They were, however, wearing no air of martyrdom.'[11]

Dr Inglis would have welcomed her friend's help; but four days later Dr Hutchison was ordered on to Kevavara in Hungary[12] where she and her companions were to be kept closely guarded for three months before being repatriated in mid-February.

The standards of behaviour of the women at Krushevatz were under constant strain. Attempts to persuade them to 'go out with' German soldiers or to work in what Dr Corbett modestly termed 'a hospital for the encouragement of vice'[13] were easy to resist; the pressure from within, harder. Constant petty illnesses troubled them: a poisoned thumb, a bad foot, influenza, dysentery; to keep at work was a struggle, to refuse tiny luxuries, a drink of milk, an hour in bed, became a painful point of honour. Off duty they filled their time with walks and visits to Serbian families. They had all cut their skirts several inches above the ankle, shorter than they would have thought modest a few months previously, but the mud was awful. Not all had good rubber boots, for the equipment department in Edinburgh never really grasped the facts of Eastern European mud, and wet feet all day and every day were the rule.[14]

Around them, misery increased. Old men could die of exposure and exhaustion in the yard, ignored by all but the women. Mrs Haverfield came one day upon a half-witted young girl, horribly dirty and naked but for a blanket, shivering and weeping in an outhouse. Mrs Haverfield cleaned, fed and clothed her but could find nobody in the town to be responsible for her except the matron of the hospital for the encouragement of vice.[15]

As Christmas approached, the weather became milder; on some days the patients could even sit out of doors. Was the country really so beautiful, Elsie again asked herself; or was it the contrast with all the misery that made it so evident? She knew she would never forget the clear days, the beauty of the sunrise and sunset, the brilliance of the stars—any more than she would forget the overcrowded 'Zoo', or the nights when she had to thrust her sleepless head under her blanket to shut out the groans and coughing of the men in the yard or the noise of their tramping up and down all night to keep warm.[16]

Outwardly, she kept up her courage. 'Dr Inglis cured not only the physical but the moral ills of her wounded patients,' wrote one of them, Lieutenant-Colonel Popovitch (later professor at the Military Academy, Belgrade). 'Every word she spoke was about the return of our army, and she assured us of final victory. She did not speak thus merely to soothe, for one felt the fire of her indignation against the oppressor and her love for us and her confidence that our just cause would triumph.'[17]

Few, in the face of this determined confidence, ventured to express any doubts. Once, she delighted a whole ward. A German officer had taunted her. 'Serbia is wiped out; we have finished France and Russia; and now we are going to do for England too.'

The taunt anyway fell somewhat flat, for Elsie, like so many imperfect linguists, grasped everything but the one vital word; she had no idea what *zerstören* meant. Something unpleasant, probably, if it was to be the fate of England. She decided to chance it. '*Aber veilleicht,*' she began in her careful schoolgirl German, '*werden wir Deutschland zerstören.*' The delight on the face of every patient told her the shaft had gone home, even before she saw bewilderment spread over the face of the officer. Then she crept away to her dictionary to look up *zerstören.*[18]

Inwardly, however, she was deeply hurt at what she felt as England's defection. When a Serbian woman said, 'We did not expect anything of Russia for she has always made a pet of Bulgaria, but we never thought England would fail us,' it was Elsie's turn to look bewildered and have no ready answer.

Things happened which the women did not fully understand. On Christmas Eve,* without warning, soldiers visited each house in Krushevatz; the old men, boys, invalids and the few black-coated workers were rounded up. They stood about all day in the hospital compound, their weeping womenfolk coming to the fence with bits of food and extra clothing, holding children up to say goodbye. At night, they were still in the yard. As many as possible were brought in and packed on the corridor floors; miserable discomfort, but better than the cold outside. After dark, the women heard under their windows a party of their Serbian friends, defying the curfew to sing carols; the accompaniment was a background of shots as eight prisoners were killed trying to escape. On Christmas morning early, as Dr Corbett walked to the little fever hospital, she saw the civilians being marched away, a long, close-packed, black line down the road.[19]

The women exchanged tiny gifts, hairpins, pen-nibs, bits of soap. They drank to Serbia and their absent friends, sang carols, speculated where they would be next Christmas, and searched their consciences as to whether their pathetic little celebration was wrong in this land of grief.[20]

Elsie Inglis might have drawn comfort, had she known, from the news of her other Units. On December 23rd, the forty-six who had set out on the Great Retreat seven weeks earlier, arrived at Southampton, carrying each her bundle of blankets, her water bottle and a bread-bag that had once been white. All else had been given away or stolen.[21]

On Christmas Day, too, the first remnants of the Serbian Army which had escaped via Salonika landed in Corsica; and a Scottish

* December 24. The Orthodox Christmas came later.

Women's Hospital Unit was with them to nurse back to health men and boys broken by war and privation.[22] In Salonika also, where thousands of Allied troops were now virtually penned up, the S.W.H. Troyes Unit with the French had established a tented hospital, which till the end of the war they ran for the Serbian and Allied armies.[23]

December 26th was sunny. Elsie had an hour or two to spare and took her paintbox out. 'There is nothing nicer than having sketches of places you have been at at various times' her father had written when she was a girl in Paris. Could he ever have imagined the circumstances in which his favourite child now found herself? Although no sketches have survived, the little paintbox was among the few things she kept with her always; it is to be seen, its paint-pans deeply dug into, in the Imperial War Museum along with her uniform with its faded medal ribbons, her stethoscope, watch, pen, hypodermic, pharmacopeia, and book of prayers, and one small dilapidated handbag to carry the lot.

By now, repatriation was spoken of. The women were offered it, and on December 28th twenty of them departed by lorry.[24] Although many patients had been evacuated, newcomers still arrived and by mid-January the hospital still had its optimum four hundred. There was however an air of unrest. Without supervision the orderlies lazed; to get windows cleaned or an incinerator lit might involve an hour's argument. The two women who had run the laundry had gone home on December 28th and Dr Inglis and Mrs Haverfield were forced to take it over themselves 'with the energy of 20 horse power apiece', as Dr Corbett said.[25]

Dr Inglis, Mrs Haverfield, Dr Corbett and a few others hoped to remain as long as possible; they now believed the Allies might come in the spring, and wanted to be ready. They buoyed themselves up with every possible argument, rational or superstitious; even the wearing or hoarding of one's last clean collar became something that might bring, or delay, the day of deliverance. On January 23rd they scanned the flags put up to celebrate the German victory in Montenegro (which gave the Central Powers domination over all the Balkans) and deduced correctly that neither Greece nor Roumania had yet joined the Central Powers. After this, however, Elsie gave up hope of the Allies' arrival. She still refused to believe that Serbia had been uselessly sacrificed; she preferred to think that it must all be part of some deep scheme for weakening Germany on other fronts.[26] She decided now to accept repatriation if offered and to try to return to Serbia via the south with another Unit.

On February 7th the women learned unofficially that the whole hospital, staff and patients, was to be transferred to Belgrade; and Elsie was approached by Mrs Haverfield who revealed that with Vera Holme and Dr Corbett, she had formed a private plan to go to ground in a peasant cottage, concealed by local people, ready to emerge when the Allies came. It was hardly a scheme which a head of a hospital could officially approve. But half amused, half almost envious, Elsie promised them stores to remove to their hide-out in the village of Bivolj.[27]

In the next two days, the hospital was emptied of its last inmates: the chronically wounded put on commission and sent home, the sufficiently fit removed to Hungary. About one hundred remained who could not recover for months, when Dr Inglis was formally notified she was to leave.

With Mrs Haverfield, who spoke fluent German, she hurried to the Austrian H.Q. They were received by a young A.D.C. who confirmed the order.

'What then is to happen to our patients?' Elsie asked.

'That is no business of yours.'

The women were aghast, and suggested that having attended the men for many weeks, they had a right to be concerned. Their protests were brushed aside. 'It is not your affair; you must leave it to us,' the A.D.C. said brusquely. 'After all, we are not barbarians,' he muttered defensively.[28] The women had to leave, but their protest had registered. Although some patients made the arduous journey to Belgrade, the worst cases were sent over to the Austrian hospital in Krushevatz.

When they had gone and the staff were packing, Mrs Haverfield and her two companions slipped away to their hide-out. They had to remain in concealment several days, for the Unit was unexpectedly ordered to remain where it was. When the final move was again ordered, on February 11th, Dr Inglis sent a message to the three in hiding; probably she guessed that their absence had been noticed. But her message was misunderstood; when the Unit's departure hour had passed, the three in hiding began to feel safe, and went to sleep.[29]

Late that night they were awakened by loud knocking. Dr Inglis with two Austrian guards was outside. 'You have to come at once,' she cried to them angrily. 'I am here with an armed guard. There is no time to waste. Bring only what you can carry.'

They were all used to Dr Inglis's wrath and none would willingly have drawn it on herself. But what had gone wrong?

'Are you,' one of them ventured to ask, 'really cross? Or are you pretending because the guard understands English?' Dr Inglis smiled strangely. 'I was not putting it on,' she said quietly with an odd glance. Most probably, she had some reason to fear reprisals on the villagers of Bivolj. In this little village of a single street where the stucco houses were all confusingly alike she had, she told them, broken the window of another cottage in a mistaken effort to attract their attention. The way to the station was enlivened with some rather forced chaff from Mrs Haverfield on the subject of militant suffragette tactics. If they had not laughed, they might all have wept to leave Krushevatz.[30]

By two o'clock next afternoon, after an uncomfortable journey under an Austrian guard with fixed bayonets, in two open cattle trucks and a third-class carriage, and with no food but tea, bread and biscuits, they reached Belgrade, and waited in the station the rest of the day. Late that night Dr Inglis got the chance of buying everyone a small plate of meat and potatoes before dossing down on the floor of the waiting-room, the eight guards and their charges all together.[31]

After Dr Inglis was in her sleeping bag, she was aroused by the Austrian officer, who himself guarded the door all night. Word of the Unit's presence had spread in Belgrade; a Serbian woman was asking after her husband, one of their patients at Krushevatz. If they would use German, so that the officer might understand, they could speak together.

Elsie reassured the woman. Her husband would recover; he had been moved to the Austrian hospital in the town. The wife grasped the little doctor's hands. '*Vrlo dobro?*' (truly well?) she asked. Elsie glanced apprehensively at the officer, then '*Vrlo, vrlo dobro*', she said, smiling. When she glanced again, the officer was smiling too. His Serbian was like her own, just equal to that simple statement, she decided. She was deserting Serbia; but at least, she consoled herself, the last Serbian she spoke to was left a little happier.[32]

Next day they reached Vienna. The American Minister in Berlin, representing British interests, had arranged their repatriation. They were kept a few days for security reasons, then sent to Zurich. It was a shock there to emerge from their four months' isolation and learn, in a long briefing from Sir Cecil Hertslet, the British Consul General, the true state of the war; that the Western Front was static, an army immobilised in Salonika, the Dardanelles given up; that so little help had reached the Serbs. 'Our hearts were sick,' said Dr Inglis, 'for the people we had left behind us, still waiting and trusting.'[33]

She arrived home in England on February 29th. To her friends, she was much changed. Hardship had left its mark; she was thin, pale and hollow-eyed.

The perceptive saw something else: a look on her face, said Lady Frances Balfour, as of one whose spirit had been pierced by a sword.[34] And Mrs McLaren believed that, in sharing the tragedy of Serbia, her sister's heart had broken.[35]

CHAPTER 16

Only Dr Inglis's closest friends realised what she had suffered. What she regarded as England's defection* had struck even deeper than the tragedy of Serbia.

'Patriot' was to be the last word chosen for her epitaph by those who knew her best. It was no facile, flag-waving, my-country-right-or-wrong patriotism. She had been bred in the tradition of trusteeship, the belief that 'our highly-favoured England' must not fail the stringent obligations of that position. Now she had to accept that England had failed those who depended upon her. If it broke her heart it also imposed what she conceived as a personal responsibility to make amends.[1]

The characteristic of heroism, says Emerson, is its persistency; all men have wandering impulses, fits and starts of generosity. Elsie Inglis was cast in the heroic mould. Having chosen her part she abided by it to 'the last defiance of falsehood and wrong and the power to bear all that can be inflicted by evil agents'.[2]

Most of the repatriated women took a holiday. Mrs Haverfield took six weeks, bringing her nicely to the end of the hunting season. Dr Inglis took no rest. Even on the way home, she attended a Paris conference on aid to Serbia. Her voice was heard with respect in such gatherings and the S.W.H. had more than once set the standard for larger organisations.[3]

She was full of plans for a Unit with the British forces in Mesopotamia, for another Unit commanded by herself on the Salonika front, where the Serbs were expected to take the field later in the year. She wanted also to increase the British people's understanding and sympathy with Serbia, and this at least could be attempted without delay.

In March, with Alice Hutchison, she addressed a large meeting in Glasgow. The *Bulletin* wrote of a 'bright-faced little woman in a grey uniform who spoke modestly, almost shyly, of her work

* Serbia had of course been guaranteed by Russia and France, and not by England, who had become involved in the war through her guarantee of Belgium.

among the Serbians and referred to the risks she had run as if they were everyday and commonplace'.[4]

The return of the 'Scottish heroines' stimulated the flow of funds. By April there was £104,000 in hand; an X-ray car was given by the Cavell Memorial Fund, being the first to be made in Scotland.[5]

On April 3rd, Elsie was guest of honour at a reception given by Lady Cowdray at which Crown Prince Alexander and Pashitch, the Serbian Prime Minister, in London for diplomatic conversations, were present.[6] Although the Prince had been her neighbour at Kragujevatz, although their electricity had come from a single inadequate source so that when the hospital X-ray was working overtime the Prince's headquarters might have no light,[7] this was their first meeting. Alexander had spent much time travelling and organising, and had also been ill during the summer.[8]

He now decorated Elsie with the Order of the White Eagle, the highest honour his country could bestow. 'The Serbian nation,' he said, 'will never forget what these women did.'[9]

Next day she addressed a large meeting at the Criterion Theatre. She had some bitter things to say: how Serbians had remarked, 'Now England has her teeth in and she'll never let go,' to which she had replied, 'No, they'll never let go'—'and I wish I could have added "they'll never muddle".' How another Serb had said, 'We are fighting for our liberty. I wonder what Great Britain is fighting for. I think it must be for sport.'[10]

For once, her personal reticence was broken. Curcin contributed a paper on her work, and Elsie could not evade personal applause. 'If I have been able to do anything,' she said quietly, 'whatever I am, whatever I have done, I owe it to my father.'

Four days later she went to Austen Chamberlain, Secretary of State for India and a member of the War Council, with a proposal that her organisation, having now thoroughly proved themselves, should supply and maintain a fully equipped and staffed hospital for two hundred in Mesopotamia.[11]

The Mesopotamian theatre was the responsibility of the Indian Government. Only guarded reports had appeared of medical conditions there; but Elsie had learned from private sources how badly the troops were served. So appalling was the situation, that when the official report was published in June 1917, public indignation was to sweep Austen Chamberlain out of office.[12]

One writer to *The Times* called the medical breakdown 'the greatest scandal that has occurred in our Empire for at least half a century'. The Mesopotamian Report of June 1917 declared that in the medical sphere it was 'impossible to refrain from serious censure of the Indian Government for the inadequacy of the preparations'. Standards of care of the wounded were such as Miss Nightingale had found in the Crimea and Elsie herself in Serbia, with men badly wounded and unable to move left in their clothes and with no attention whatever for as long as ten days. It was by no means unusual for ten times as many men to be laid low by sickness as there were battle casualties.[13] Numbers of the medical corps itself were invalided. So slack too were ordinary health precautions that General Maude was actually to die from cholera in the same house in which his German opponent, von der Goltz, had died from the same disease shortly before.

But of all this, little was suspected by the general public in 1916 when Dr Inglis made her proposal to Chamberlain.

Although Mesopotamia was the responsibility of the Indian Government, Indian resources, owing to an earlier economy wave, were inadequate for full-scale war. The War Office was supposed to supply additional needs, but liaison was almost nonexistent. Not only were the young army doctors sent out, totally inexperienced in such diseases as cholera but, as we have seen, often those who trained them had never seen a case either.[14] It was a situation in which women like Alice Hutchison, with experience both of tropical diseases and war casualties, could have saved lives.

Chamberlain received Dr Inglis kindly. He was noncommittal, but passed her on to a Captain Padham at the War Office. In view of the official strictures later passed upon the Indian Government and the virtual exoneration of the War Office,[15] Dr Inglis's experiences are decidedly revealing.[16] Medical care in the field was not the only thing to have remained unchanged since Miss Nightingale's day. The War Office, too, had not changed its spots.

Padham was as cordial as Chamberlain, and outlined the arrangements between India and the War Office. He was in charge of a department which received requests from the Indian Government; it was his business to supply them. He thought he would be going beyond his duty actually to *offer* anything. Even this he declared himself willing to do if General Russell, in charge of medical arrangements at the War Office, approved.

He took her to the General, who agreed that should the Indian Government ask for a women's hospital, he would certainly send it. But duty was duty, and he would be exceeding his duty to offer one.

Dr Inglis swallowed her disappointment. The difficulty must be worked away. 'Then I understand,' she said as she left, 'that the offer of the hospital must be made to the Viceroy.'

An official telegram was at once sent to the Viceroy: 'Scottish Women's Hospitals offer unit of 200 beds for Mesopotamia. Fully staffed and equipped. All expenses paid. Please apply General Russell, War Office.'

The Viceroy was Lord Chelmsford. He had taken over a few days earlier[17] from Lord Hardinge, who was, with somewhat suspicious promptitude, rewarded with the Garter for his own work for India's war effort. To Lord Chelmsford, Lady Cowdray, who knew him personally, also telegraphed privately, offering the hospital.

No reply had been received when, about the middle of April, Dr Inglis departed for Corsica to inspect work by the S.W.H. for Serbian refugees there. She returned on May 1st to learn that during her absence Pashitch, the Serbian Prime Minister, had asked for a further hospital for his soldiers. She wanted to comply, but the Tommies dying in Mesopotamia, and unnecessarily, had first claim. 'I cannot bear to think of them, *our boys*,' she said to Mrs McLaren. Moreover, Lady Cowdray had had a telegram from the Viceroy: 'Government of India much appreciate offer of Scottish Women's Hospital for Mesopotamia, but offer should be referred to C.I.G.S. War Office.'

Dr Inglis hurried to Captain Padham. He was still kind, still doubtful. The telegram, he felt, was not a request, but was carefully worded to shift responsibility for refusal on to the War Office.

Again he took her to General Russell. Again she met a stonewall politeness. The telegram was *not* a request. That was the General's view. He had nothing more to say.

She hastened to Lady Cowdray, who again telegraphed the Viceroy: 'After making inquiries find it necessary Indian Government should apply for Scottish Women's Hospital to Imperial General Staff War Office. Will you do this and cable me at same time.'

Two days later, on May 3rd, Lady Cowdray received a letter

from a legal member of the Viceroy's Council, written on April 13th, over two weeks before Dr Inglis's second interview with Padham and Russell. 'I duly received your cable [it read] about the Scottish Women's Hospital for Mesopotamia and sent it on at once to the Army H.Q. Medical Branch and I hear from the Chief of Medical Services that the offer has been gladly accepted, that they have wired to the C.I.G.S. at home stating the offer, their intended acceptance of it, and asking for particulars of the accommodation the hospital will provide. He has also wired the G.O.C. in Mesopotamia informing him of the offer and of the action he has taken. This will, I hope, be quite satisfactory. The offer is a splendid one and will, I am sure, be of the greatest service to the Army in Mesopotamia.'

This was Dr Inglis's first intimation that an actual request had indeed been made by the Indian authorities. It was puzzling? Why had not Russell mentioned it to her?

Two days later came the Viceroy's reply to Lady Cowdray's second telegram: 'Application for Scottish Women's Hospital was made to C.I.G.S. and following reply was received, begins, Can send you all the hospitals you may require you should not accept others as long as we can supply.'

The weekend intervened before Dr Inglis could renew her attack. On Monday morning, May 8th, she was at the War Office again armed with the Viceroy's communications. Padham was courteous as ever. The Indian Government's request ought, he told her, to have come to him. Yet this was the first he had heard of it. Strange! However, perhaps no real harm had been done; he thought that by now the Indian Government had anyway all the hospitals they needed. Again he passed her on to General Russell.

Russell, cornered, admitted that yes, the Indian Government *had* asked for a Scottish Women's Hospital, and that yes, the War Office *had* sent the telegram of which Dr Inglis had a copy. No, he could give no reason for the War Office's side-tracking of the Viceroy's request; except that as long as the War Office had hospitals of their own, they should use them.

Dr Inglis was more angry than she had ever been in her life, but controlled herself to speak calmly. It was, she declared, time to raise the whole question of the War Office's refusal of services which medical women could give the country. Inexperienced young men, she pointed out, were being sent out, while women who were widely experienced, first-rate surgeons, and had proved powers of organisation, were refused the chance to serve. The question would also have to be raised, as to why the Scottish Women's Hospitals, which had proved themselves efficient, well-organised, well-equipped and well-staffed and would cost the tax-payer nothing, were refused for service with the British Army when they were gladly accepted by Britain's allies.

The General listened; and, perhaps, congratulated himself that this tiresome, aggressive little person had missed the real point. She had enough evidence, had she realised it, to have blown the gaff, a year before public opinion called for the Mesopotamian Report, on the total failure of the War Office to support the Mesopotamian campaign. She had concentrated instead on the politically inexplosive subject of women doctors. Now, with luck, awkward questions might yet be averted. When she had finished, he coldly suggested that she put the whole case in writing and send it to the Secretary of the War Office.

And the Secretary of the War Office was, of course, Lord Kitchener. If 'K.' looked coldly upon women, he looked even more coldly upon Mesopotamia, as *The Times* commented later that summer.[18]

Was Kitchener the whole explanation of the attitude of his department? Or was the War Office determined, now that the Nightingale had at long last died, never again to have such a woman round its neck? Or was there another explanation?

At that very moment, an obscure writer in a Wiltshire cottage was preparing a new study of Miss Nightingale. 'She moved naturally among Peers and Cabinet Ministers—she was one of their own set ... What kind of attention would such persons have paid to some middle-class woman with whom they were not acquainted, who possessed great experience of Army nursing ... ?' Lytton Strachey was asking himself and two years later was to ask his readers. The question is pertinent.

Her friend Lady Cowdray might be on telegraphing terms with the Viceroy, her other friend Lady Frances Balfour in the habit of lunching at Downing Street, but essentially Elsie Maud Inglis, possessing the fire, the drive, the organising ability, the vision of a Nightingale, and with even greater practical experience and personal courage, was at one remove from real power.

It was a gap that was unbridgeable.

There remained Britain's allies. At Royaumont the steady, valuable work continued. At Salonika the Unit under Dr (later Dame) Louise McIlroy was caring for hundreds of French, and there, too, Miss Edith Stoney the physicist was repairing the X-ray installation aboard British hospital ships whose own staff had insufficient knowledge to do so, and was operating the only X-ray equipment in Salonika itself.[19]

A Scottish Women's transport column was being prepared for work with the re-formed Serbian Army, the first organised motor transport this army had ever had; and a tented hospital was being assembled for them, commanded by Dr Agnes Bennett, an Australian who had been among the first students at Dr Inglis's Medical College for Women years before; it too was the only hospital the Serbian Army had of its own.[20]

All this cost money. Meetings were planned, appeals made; Miss Burke made a transatlantic trip, and Mrs Abbott was packed off on a speaking tour of India with hardly more ceremony than she had once been despatched to speak at her first suffrage meeting.[21] The office was at full stretch, but Dr Inglis's energies still overflowed. She conceived a further idea, a Kossovo Day Campaign, celebrating the Serbian national festival and educating English public opinion about their neglected ally. By May 18th she was hard at work with Curcin and Mrs Haverfield as her lieutenants. Hundreds of pamphlets, mostly historical, went to schools, scores of lectures were arranged, exhibitions planned. The press was roped in—G. K. Chesterton wrote in the *Daily News*, Sir Arthur Evans, the discoverer of Knossos, in *The Times*, Henry Nevinson in *The Nation*. Society hostesses held meetings and twelve thousand schools gave special lessons.

Large sums were raised, but money was not the first objective. She wanted British understanding, British prayers, for Serbia. The Church of England announced July 2nd as Serbian Sunday, and on July 7th the Archbishop of Canterbury addressed a special service at St Paul's.[22]

The question has been raised, and should be answered, how far was all this, and Dr Inglis's role in it, politically motivated?

Much political activity over Serbia was taking place in the summer of 1916, with Alexander and Pashitch working for a pan-Slav alliance with Serbia dominant, while an émigré body, the

Yugo-Slav Committee, lobbied for a federal state in which Croats, Slovenes and Serbs would all be equal. It has been suggested that the Serbian Relief Fund's work and the Kossovo Day Campaign, ostensibly non-political, were actually politically motivated.

There is certainly no evidence that Elsie Inglis had any political aim in view.* She alone was the driving force of the Kossovo commemoration; the following year when she was elsewhere, it was marked by one single public lecture. Certainly Seton Watson and Dr Curcin both believed Dr Inglis to be a convert to the idea of South Slav federation which they themselves supported. Seton Watson even convinced himself that this insular British woman was somehow or other a 'true European'.[23] It is hardly a viewpoint which finds confirmation in her reported speeches or is borne out by her writings and I have been assured by the late Sir Frederick Whyte who was closely associated with the Serbian Relief Fund that 'her interest was Serbian relief, *not* politics'.[24]

'These poor little people, our highly-favoured England *must* help them' was her attitude; and she certainly had the island race's usual difficulty in distinguishing between the various branches of the Yugo-Slav nation; they were all 'Serbs', just as all branches of the Orthodox Church were Greek to her. One political aim she did pursue, inexorably, inflexibly: to prove women worthy of the vote.

In July, Pashitch made another request. Two Serbian Divisions were being recruited in the south of Russia from Austrian Slavs who had deserted to the Allies. The Serb Army in Corfu was supplying officers: Jivkovitch, whom she already knew, had started for Odessa as early as March. Could the Scottish Women's Hospitals supply medical services?

The financial problem at least solved itself. The London Committee announced it would pay for two field hospitals of one hundred beds, a transport section, and a staff of seventy-five. Although the source was not revealed, it is probable that Lady Cowdray, the Committee's treasurer, personally paid for it. She was an enthusiast for romantic royalist Serbia as well as for Elsie Inglis: and though she openly subscribed large sums for good causes, she could and did subscribe nearly ten times as much to the same causes anonymously.[25]

Now recruiting for the Unit to Russia went ahead. Thousands

* Nor in my own reading of the files of the Serbian Relief Fund have I come across any such evidence about that body.

of women had been absorbed into war work but there was still a plentiful supply of adventurous souls.

The daughter of a Royal Mail steamship commodore, turned down because she did not look strong, re-applied each week until she was accepted. A driver for the Metropolitan Missions, lunching at a women's club, overheard Mrs Haverfield at the next table say 'I must have drivers to work with the Serbs'; Miss Hedges was with difficulty persuaded to finish her coffee before volunteering. The granddaughter of Dr Inglis's friends Sir William and Lady Muir begged to go—and was taken to tea at the Admiralty by her mother, who requested Lord Jellicoe's personal assurance that Russia would be perfectly safe. What he said is not on record, but Miss Arbuthnot eventually got her way.[26]

Another volunteer at this time—she was however sent to Royaumont—was a certain Alina Dolling,* a young Canadian musician whose husband had been killed in Flanders and who like many others was gallantly trying to fill her empty life. In 1935 she was to achieve a special type of notoriety when she was tried at the Old Bailey and, acquitted of murdering her third husband, tragically and spectacularly committed suicide. She is better known to criminologists as Mrs Rattenbury.

Several of Elsie Inglis's associates in Serbia volunteered again —Dr Chesney and Dr Laird who had been through the Great Retreat; Dr Corbett, Mrs Haverfield, Miss Holme; and Dr Lena Potter who had worked with Serbs in Corfu. They had all lost their hearts to Serbia. Mrs Haverfield, indeed, gave an interview to the *Lady's Pictorial* in which she was sufficiently carried away to say that Serbs would concede voting powers to women without demur because 'a man like the typical Serb, who loves the birds and the beasts and flowers—a man of the stamp of St Francis of Assisi—understands the woman question, not because he has studied it, but because the simplicity of his nature and his disposition makes all clear to him'.[27]

At last the party was ready. Dr Inglis had under her four doctors, an administrator, a radiographer, a dispenser, seventeen nurses, sixteen orderlies, several cooks and laundresses mostly from the staffs of domestic colleges. 'Healthy wholesome bricks of girls' was her verdict on them, and 'very nice and capable, though there are one or two queer characters!'[28]

* More often given as 'Alma Dolly' but the name is 'Alina Dolling' in the normally meticulous records of the S.W.H.

Mrs Haverfield, in command of the transport, had eight ambulances, two kitchen cars, one repair car, four lorries and three touring cars with a staff of chauffeurs and cooks. There were fifty tons of equipment.

The preparations had occupied July and August. Dr Inglis found time, however, to attend on July 10th a meeting at Seton Watson's house at which the Serbian Society was formed to work for a Yugo-Slav state, a political aim indeed. Her involvement, however, was nominal; more than six weeks before the inaugural meeting she had left London never to return, and when *The Times* on September 28th listed the executive, hers was not among the names.

She also found time for old friends, including some with whom she did not now see eye to eye. The Pethick-Lawrences had often stayed at 8 Walker Street during the suffrage campaign. But now they were pacifists, fighting a by-election on this issue, and Mrs Pethick-Lawrence was passing through Edinburgh to speak at Dundee. It was a time when anyone who dared to breathe the word 'peace' was denounced as a traitor, at least by those who had never been anywhere near the front; a time, said Emmeline Pethick-Lawrence, 'when one's nearest and dearest failed to understand. But *she* understood. And she broke into a busy morning's work to come down to the train to shake my hand. What we said was very little; but the look and the handclasp were sufficient. We knew ourselves to be serving the same God of Love and Mercy, and that knowledge made the bonds between us indissoluble.'[29]

There was time, also, for a short reunion late in August with her family, at Leven on the coast of Fife; for games with the younger ones, for walks and comfortable talks with the elders. They were deeply concerned about her. Her health had failed to improve. In fact it was now known to her, and to Mrs Simson and Mrs McLaren, that her disease was not merely the result of overwork and the hardships of imprisonment. It was malignant. Unless it could be arrested, she was a dying woman.[30]

If they tried to persuade her to abandon her project, to stay at home for treatment, she would have none of it. In conversation with Mrs McLaren she referred again to the episode in Notre Dame in 1914. For the moment forgetting everything else, she said, with a keen glance and half-humorous smile, 'You know, I would awfully like to know what Joan was trying to say to me.'[31]

She did not forget the problems in Edinburgh. Taking her farewell of The Hospice, she begged the committee not to let the work suffer in her absence.[32] A great recruitment of medical women students had been stimulated by the war—there were now four hundred of them in Edinburgh alone. Dr Inglis greatly hoped, she said, that at The Hospice 'they should come into such close contact with the problem of unnecessary suffering of mothers and deaths of infants, that the solution of these problems would be their first aim in professional life'.

She returned to London for the final preparations. It was an exhausting business. Most of the party was already assembling at Liverpool and Dr Inglis, remaining in London to address one more meeting and collect some late equipment, was very tired. Did some deep unconscious streak treacherously take over for a moment? In the afternoon, she came in to the S.W.H. London office. 'May Curwen, I've done a dreadful thing,' she announced to the startled secretary. 'I've left all the passports somewhere, and I don't know where. Now here is a list of all the places I've visited. I want you to go at once and call on each of them till you have found the passports. And now as I know I can trust you to find them, I shall just take a snooze.' And she did. Naturally the passports were found. Who could fail such a woman? Certainly not the future Dame May Curwen. For Dr Inglis *meant* to go to Russia.[33]

On the afternoon of Sunday, August 27th, she spoke at a huge Trafalgar Square meeting to raise funds; equipping the Russian party had left a balance of only £17.[34] Then she left at once for Liverpool. A new electoral Bill was expected, to meet the case of men moved about by war service, and the suffragists fully believed their claim would also be recognised. 'When we return, women will have the vote,' Elsie said confidently to a friend seeing her off at Liverpool.[35]

They left the Mersey on the night of August 31st. And even while they were tossing in a heavy sea off the north of Scotland, the Serbians with whom they were to work were moving into action against the Bulgarian Third Army, which had invaded Roumania.

CHAPTER 17

When Dr Inglis sailed for Russia she was—could she have known it?—facing the biggest task of her life.

Paradoxically, it was to be the work already accomplished in Serbia itself, that would become the publicly-lauded part of her life. It had, indeed, won her 'an imperishably glorious name'. In Russia she was to face again in harsher form the same challenges, and to overcome them more triumphantly.

On September 10th she arrived at Archangel after a voyage of storms and submarine alarms (in this same North Sea Kitchener had been drowned the previous June after—it was then commonly rumoured—a submarine attack).[1] Archangel, a picture-book town with its towers of blue, red, green and gold, its toylike wooden houses on a flat shore with scrub, baby pine and silver birch growing to the water's edge, had the curiously impermanent air which resulted from its sudden expansion, at the beginning of the war, from 5,000 to 20,000 inhabitants.[2]

She spent the day ashore. Cut off from news since Liverpool, she now heard for the first time of the enormous casualties suffered by the Serbians in the defence of Roumania's Dobruga territory, of how they had stood against the German-Bulgarian-Turkish onslaught for twenty-four hours, been left without support by Roumania and Russia, and lost three-quarters of their number.

This called for drastic revision of her own plans.[3] She must proceed at once to Odessa rather than going via Petrograd as planned; and she telegraphed home for vast extra quantities of ether, dressings and chloroform. Even now the full extent of the catastrophe was not made known to her, nor, indeed, realised by her informants. She had to endure two days of fêting and entertaining at Archangel, culminating in an elaborate formal send-off by a guard of honour and the entire British colony, with cheers and anthems and dancing on the station platform; the thing which touched her most, she said, was the simple, direct 'God bless you' of Captain Bevan, R.N., commanding the British contingent in the port.[4]

The journey to Odessa was worse than uncomfortable, it was meandering and slow, although the railway staff had been ordered to expedite them. Dr Inglis had an interpreter, but could seldom resist jumping down herself to harangue the railway staff in forceful English when there was delay. She *meant* it to be effective, and was amused when her interpreter reported overhearing an official remark after one such episode, 'There will be a great row tomorrow if this train isn't got off quickly!'[5]

After nine days they reached Odessa, and another magnificent formal reception. Next morning Dr Inglis called upon Jivkovitch, the 'Iron General', whom she knew from Belgrade the year before. From him she heard at last the full story of what had happened in the Dobruga.

'It was very pathetic to realise how much we were needed,' she reported. 'He told me that there were 1,000 wounded from the First Division in Odessa, and he seemed inclined at first to keep us here to take charge of them. He suggested that our Motor Transport should be sent on at once to the 1st Army. I told him that I was ready to do whatever he wished, but I pointed out that if our transport left us we would become practically a stationary hospital and that we were not equipped for this. I therefore suggested that the British Red Cross Unit which was close behind us should be kept for this work ... and that as field hospitals are immediately necessary with the First Division we should go on.'[6]

Dr Inglis had once remarked, apparently without vanity but certainly with supreme self-confidence, that when she yielded her own convictions to the opposition of others, the result was unfortunate.[7] It was a highly subjective way of saying that over her own decisions there was no jobbing backwards. There is no sign that she ever later asked herself whether Jivkovitch might not have been right; whether she might not have done as useful work, and done more of it *for Serbs,* had she agreed to remain in Odessa. Had she been capable of asking this question later, she would not have been the woman she was.

In any case Jivkovitch knew her of old, and when she suggested going on to the First Division at the front, he, like so many who had dealings with her, 'immediately saw the reasonableness of this proposal',[8] and contented himself with getting her to make certain arrangements in Odessa for the reception of the Red Cross group coming out just behind her. She also telegraphed to ask her own Committee to supply yet another base hospital for the Serbs. 'I know you have your hands full,' she wrote, reinforcing the telegram, '... but I also know that if the people at home realise what their help would mean out here just now we would not have to ask twice. I only wish they could see the Serbian Force here—such magnificent fighting men—worth helping only for the sake of the war—and a thousand times more for their own sakes—for after all we all have men at the front who matter more than anything, and think what it would be like to send whole divisions out with two little field hospitals each.'[9] 'I wish,' she wrote to Mrs Simson, 'we were each six women instead of one.'[10]

They did not send another hospital. The sights she set her Committee were too high, and all along her work in Russia was to be hampered by the impossibility of communicating to those at home in England her own sense of urgency.

Before she could leave Odessa for the front, she had to endure four more days of fêting, with more invitations than her party could accept. She described their reception at the Serbian officers' mess: 'The whole Mess of 200 men rising when we went in and cheering till we were nearly deafened. General Jivkovitch came in for part of the evening and there were songs and dances. We sang all the National Anthems beginning with the British, and the list included three anthems which we had never heard before, the Croatian, the Bohemian and the Czech,* all three especially the last, being most rousing tunes.'[12]

At a Gala at the Opera, the Unit was inspected by Grand Duchess Marie Pavlovna, aunt of the Czar, who had made Red Cross work her concern. The wooden-tongued Elsie marvelled: 'How she could say something different to everybody, I don't know. But she did.' And when the orchestra played 'God Save the King' and the whole audience rose and cheered, 'I can tell you I felt quite chokey' Elsie told Lady Ashmore in a private letter.[13]

On September 24th they left for Megidia. The journey to Reni on the Danube, where they would transfer to boats, was said to take six hours normally. Dr Inglis was warned it would be twenty-four in war time. In fact they were three days and four nights in the train, meandering gently along a single-line track through the endless steppe, stopping at toy-like villages where she had time

* Until the creation, later, of the Czech Division, about 400 Czech volunteers were attached to the Serbian Division.[11]

to attend church and make friends with small children, while the train fuelled or traffic in the opposite direction went interminably past. To add to her impatience, at each stop they heard, 'You are needed there at the fighting', and 'They are awaiting you anxiously, sisters'.

Reni proved to be a town 'rather like Crewe'[14] on a pleasant stretch of the Danube with, away to the south, a hazy line of hills reminding the Scots of their own Lowlands. A steamer was waiting; impatient of delays Dr Inglis had contrived to send Mrs Haverfield ahead, and she had luckily encountered a former acquaintance of the hunting field,[15] the genial, worldly Admiral Visolskin,* commanding the Danube Russian Flotilla, who gave all possible help and invited her to dinner, for he was a great host and a raconteur who revelled in a new audience.

The fifty tons of equipment were quickly transferred to the steamer and they left Reni in the evening of the 29th. Leaning over the rail, some of the women wondered if there would ever be real work to do? They were answered by a shadow or two swirling in the Danube, swept by the river on a tide of indifference, shadows which as they came nearer were seen for what they were: dead men, in the blue-grey of the Austrian Army.[16]

Disembarking next afternoon at Csrnavoda, one hundred miles up the Danube and the port for Megidia, the Russian headquarters, Dr Inglis was welcomed by a Russian officer sent to escort her party. He turned out however to be a polyglot soldier of fortune from Belfast, Bryson by name,[17] who had enlisted in the Russian Army at the outbreak of war. He had a train waiting and got them all to Megidia late that night. At breakfast next morning in the Russian mess, Dr Inglis was greeted by the commanding officer, General Grutskoffsky. She had, he told her, arrived in the nick of time. An offensive was to begin that day. He spoke of the Serbs' heroism earlier that month. *'C'était magnifique, magnifique,'* he kept repeating. *'Ils sont des héros.'* Elsie Inglis reflected bitterly that that was when her Unit should have been there—and could have been there, had the business of equipping and

* Visolskin was commonly said to be the natural son of Alexander III to whom he bore a strong facial resemblance; he was on the closest terms with Nicholas II whom in conversation he would *tutoyer*. Stanojevitch, p. 97.

getting away only moved at what she thought a reasonable speed.[18]

'I do hope the papers at home have realised what the 1st Division did and how they suffered,' she wrote to Mrs Simson. The papers had not. The Russians, indeed, hushed up a tale so discreditable to themselves. *The Times*,[19] getting its information in Petrograd,* gave the Serbian story two inches; and General Knox, the English military attaché and certainly a man to honour courage, made in his diary only very brief reference to the affair.[20]

Elsie was offered a barrack for her hospital, but before accepting it insisted on consulting Colonel Hadjitch, commanding the 1st Serbian Division, at his H.Q. five miles from the front. Though he put aside the maps which were engrossing him, and attended to her politely, deferentially even, she soon saw it was no use talking to him of field hospitals. 'The ordinary male disbelief in our capacity cannot be argued away. It can only be worked away,' she wrote of this later.[21] So a base hospital it must be, in the Megidia Barrack; and it was arranged that Mrs Haverfield's transport should bring in the casualties.

Two days later the first patients arrived, and the rush went on for days. The men were pouring back in hundreds.

'More than half our patients were Russians,' she wrote on October 26th, when she at last had time to report at length (it was received in London only on December 13th), 'and we had two Roumanians ... Our Serbs, as always, were grateful and trusting, but the Russians could not at all understand the situation. They were very reluctant to come to the operating room and grumbled to the numerous officers who came in and out. One of the officers, quite a boy, sent for me and said brusquely that the men were not getting enough food. I thought it time to stop it, so I said quite firmly that there was ample food, that I would like him to remember that we were a Serbian hospital and that the diet was on Serb lines, though I was more than willing to take in Russian soldiers, but if they did not like it they need not come. In quite a different tone he said the Russians always wanted *kasha*, a kind of bean porridge. So I said if that was the only difficulty *kasha* they should have ... The Russian sisters in the other barrack most

* *The Times* correspondent in Odessa at this period was their famous man, Bouchier, who had long been stone deaf, was now approaching retirement, and had always had strong Bulgarian sympathies.

kindly allowed their cook to teach ours how to make *kasha* and I went down to the Russian headquarters and demanded *kasha.* The dear little Russian sister put her finger on another sore point. "They do not love open windows and they do not love to be so clean." But on these two points we were adamant and it was very interesting to see how human nature accommodated itself. Gradually the faces began to smile and the inquiring [inspecting] officers used to turn to us and say "He says everything is good. The only difficulty is the language". One boy who had his arm amputated said "It is so good here I am in no hurry to go back to Russia." '[22]

After only two days Dr Inglis was asked by the Serb H.Q. at Bulbul Mic to open a field dressing station there. Male disbelief had been worked away; at top level at any rate. Dr Stanojevitch, with whom the women actually had to work at Bulbul Mic, was privately unenthusiastic; he considered the equipment too cumbersome and impractical for a field hospital and that there was far too much attention to the personal comfort of the staff.[23]

Dr Inglis herself remained at Megidia for three weeks. Weeks of rumour and counter-rumour, of armies marching past in brave array and retreating in a disorganised rabble; of air raids, smoke screens, the sound of guns; of wounded pouring into the hospital, of beds packed closer and closer together; weeks which drew the oddly assorted members of the Unit into a comradeship of work and mutual trust such as only those few who had been in Serbia had known before.

On October 20th came the order to evacuate the hospital. They moved out all the patients and began packing. The main party of women, (as we have seen in Chapter 1) with all the equipment, were to go back as far as Galatz under Dr Catherine Corbett; Dr Chesney's little field hospital was retreating by horse-transport with the still-grumbling Stanojevitch, and Eve Haverfield would bring the motor transport through. On Sunday afternoon, October 22nd, Dr Inglis watched the last of her own party, from whom she hoped to form another hospital farther to the rear, drive off from Megidia, some in an ambulance, seven perched precariously atop a borrowed Russian Air Force lorry. When everyone else was out, she climbed into her staff car.

In the disordered countryside, with refugees crowding the roads, lorry, ambulance, and her own car were quickly separated and Dr Inglis became exceedingly anxious. She remembered too well the fate of the excellent Mrs Toughill. Her anxiety did not, however, prevent her sleeping soundly that night on a bed of straw at Caromarat, the little village which was the new Serb H.Q.; she had not rested for more than forty-eight hours and in any case, was seldom inclined to lose sleep when she knew she had done all that anyone could do.

In the morning, learning that the rest of her party was at Suragea, the Russian H.Q., and setting out to collect them, she saw the refugees by daylight. The scene was as confused and panic-stricken as it had been the night before. Constanza, thirty miles away, fell to the enemy that day, and already the villages in the area were deserted, the roads thronged. 'One thing seemed, somehow, so pathetic,' she wrote. 'There was a piano perched on a cart, and on the cart in front of it a gorgeous red sofa, and the anxious little housewife. She must have taken such a pride in her little house and there it was all broken up around her. In another cart there were two fascinating babies of about three years old, with pillows and rugs around them sitting up looking at everything.'[24]

Having found the girls, she decided to send them, too, right back to Galatz; she herself would remain and work with Kostitchi so far as possible. Descending upon Russian headquarters she obtained the promise of transport to move the girls, and settled to wait until it should arrive, promising to join up with Kostitchi later.

She waited hours. It was a strange, disorganised day. Faces they knew, Serbian or Russian officers, appeared at the windows of passing cars, greeted them—and passed on. No one thought of stopping for the women. All around was a panic retreat. Once she enquired anxiously of a passing officer about food for her orderlies; he pulled a chicken bone from his pocket and gave it to her, while another similarly produced some bread. Hours passed. The Russian transport never came. The noise of gunfire was constant.[25]

Late that afternoon, a girl exclaimed, 'Why, there is Mr Bryson.'

Bryson was an odd fish. Some of the women suspected him of some strange double game of his own. But no one could have been more welcome than the wandering Irishman just then. A man, a fellow-countryman, who spoke one's own language and could be assumed to share one's sane, British assumptions about life.

Bryson was unshaven, exhausted, and with a box full of despatches to send off. But when, having heard Dr Inglis's story, he promised to return and help, she at least knew he would do so.

He did; stopped the first lorry to pass, and ordered it to Ghersova, the nearest Danube port, from which boats could be boarded for Galatz. The driver demurred nervously and Bryson struck him twice upon the face. He argued no longer but his fury was hardly lessened when, having loaded up the women's belongings, he had to unpack them again because someone needed a skirt to cover her khaki driving breeches and satisfy—even in a panic retreat and in darkness—Dr Inglis's sense of decorum.[26] But he got them to Ghersova where next morning they caught a barge and—ministering to the wounded on board as they travelled—sailed for Galatz to join the main party.

After the lorry commandeered by Bryson had left, Dr Inglis, with her own two vehicles and a handful of the women, herself went after Kostitchi in the dark. She soon overtook his horses, but when the track brought them to an insecure bridge 'which Miss Onslow quite rightly absolutely refused to take in the dark and risk the cars and all our lives', Kostitchi was enraged and a heated argument ensued. He was not always an easy man to work with, Dr Inglis was coming to realise. The argument was still going on when out of the dark there emerged Dr Chesney and her party, in another of the inconsequential, dream-like, or, as Elsie put it, 'the Alice-in-Wonderland' encounters of the day; they, too, were trekking north with the Serbian H.Q. as part of a disorganised retreat. After they had disappeared into the darkness, Elsie again turned to Kostitchi, and, though he was this time persuaded to take his own horses on, with her promise to overtake him as soon as it was light, he had the last word: 'It is never any use arguing with a woman.'[27]

Her own little party camped by the roadside, and a strangely pleasant camp-fire picnic followed. Elsie Inglis glanced up. 'But this is the best of all. It is just like a fairy tale,' she exclaimed. The women followed her look; groups of soldiers were standing there motionless, holding their horses, and gazing at the women through the drifting wood smoke. The firelight had drawn them, but to see nine women laughing and chattering, alone, and within earshot of the guns, the distant sky red with burning villages, was beyond their understanding. They melted away again into the dark, and the women, rolled in blankets, waited for day to break. Then they set off across the bridge.[28]

They were still fourteen miles from the rendezvous with Kostitchi when petrol ran short. Determined to keep her word to him, Dr Inglis ordered her driver to make for Ghersova to get supplies. There, the only petrol left was *benzine lourde,* impossible for her cars. Colonel Hartsoff, chief of the Russian Medical Department, urged that she too make for Galatz. Megidia had fallen, so had Constanza, the situation was desperate. She still would not abandon Kostitchi, whom she pictured waiting in reliance upon her. She was begging the loan of horses to go to him when Dr Cartonerts* of the Roumanian Medical Department arrived. He had heard she was in the town, and the Scottish Women's work was by now famous. He asked her to send her cars back into the threatened area to pick up some three hundred wounded men he had out there. When it appeared that he too could provide only *benzine lourde,* she had sadly to say that she could not go. It was, she wrote later, 'most awfully hard to do'.[29] Was there any other way to help? she asked. Cartonerts told her hundreds of wounded were passing through Ghersova, being now the only outlet from this area of the Dobruga to the Danube barges connecting with the railhead. A dressing station would greatly relieve the situation.

Thankfully she agreed. This was the work she had come to the Eastern Front to do. The cars and drivers must be sent off to keep them out of enemy hands. Then, asking for three volunteers to stay with her, she set up her dressing station. And when Kostitchi himself arrived, she was able to abandon any guilty feeling that she should somehow, *somehow,* have gone back into the Dobruga for him.

All that day, much of the night, and the whole of the next day, the four women toiled in the wharfside dressing station; and organised a canteen for the wounded.[30]

Towards evening on the Thursday, the stream of wounded eased off. All civilians had left Ghersova hours before and now the four women noticed that the little town was strangely quiet. The ambulances full of wounded were no longer arriving. All the patients had been despatched to safety by boat. Miss Gerald-

* Dr Inglis's spelling. More probably Costinescu.

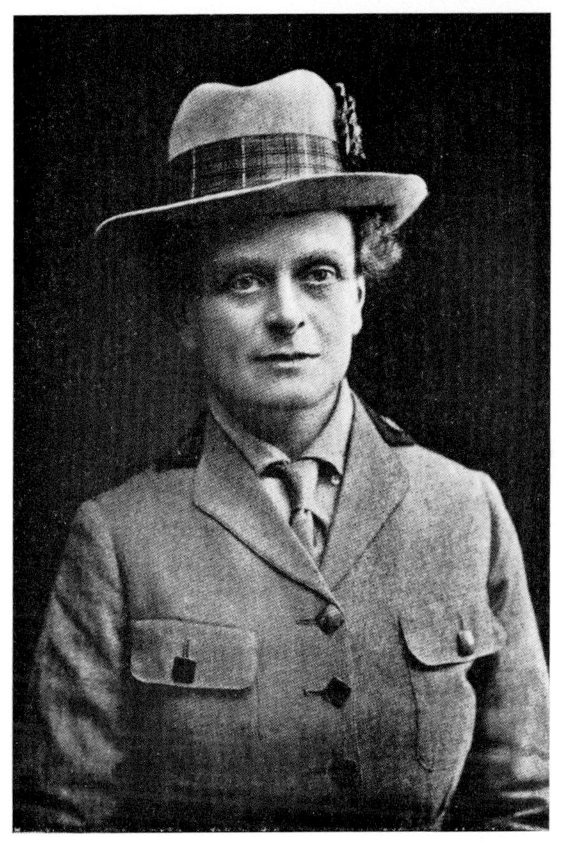

Elsie Inglis in 1916.

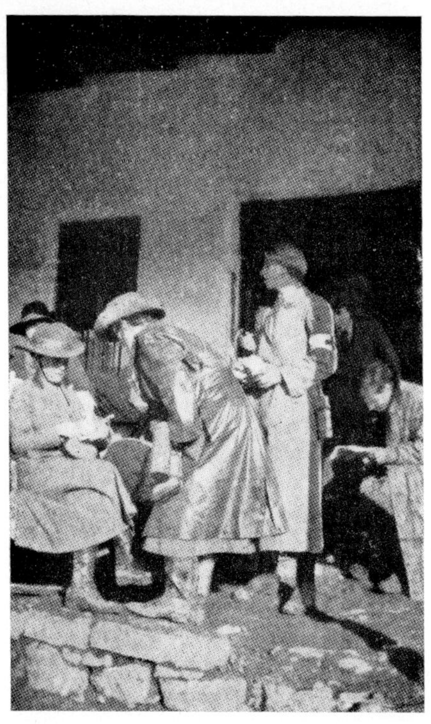

Left Elsie Inglis (seated left) and companions during the retreat in Roumania.

Below Elsie Inglis (left), riding astride for the first time, at Reni in May 1917.

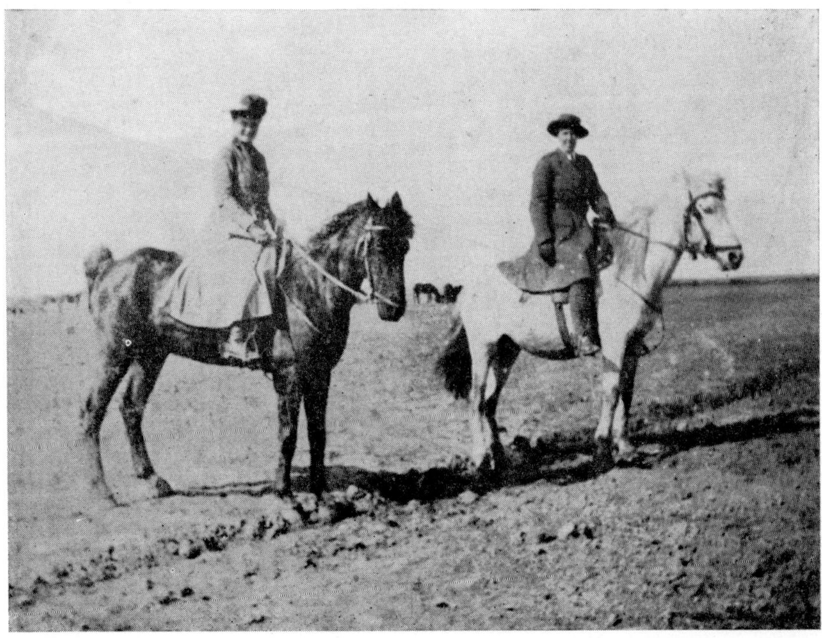

ine Hedges found herself sitting alone with Dr Inglis. For the first time for many days they had nothing immediate to do.

'The ambulances have gone,' said Dr Inglis quietly. 'I wonder why they left?' Then, after a pause, 'Do you think they were afraid? They can only kill us.'

But she had long ago discovered that she was afraid of *nothing*. Now, suddenly, both women realised they were extremely hungry; and that the sacks on which they were perched were filled with sugar. A twinkle came into the little doctor's eyes. 'Do you think we might take lumps?' she asked. Miss Hedges thought they might. 'And we're alone,' Dr Inglis added, decorously. 'We're alone. We may smoke.'

They sat, smoking. At Dr Inglis's instigation, one of the women searched and found in a deserted house some ingredients for a meal. When Cartonerts arrived, declaring they must leave at once, that nobody could say which boat would be the last, Dr Inglis refused to be panicked. 'Bring on the stew,' she ordered. Only when they had eaten, did they go aboard.[31]

On the steamer, moving down the Danube, Dr Inglis had time to take stock. She sat down to write a report for her Committee, the first she had had time for since leaving Odessa. Only then did she realise that it was October 25th. 'And here we are in full retreat again. On October 25th last year we evacuated Kragujevatz.'[32]

This time, however, at least all the wounded for whom she was responsible had been sent out of the danger, ahead of her.

CHAPTER 18

A snapshot[1] taken during the journey down the Danube shows Dr Inglis sitting with a party of Roumanian officers. Thin and hollow-eyed, yet oddly youthful-looking, she sits straight-backed and neat, with hands folded in her lap and a composed smile; wearing the curiously touching air of a very good little girl.

She spent most of the journey writing her report. She had heard from the Roumanians on board, she wrote, 'their side of this woeful story. Until then we had only heard the Serb and Russian side.' She already had come to recognise the asperities existing between the three nations, but commented with satisfaction, 'There is one thing that everyone agrees about and that is that the Serbs have behaved magnificently.'[2]

'One does not see much of the glamour of war from this end,' she wrote in the same report. 'It was terrible to have those broken men pouring in ... We had four Serbian officers in the last two days and their despair was dreadful. "You can save Serbia," one of them said to me, "but what about the Serbian nation?" Their Division had gone into action so hopefully and only a wreck was left. My German wasn't good enough to even try and comfort them so I could only sympathise. They do love their country so.'[3]

It was to be her destiny to play an important role in saving the Serbian nation. But before that could happen her spirit must be tempered further, tempered until she *knew*, as a fact repeatedly experienced, what she had always felt instinctively: that *nothing* had power to deflect a course of events determined by her will.

The first apparent setback came almost at once.

At Braila was the celebrated Russian bridge of boats across the Danube, the only crossing place below Csrnavoda with its 12½-mile girder bridge. And just now the bridge of boats was in operation, effectively closing the Danube to water traffic. Providence was certainly against them, the women concluded, dragging themselves reluctantly ashore. Near the quay they met some of the Transport, and while the whole party was snatching a meal, the Mayor of Braila, a Mr Szarderry,* arrived. Could the English Sisters, he begged, come and help? There were more wounded in town than the army doctors could deal with.[4]

Dr Inglis went with him at once. She found a problem bigger even than that which Florence Nightingale found at Scutari. In the town were more than 8,000 wounded men†, with seven doctors, only one a surgeon. Perhaps, she reflected, the hand of providence had not altogether slipped. 'We just turned up our sleeves and went in,' she wrote to Mrs Simson later.[5]

Of fully trained women she had on this first evening only herself, Dr Potter and Sister Edwards, but most of the Transport girls had been V.A.D.s and they were pressed into service.

'That first night', she wrote, 'we all turned to in that hospital ... the people here had been working thirty-six hours without stopping. The women of the place had turned out splendidly but of course they are not trained ... It was just a case of going on dressing blindly, and the wounded coming in, and in, and in.'[6]

Since all the equipment had been sent to safety at Galatz, no operations could be done, but through the night they worked at dressing. Next morning, Dr Inglis went round with the Mayor to survey the rest of the town, and seeing the need she agreed to his request to open a proper hospital. 'The Roumanians', she wrote, 'have organised really finely but the flood was too great for anything ... there were still men lying about in empty houses with their uniforms on and the horrible smell of sepsis from their wounds.'[7] That afternoon she opened another dressing station in an empty school, where the less badly injured could be dealt with before being moved back to Galatz or farther.

Over the permanent hospital a difficulty arose. The only suitable building was one where a Roumanian woman doctor had been working for a month almost single-handed; Szarderry's proposal was to turn her out in favour of the well-staffed and well-equipped Scottish Women's Hospital.

Dr Inglis, to whom the solidarity of womanhood was a first principle, objected; and although Szarderry protested that the two of them would never agree, she persuaded him to accept her proposal to share the premises with the other doctor. She knew she was right, and Szarderry, like so many others, saw it was useless to argue.

* Dr Inglis's spelling.

† Sometimes given as 11,000. 8,000 is the official figure compiled later.

Before they could move in, equipment must be fetched, and on a flying visit to Galatz, Dr Inglis found that part of the Unit which had preceded her from Megidia, under Dr Corbett. She ordered them all back to Braila. On enquiring for her equipment she learned that, on advice from the British Consul, her administrator had removed it all to safety miles away to the north. Between anger and derision at 'the scuttle', she ordered it back; not even the Germans, she declared, could cross the Danube without some days' warning.[8]

When she returned to Braila it was immediately evident why Szarderry had not wished to put them with the Roumanian woman doctor. 'Some lovely ladies were hovering around when we arrived. I'm afraid we turned them out. It was good for the work even if bad for the Entente!' recorded one of the orderlies, Miss Yvonne Fitzroy, in her diary.[9]

There was no time to indulge in outraged prudery. So great was the number of the wounded that it was several nights before any of the Scottish women got more than two or three hours' sleep. By October 31st Dr Inglis had opened her own theatre and wards and they worked under high pressure for several weeks. 'The Unit as a whole has behaved splendidly, plucky and cheery through everything and game for any amount of work', she wrote to Mrs Simson on November 11th. '... Personally I have been awfully well and prouder than ever of British women ... It is a comfort to feel you are all thinking of us.'[10]

The authorities found them quarters and took trouble over rations and other arrangements. The house, Dr Inglis wrote, was 'quite clean and nice big rooms and beds and a table in the dining room and chairs. But we were perfectly comfortable. More is not really necessary and they took a lot of trouble to get us that.'[11]

Although the first lot of lovely ladies had gone similar difficulties, and others, arose with the Roumanian woman doctor. The Mayor had been right; their ways would never agree. 'Our methods, penchant for open windows, etc., have made a decided difficulty,' Dr Inglis went so far as to admit, discreetly, to her Committee towards the end of November. 'But we were determined to make it work, and we have made it work quite well ... However, we learn, and I shall not attempt a hospital under other management again.'[12]

Other difficulties were also arising. Because of cholera in the town, the country folk refused to bring in supplies; on some days both meat and wood failed entirely. Dr Inglis never complained in her own person, but a letter on December 1st, making excuses for one of the Unit who had found the strain too much, tells the story. 'It is a very hard life, discomfort, irregular meals. Above all the food is a real difficulty here. Tough meat and very little choice ... Do help her all you can ... It was not she who wanted to give up this job. I made her.'[13]

To add to the difficulties, the weather was excessively wet. Rain, in fact, saved the Allies, turning the unmetalled roads of the Danube Basin into rivers of mud, hindering the German advance and enabling Roumania to stage a counter-attack in Transylvania;[14] it was from this that the wounded were pouring into Braila.

The work of the hospital, the physical and emotional strain of the operations and dressings, the rubs with the Roumanian woman, were not Dr Inglis's only worries. The leadership of her group of high-spirited and enterprising young women was no easy task. Many had obeyed at first only because she was stronger than they. And though the experiences of the past few weeks had brought many of them to see that her authority in fact sprang from a selflessness that was an example to them all, that she was a woman who would never in any circumstances fail the cause she followed or those who followed her—nevertheless, a few of the 'queer characters' were now failing her.

One—she spoke Russian and had been extremely useful, too—'ran away from her job' in a panic and added to her enormities by talking 'extraordinary rubbish' to the press. Another had turned out 'quite useless'[15] and been thankfully passed over to the short-staffed British Red Cross party under Dr Clemaud which had followed them out. Even Mrs Haverfield was being difficult again. This time it was the young Serbian medical director of the Field Hospital with whom she could not get on; and she had gone over Dr Inglis's head and complained to the High Command at Salonika about him.[16]

Dr Stanojevitch was very young. He was autocratic. He was not in the least like St Francis of Assisi. He disapproved entirely of too much comfort in hospitals. And he knew nothing about motor transport, and expected, said Mrs Haverfield, impossibilities. There was a stormy interview at the Serbian H.Q., only saved when Elsie noticed a twinkle in the eye of Colonel

Popovitch, the Chief of Medical Staff. Not that Kostitchi, her own director, had been easy to work with either, she wrote privately to Lady Ashmore next day. 'But,' she added (very much the daughter of Inglis Sahib), 'it is so silly to quarrel with these poor little men—peasants in the last generation. The point is to work with them and manage them. They are doing their bit as well as they know how—and we can see how difficult it is for them. After all we came out to help.'[17]

There had also been, earlier, another failure, and by her own staff, to live up to her standards. Swearing, to her, was 'far more disgusting and disagreeable' than spitting, but 'I am sorry to learn from a private letter, that the Committee has been told about the disgusting habit of swearing which some members of the Unit had adopted'[18] she wrote in December. To Mrs McLaren she wrote more freely. 'My dear—do you suppose for one moment that I should allow either men or women to swear for whom I was responsible. I never even heard of the disgusting habit until just before we left Megidia and I spoke to Mrs Haverfield about it at once. She had heard nothing of it—nor Miss Onslow. But once I had discovered it I got any amount of evidence, and you may be quite certain the Transport did not escape. I had them all up and gave them the worst talking to they have ever had in their lives—and the rest of the Unit caught it for not having stamped it out... Sister Edwards actually said to me that she thought I approved because I evidently liked that sort of girl. I told her I had never been so insulted in my life, that because I like the modern healthy out-of-door girl with her energy & resource & independence I should approve of language that I would not tolerate in a coster, was an impertinence. Well, you need not be afraid of that special sin any more, but as Eve [Haverfield] and I said "What will they do next without our knowing?" In Serbia they flirted. Now apparently they don't flirt—but they break out in a new direction. And they are so splendid all the time—the wretches! Our naughtiest girls in Serbia were some of those who had worked right through the typhus ...

'And these girls have been such bricks too ... This same naughty Transport has been doing simply magnificent work during the retreat. They were right in the thick of it ...'[19]

Such was the force of Dr Inglis's dressing down that it has proved impossible to persuade any of the few remaining of those who received it, to remember precisely which expressions brought her wrath on their heads; though Mrs Haverfield had a year before lamented (not in Dr Inglis's hearing) her paucity of Serbian swear words and in particular had thought a translation of 'damned fool' might be useful.[20] And a few months before the outbreak of the war, *Pygmalion* had shocked and delighted the London theatre public.

Dr Inglis's severity had its roots not only in her own Victorian prejudices, but also in the determination of the older suffragists to prove that dignity, and gentleness, and womanly refinement, need not necessarily, as the 'antis' averred, be sacrificed with emancipation. Women had to be able to face hardship, difficulty, danger, yes; and they had to be able to do it without abating one iota of womanly sensibility. She had also the reputation of the Unit to consider, in a part of the world where nurses were still more commonly 'lovely ladies'.

One specific problem of this nature had already cropped up. It worried Dr Inglis more than all her professional problems of running the hospital could do. On November 3rd she wrote from Braila a confidential letter to her Committee about 'a very uncomfortable incident ... one of the Transport has left us and is going about dressed like a man—sitting in restaurants, smoking, and talking to anybody and everybody'.[21]

This, too, had begun at Megidia, when the Russians quickly summed up the situation, advising Dr Inglis to send the woman home, for the sake of all their reputations. This was beyond her legal powers. With persuasion she was for once unsuccessful.

The woman in question had been widowed in singularly distressing circumstances and was now, as a Roumanian specialist later diplomatically certified to get her put under supervision, 'suffering from a maniac excitability which renders her dangerous to public order'.[22] She dressed as a man, flourished whip and revolver, demanded to lay her grievances before royalty, actually got into the palace at Bucharest and borrowed money from a lady-in-waiting, 'flirted' with Roumanian girls and generally made herself a scandal to the whole Red Cross. 'I am sure the Committee would not wish us to shirk the responsibility. After all, she came out with us', wrote Dr Inglis.[23]

Not shirking the responsibility was to cause her anxiety until the following April. She telegraphed begging the woman's own people to come and take charge; she personally guaranteed travel expenses home; she wrote endless letters, made trips to Bucharest, often at highly inconvenient times, to consult the British Minister, Sir George Barclay, and distinguished neurologists. At one time so many telegrams were being sent home about the case that official war messages were seriously delayed, bringing Barclay a rap over the knuckles from the Foreign Office.[24] And worst of all, Sister Edwards, 'one of our best nurses', had to be taken off duty and given the charge of this one woman. Elsie wrote from Bucharest on November 20th that this whole episode was 'the worst thing that has happened here'.[25]

There were money worries. After her administrator had gone home to address meetings, raise funds, and return with some much-needed stores, Elsie discovered to her dismay that the accounts had all along been neglected.

Generous and even casual where her own possessions were concerned, she was punctilious about other people's, but now at over fifty found it no easier to look after money than when, as a girl, she had resolved, 'I must devote my mind more to the housekeeping'. Somehow, she got accounts drawn up retrospectively. 'But', she wrote to Lady Ashmore, 'if money is not to dribble away it must be watched every minute—must it not?

'Now I cannot manage money. I'll do my best while I am without an administrator, but I confess that in addition to managing the Unit and doing surgery, the prospect of doing what I loathe —looking after money—nearly appals me! ... I wish the Committee would immediately send me an administrator ... I know exactly the woman I need—a gentlewoman, tolerant of other people's views, good at managing money—and who can talk French well ... whoever comes *must be strong as a horse*.'[26]

The financial situation was indeed complicated. There had been difficulty at the start over their account being transferred from Petrograd to local banks. Then, £1,000 had been changed into Roumanian currency on a rapidly falling exchange so that one quarter would be lost when re-converted to roubles; worse, the money had not been made payable to Dr Inglis, and she could not get at it until the mistake was cleared up. 'The Consul is wiring about it. If it is not a mistake he will have to draw on the Foreign Office for us as he did before', she wrote on December 19th, 'and the Committee be obliged to pay it in England ... I am sorry about it all. Mr Watson [a British merchant in Galatz] says he thinks that a far better way would be for us to draw by

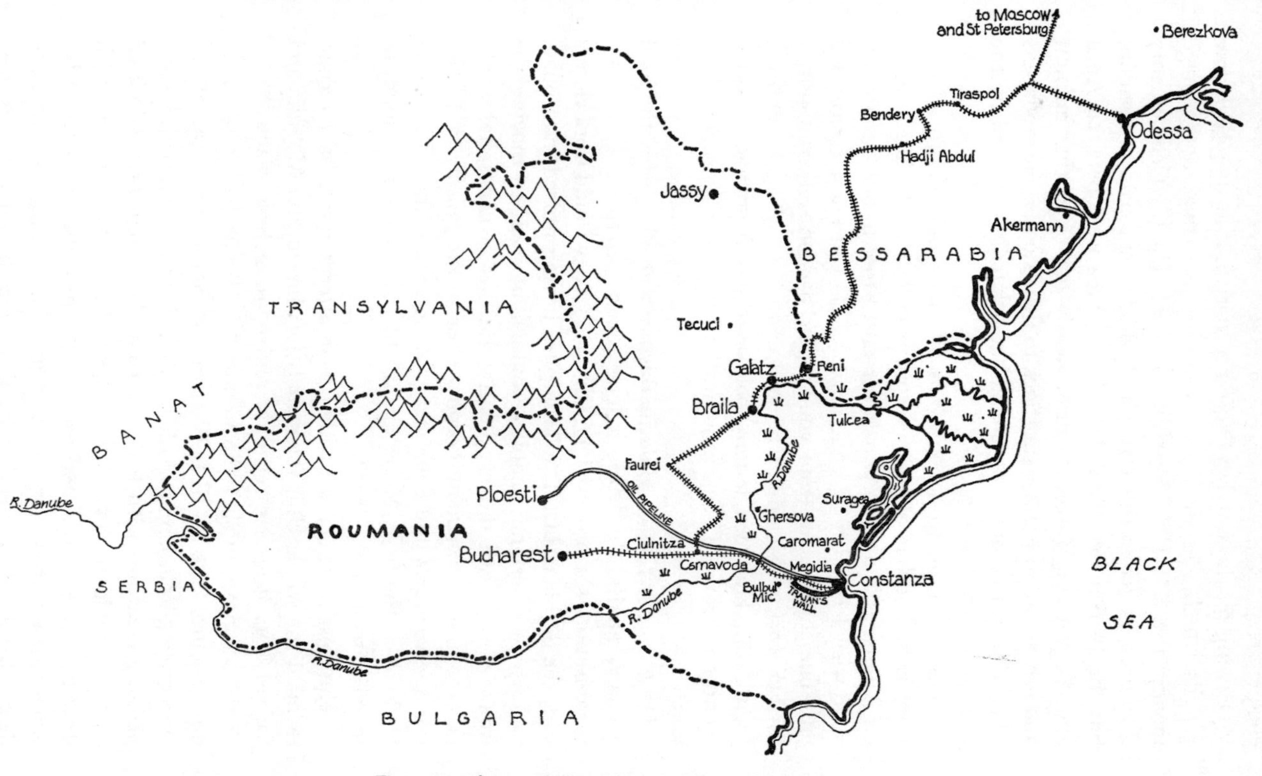

Roumania and South-east Russia 1916–17

cheque on a London bank. Any bank will cash an English cheque.'[27]

Drawing on the Foreign Office was not without its pitfalls too; pitfalls which, despite Elsie's plea that she could not manage money, the S.W.H. successfully avoided. Up till October 1917 they drew £1,400 in this way, all of which was repaid in London; but the British Red Cross Unit in the area were between April and August 1917 forced to draw nearly ten times that amount and it came as an unpleasant shock to their London headquarters when the full account was somewhat belatedly rendered by the Foreign Office.[28]

Communication with home was all along difficult. In all this time, Elsie had had almost no word from home. She left London on August 27th and on November 14th wrote to her Committee, 'I do wish I could hear some news ... Do you know I have had only one short letter from you?'[29] She had no sign of approval for her work at Megidia, Ghersova or Braila. It was not entirely their fault. Her own letters took anything from one to three months to travel. The communications lag was a constant hindrance.

On November 20th, while in Bucharest dealing with the mad woman's affairs, she wrote a long report describing certain reorganisations she proposed. Dr Chesney's party would work closely with the Serbian H.Q. The Transport, having proved inadequate to keep two hospitals mobile, would limit itself to moving the wounded, which it did excellently; and her own hospital would become more permanent, keeping close to the railway and holding reserve stores and equipment. 'All reserve stores will be kept far back at the base. Never again will I risk such an amount of material so near the front.

'The Russian H.Q.,' she added as an afterthought, 'have recommended the whole Unit for medals for the work at Megidia and Bulbul Mic. We were certainly under fire at both places.'[30]

All this time nursing the wounded in Braila had gone on at top pressure. The Scottish Women had borne the brunt of the emergency. Roumanian patients they found 'unattractive complaining creatures with little self-control', though they admitted that the male students who helped the military doctors with dressings were 'devils, and torture the men quite unnecessarily'. Roumanian nurses were 'very young but amazingly self-confident'; 'for all their emotionalism, the real horror seems to pass them by completely'.[31] The Roumanian nurses apparently admired the Scottish Women but were puzzled by their professionalism and lack of feminine airs and graces; and not above the occasional feline jibe. 'One of them said what they loved about us was our "simplicity",' Elsie wrote. 'We wondered what "simplicity" could mean and Dr Corbett suggested it must be our *boots*!'[32]

By the time the flow of wounded had steadied to manageable proportions and the Roumanians had drafted medical reinforcements into the area, the situation was again threatening. Between November 23rd and 25th Mackensen put five divisions across the Danube. On the 26th it became clear that Bucharest was threatened and the government moved to Jassy.

In the Scottish Women's Hospital once again they were putting two beds together and three men in them, but could not find enough room. Once again there were rumours and counter-rumours. Dr Inglis on November 21st was approached by the Russians. Now that the Roumanians were organising their own hospitals so much better, and the Serbian Divisions out of action and re-forming, could she provide the Russians with a hospital for their new offensive?

She appreciated the compliment but was anxious over her commitment to the Serbs. She had a week earlier seen Popovitch of the Serbian Staff and told him she was anxious to return when the Serbs needed her. He already had at his H.Q. in Bessarabia, Dr Chesney's hospital and the Transport, who had had some remarkable adventures of their own during the Dobruga Retreat.

On the Russian assurance that any commitment she entered into with them would be purely temporary, she agreed to work for them while the Serbs re-formed. The Russians were generous allies. There was to be an allowance of 3,000 roubles for rations and wood, with more money when needed, and unlimited petrol for the Transport; and best of all from Dr Inglis's personal point of view, a Russian Sister attached to keep accounts and deal with language problems. 'It is very comfortable working for a big nation', she wrote on November 27th, 'tho' I love the little ones!'[33]

Hadjitch, the Serb commander, when she saw him, however, was not pleased. She could only reiterate that the moment the Serbs went into action her hospital would return to them; and she arranged for Dr Chesney's little group at the Serb H.Q. at Ismail to be increased in size.[34]

When she saw Ilneachenko, chief of the Russian Red Cross, on December 4th, he told her that the most useful thing she could do for him would be to form a field dressing station at Ciulnitza.

Now Ciulnitza is far to the south, on the oil pipeline from Ploesti to Constanza and on the Bucharest-Csrnavoda railway. Was Ilneachenko ignorant that two German armies were then racing for Bucharest, which fell the next day?[35] Was it all characteristic Russian muddle? Could there have been some more sinister reason for his order? Elsie's own dry and discreet retrospective comment, after it was all over, was that it was 'a funny mistake'.

For hardly had she arrived at Ciulnitza with her Unit, on December 8th, when fresh orders came; they must leave directly. She now learned for the first time of the fall of Bucharest three days before. All communications had been cut and the army was falling back. Gloomily she assembled her party at the station. The danger was great, but the food problem was immediate. They had come unprovided with anything above one day's rations, and nothing was to be obtained in Ciulnitza. To add to the anxiety, five of the party were coming separately, by car.

In one of those strange encounters which can happen in war, Dr Inglis found in the village a squadron of British and French pilots attached to the Russian Air Force; they had flown into the district from Salonika. Once again, when her own countrymen promised help, she knew they were to be relied on, and asked them to trace and turn back the car party. The encounter was as reassuring as the earlier meetings with the 'wild goose' Bryson, and that settled, she prepared to leave.

All afternoon the women sat in bare railway trucks at the station. Train after train crept out loaded with refugees and soldiers. Word came that the order had been given to destroy the railway and the station at five. Still their Red Cross train did not move.

With a French air officer who had begged a place, having been unable to get on any other train, Elsie watched the Allied flying machines, three British and five small French ones, loop the loop in salute before disappearing into the darkening eastern sky. Then, just before five, eight trucks of ammunition were hooked on to the Red Cross train by order of a Russian officer with a disregard of international convention amounting to panic.

Even after some of the petrol in the station had been set afire, Dr Inglis saw him harangue the station commandant; he had to threaten to blow the man's brains out before the train was moved. 'As a matter of fact everybody's nerves were very much on edge', she wrote with the scorn she always had for those who gave way to even justifiable fear. 'We had a French airman on board ... and he and we enjoyed the situation thoroughly.'[36]

Suddenly, huge flames were seen leaping up beside the engine. A young and dashing Roumanian officer, who was helping the girl orderlies to prepare some food in their wagon, hurried to investigate, then came running back shouting to them to close the doors as the train began to move. They hauled him in and slid the wagon door closed, while the train with its load of explosives passed within a few inches of what proved to be a blazing oil tank.

When, safely past, they looked out, the horizon too was in a blaze; oil, granaries, haystacks, all had been set alight and burned with a terrible beauty. Men, women and children were running alongside the train, trying unsuccessfully to pull themselves into the overloaded trucks; as the train drew away they settled to a dreary, dogged tramp, the tramp of the eternal refugee, with the blazing sky as background.[37]

That night, all next day, and until midday on December 11th, they were in the train. The line was single track, and at each tiny station there were long halts while troop trains passed in the opposite direction. The guns could be heard, enemy planes flew overhead with the dual purpose of reconnoitring and bombing. It was freezing hard, and owing to the length of the train there was no heat. The women were also desperately hungry. Once again, Dr Inglis's luck—*was* it only luck?—held; at a tiny wayside station she somehow found a goose, a duck, a hen and half a pig. 'Not half bad' was the Unit's verdict.[38]

They reached Faurei, having taken over sixty-eight hours to travel seventy-five miles, only to find the telephone line cut. Dr Inglis decided to make for Braila and, now on a main line, progress was quicker. They arrived late the same evening.

Braila was in uproar. But there Dr Inglis learned that the car party was ahead of them; it had had a serious accident and was being towed to Galatz by oxen. She was moved to anger at the discovery that four sterilising drums had been lost during the car party's wanderings: Mrs Milne had failed to stick to the equipment and had trustingly put them on a train unsupervised. 'I suppose it was a little difficult to decide what to do; but ... I confess I was a little annoyed to think we should have lost some really valuable things of that sort in such a stupid way,' she wrote with characteristic understatement.[39]

At Braila next day they met more fellow countrymen. Colonel Norton Griffiths, M.P., was touring the area, at the request of the Russians, methodically wrecking the oil installations.[40] From his British staff they learned that it was touch and go whether the Russians could hold the German attack, and the following evening December 13th, having conferred with the authorities, Dr Inglis announced that the Unit would move back to Galatz next morning. Such was the congestion on the railway that although the two places are less than twenty miles apart, it was late afternoon on December 16th before they reached Galatz.

'This has been our second retreat in less than three months', she wrote when she arrived, 'and the Unit has behaved with its usual good temper and cheerfulness ... I think [this] has been the most uncomfortable retreat I have ever experienced; and I feel that I am becoming an old hand at them now.'[41]

Galatz seemed safe for the moment, and Dr Inglis was shown a building she realised would make a very good hospital. She now had most of her Unit collected together, even including the members of Dr Chesney's group who had been mustering in the town ready to go where the Serbs wished.

By December 18th, however, they heard that Braila itself was threatened; if it fell, Galatz could hardly be held, and they must prepare to retreat to Odessa. They spent the whole day packing, while Dr Inglis tried to sort out the currency situation, wrote urgent letters about the wretched mad woman at Bucharest, and prepared a long report for her Committee.

She was engaged upon this last when she received another message.

A pencilled postscript at the foot of her report reads, 'Have had orders after all to stay here. Very glad.'[42]

CHAPTER 19

Dr Inglis was taking a risk in agreeing to stay in Galatz. She informed her Unit of it. The best of them were solid behind her. 'We are to stay. The Russians say they will not take the responsibility of getting us away [later] but nevertheless would like us to stay. Am glad',[1] Miss Fitzroy wrote in her diary. If some others were less glad, well, they were more afraid of Dr Inglis's scorn than of the Germans.

The next day or two were quiet. It even began to look as though Galatz might be saved. Sections of huge Russian guns, some drawn by teams of twelve oxen, passed the hospital on their way from the quays to the town's outer defences. Food was plentiful, the town market attractive even.

On December 21st the women learned for the first time, from a local family with whom some of them were billeted, of the fall of the Asquith Coalition and the formation of Lloyd George's government (which had taken place two weeks earlier). Elsie commented to her niece Eve Simson in her next letter: 'What did happen over the change of Government? I do hope we have got the right lot now, to put things straight at home, and carry through things abroad. Remember it all depends on you people at home. *The whole thing depends on us.* I know we lose the perspective in this gloomy corner, but there is one thing quite clear, and that is that they are all trusting to our *sticking* powers. They know we'll hold on—of course—I only wish we would realise that it would be as well to use our intellects too and to keep them clear of alcohol.'[2] It seems she had already realised that there was little to be hoped for from either Roumania or even from Russia itself.

The building she was now given for a hospital in Galatz was not the good wooden building she had first seen, but was in a dark and dismal slum between railway station and quays. It was, she said, determinedly looking on the bright side, 'in many ways more satisfactory as the wounded were coming back by barge'.[3] It had once been the Scola Pappadopol and had accommodation for reception room, bathroom, dressing-room and theatre, as well as wards for one hundred beds; but no light and —they had come to expect this—no drains. The stoves were, as usual, wood-burning; and the hospital was able to get a plentiful supply through the good offices of Sister Marie, the remarkably pretty little Russian nurse now attached to them; she had turned out to be hopeless at accounts but had—she told them—several brothers in the army; certainly she seemed to know personally a great many officers out of whom she was adept at coaxing supplies.

The equipment was brought down by ox wagons, and even as they installed themselves they learned that Ilneachenko had ordered the British Red Cross unit under Dr Clemaud, to leave the town. It went the same night, the 22nd, taking with it the Scottish Women's personal kit.[4]

The Scottish Women's Hospital was now the only hospital of any kind left in the town.

Christmas Day was a curious day. Only the Russian orderlies worked, stuffing mattresses with straw. Everyone else was rather too obviously cheerful. Some must have remembered the previous Christmas, when, prisoners at Krushevatz, they had kept up their spirits by playing 'this time next year'. Could their wildest imaginings have possibly foreseen the circumstances in which they now found themselves? To keep up their spirits they sang carols and dressed up for tableaux in which their 'Dr I.' benignantly appeared attired as a knight, in a cloak and, yes, *breeches* —to enormous applause, for they all knew her views on decorum in dress.

Next day came the first night Zeppelin bombing raid. Ilneachenko, visiting them, told Dr Inglis it might be days before it was clear if Galatz could be held; and gave her a written order to stay 'till the last moment'.[5]

By December 30th, the hospital was ready; even to Dr Inglis's eye, it looked satisfactory. Then, in a sudden rush, the wounded began to arrive. They came from the Braila area and from the Dobruga itself. Within an hour or two the hospital was full. In the glimmer of oil lamps and candles, Dr Inglis herself examined every patient on arrival, sending those in need of dressings to the other doctors, while the rest went direct to the bath. Before long, however, the rush of helpless men forced her to abandon such an orderly reception.

By next day, the wounded were pouring through Galatz at over a thousand a day, and the flood continued for nearly a week. All the most serious cases went to the Scottish Women's Hospital; men who were by any possible reckoning fit to do so, went straight to the evacuation barges for Reni or Odessa. Even so, before long all order or method at the Hospital became impossible.

At first, they tried to record each case; but so many were delirious, unconscious, or dying, that it could not be done. 'If they die, I suppose no one ever discovers who or what they are or where they come from. And I suppose their families just go on—waiting', wrote Miss Fitzroy.[6]

By the second afternoon, Elsie was at work in the theatre. Already she had worked a full twenty-four hours supervising admissions and dressing wounds. The numbers awaiting operations were far more than she and her colleagues, Drs Potter and Corbett, could hope to keep pace with. Once again, providence was on her side.

There was at work in this area a British Armoured Cars Division commanded at this time by Commander Reginald Gregory, R.N.,[7] himself a qualified Danube pilot, and manned by petty officers of the Royal Naval Air Service. Originally sent east to operate in the Caucasus, it had found the terrain there impossible and been transferred to south-east Russia where it 'made an impression out of all proportion to its small numbers'.* The Scottish Women had first encountered one of the officers of this unit at Braila on October 28th, when he reported to the Admiralty that everyone he met had 'nothing but praise for the Scottish Women's Hospital, whose motor ambulances were the first thing to be noticed on landing at Braila'.[8] It had heroically defended Ghersova, just after Dr Inglis and her party left there, and had helped some of the Transport and Dr Chesney's group in the First and Second Dobruga Retreats. Some of its members had been seconded for work with Colonel Norton Griffiths and had met the members of Dr Inglis's party then.

Now, in all the rush at Galatz, one girl, coming into the hospital from her billet, encountered in the street Surgeon-Lieutenant Maitland Scott of the Armoured Cars. He gave her a message for Dr Inglis—could he be of help? In an emergency such as this, theoretical notions of demonstrating what women could accom-

* Sir Basil Liddell Hart, *The Tanks*, p. 20.

plish unaided were as expendable as the routine bathings and the record keeping; Dr Inglis replied that she would be very glad of his help.

So Maitland Scott and four R.N.A.S. orderlies joined the women. 'He worked with us without a break until we evacuated. He is a first rate surgeon and it was a great thing having him here,' Elsie found time, a week later, to write to her Committee.[9]

For the thirty-six hours following his arrival, the two of them toiled on, with one break of three hours in the early morning of New Year's Day. Through that day the operations and equally horrible dressings (done by Dr Potter and Dr Corbett) went on. Most men stayed only a short time and were evacuated by Russian horse ambulances to barges for Reni. Dr Inglis had to abandon all hope of nursing, or even washing, for the majority. 'We had eventually to lay down one room entirely with straw where we simply put the men in their uniforms after dressing them, and the more serious cases we gradually moved to mattresses.'[10]

She had only six trained nurses (two who would have been invaluable were now at Jassy with the mad woman) and when the theatre and night duty had been staffed, only three sisters remained for the wards. For several nights none of them got more than two or three hours' sleep. At one time, the sister in the first floor ward was nursing over ninety cases, most of them very heavy, with the help of one untrained girl orderly.

'It was a terrible experience', Elsie wrote to Lady Ashmore on January 9th. 'Every single case a bad one—poor, poor fellows. It was one of the worst things to feel that one ought to have a "special" on in at least a quarter of the cases ... and the actual dressings took so long—the wounds were so bad. And then to have to move them on when they really ought to have stayed in —to make room for the rush behind.'[11]

In the early hours of January 2nd the tide had turned. There were, for the moment, no more men awaiting operations. With Mr Scott, Dr Inglis had been operating for thirty-eight hours with only one brief rest; and she had been on duty for a full twenty-four hours before that.

Even the experienced doctors and nurses had never imagined such conditions. 'When these poor broken creatures are brought in here', wrote Miss Fitzroy, 'in the springless carts, to find, at best, a straw mattress to lie on, to have to suffer tortures which perhaps they don't understand, with all day the horror of gangrene or tetanus before their eyes and all day and all night long the smell, the confusion and the dirt—I think it is hard to realise until you have seen it the heartbreaking courage and loneliness of them all ... You thank Death whenever it comes, and often you pray that it may be quick ...

'It is no consolation to think that these men after all expect so much less than our own—they do, no doubt—but that only makes it worse. They have led grey, grey lives always and now they are dying this slow grey death.'[12]

'Galatz', she wrote when it was all over, 'has been a nightmare.'

'War is an awful and horrible thing', Dr Inglis wrote to Mrs McLaren on January 9th, completing a letter begun before the rush. 'Those poor poor fellows. I have never had such wards in my life—not one light case ... One thing one learns here & that is how very little one can do [with]. We neither undressed or bathed for I don't know how many days. One day I did not even do my hair! That is striking bedrock! ... One such pathetic thing happened. Somehow one man, a Russian, had lost his little case with his medals in it & he was crying & miserable. So I took the Roumanian interpreter up to say I would get it put right. The man said quite fiercely "Do you think I trust the word of a Roumanian?" & the poor little Roumanian said quite humbly "But Madame is English." And the poor man turned to me with such a sudden smile through the tears. So I must get him those medals—because I am English!'[13]

By January 3rd things were beginning to run smoothly. Inside the hospital there was even something approaching an air of order. But the very slackening of work was ominous; resistance to the enemy was evaporating. On this day the British consul left Galatz.

Ilneachenko had ordered Dr Inglis to stay 'to the last moment'; but when had that last moment to be recognised? She would have been anxious but for a message from Commander Gregory of the Armoured Cars, to whom she now applied as the senior British representative in the area. In the last resort, he said, he would see her safely out of Galatz. And it made, one of the girls observed to her, such a difference, to feel their own men, *Englishmen*, were behind them.[14] 'We were able really to stick on to the last minute and work with quiet minds,'[15] she reported to her Committee; and to Mrs McLaren she wrote, 'When a Scotsman says he'll see us out—I know he'll see us out! When anybody else says it I keep my eye on the means of exit myself.'[16]

On the afternoon of January 4th the evacuation officer for the town ordered Dr Inglis to leave. When she pointed out her instructions to remain till the last moment, he retorted that the last moment had come. In fact, although he did not tell her this, the Russian headquarters staff had gone, at less than twelve hours notice, that morning.[17] He would, he assured her, send ambulances to remove the remaining patients to the station at eight the next morning; several of them were anyway not expected to live through the night.

On going to arrange for Red Cross wagons to move her own equipment to the station, she found that the railway was blocked in both directions. As she debated what to do another message arrived, this time from Commander Gregory: he would take the entire Unit back to Reni that evening in the single barge remaining to him for his own squadron. (Most of his men, supplies and ammunition had been sent back days before; he had kept one squadron for the last defence of the town.[18])

Elsie decided to accept his offer; but that she and four other women should stay overnight to comfort the dying and move the survivors next morning in the promised ambulances. She was not astonished when more than half her staff came privately to beg for the duty.

Late that evening she went to the wharf to see how loading of her equipment was proceeding. While she was there, Mr Scott brought a fresh message from Gregory. *No one at all* was to stay in Galatz.

In fact the opposite bank of the Danube was now in enemy hands; the Germans could be clearly seen moving their artillery up, and a bombardment was expected within hours.[19] But if to Commander Gregory it was clear that he must get the women out, and that the barge which would leave that night was the last chance, to Dr Inglis it was equally clear that she could not leave her hospital while it contained nearly seventy seriously ill men.[20] A year ago, at Kragujevatz, she had taken a vow never again to do this.

'When they realise we are English they are nearly always

confident and friendly,' one girl had remarked at the outset of the work in Galatz.[21] Now was the moment when that confidence must be deserved to the ultimate. Men, in this feckless and disorganised land, could disappear without trace as easily as steriliser drums unless one saw to things personally. Elsie assured Scott that she and her four girls would somehow find their own way out of the doomed town. He knew better than to argue, but ruefully agreed that she was doing the only thing possible.

The barge, with its complement of Tommies,* waited until the small hours, while the women worked clearing the hospital. From that day, 'You must think we are Scottish Sisters, sir' became the ironic response of the Armoured Car men to any request for unusual devotion to duty.[22] At 2 a.m. all was ready. The women embarked, the barge cast off, and they reached Reni within a few hours.

Elsie Inglis and her four companions were left in the almost deserted port; their only companions the wounded and the dying. In the night they worked round the hospital, soothing and comforting where they could, though there was little enough they could do. It was, Gregory was to write later, 'a devotion to duty that was an example to us all'.[23]

The enemy bombardment began at five, and continued for some hours.[24] It was still going on when the last remaining patients were seen off in the Russian ambulances. Dr Inglis said little at the time, even to her sisters; the bombardment she never mentioned at all, but six months later, while writing a routine request for more blankets, her feelings suddenly overflowed at the memory of that morning: 'Those poor men, every single case horribly wounded—some of them dying—I could not put them to the torture of dressing. So we did not attempt it. We simply put on their great coats and our thick stockings and rolled them up in blankets and put them in the ambulances.

'I knew the Committee would approve,' she added, feeling she must somehow justify the fact that she herself had, for once, failed to stick to the equipment and had given away nearly one hundred blankets at Galatz.[25]

By eight all the patients were away. Shells were still falling. The women turned to consider their highly dangerous situation.

* The Armoured Car men were always referred to as Tommies by the S.W.H. They were in fact R.N. and R.N.A.S. personnel, but wore khaki for reasons of camouflage, with naval badges of rank.

Then—it was extraordinary—Commander Gregory, a naval officer of authority and experience, well accustomed to judging what can and cannot be undertaken, reacted just as others had done before: by achieving what he had previously declared to be impossible.

Now, hours after the last possible moment, somehow, from somewhere, another Armoured Car Corps barge materialised down at the wharf.

It must have come from somewhere, though Gregory's own scrupulously detailed reports, with all his barges apparently accounted for elsewhere, give no indication from where; nor do the other records of the Armoured Cars. It was simply there. It was almost enough to justify the belief firmly held by more than one of her Unit, that their Dr Inglis could indeed influence not only persons, but inanimate objects, even from a distance.

The five women were taken off in it at eight. They arrived at Reni only a short while after the main party.

'I hope you have not been anxious about us,' Elsie wrote to Lady Ashmore when she arrived. 'I expect you know by now that we always get out all right ... My third retreat! Surely the luck will change now.'[26]

Many of the Armoured Car Corps were decorated by the Russians for their courage; and some by the Russian Red Cross for their services to the hospital. While it lasted, however, it must have been a very bad few hours for Commander Gregory.

CHAPTER 20

Reni, where Dr Inglis was to remain for the next eight months, was an insignificant town which had achieved sudden importance from its position on the Danube at the confluence with the River Pruth and on the direct rail line to Odessa. The station and the barge port lay among bare, undulating, windswept acres down by the river. The strange little wooden town was half a mile to the north; to the south lay a jumble of railway lines and temporary barracks.

On January 5th the twenty-one members of the Unit were packed into three rooms they had got as temporary quarters, so overcrowded that it was almost a relief when a few days later the 'half-timers', women who had joined for six months only, left for home.[1]

It left Dr Inglis, however, short of staff. She had already telegraphed for replacements. 'Do engage them for a year and get as good a class of girl as you can,' she wrote. 'The better bred they are, the better they stand roughing it.'[2]

Although the danger was not now immediate, the sound of guns on both sides was incessant. They could see Galatz burning. It was uncertain if Reni could be held. Their physical hardships were acute. It was bitterly cold. The mud was knee deep. The only water they could get had to be brought from the Danube in carts. Since they were not now working for the Russians, they had no official rations. On two days they were helped out by the Armoured Car Corps; the little Russian nurse who was so pretty and knew such numbers of officers again proved resourceful in getting supplies.[3] And there was always, of course, porridge.

Dr Inglis left these problems to others, who usually justified her confidence. When, however, she raised with officialdom the question of work for her Unit there were vague, indefinable difficulties, and a few days later she learned that the head of the Red Cross, Ilneachenko, had been removed from his post. 'The Committee will probably not be astonished,' she wrote diplomatically, adding however, 'We were quite sorry for he had been very pleasant to work with.'[4]

The new Red Cross head was Prince Kropensky, a rich Bessarabian landowner. Dr Inglis was delighted—and probably relieved—to discover that he spoke perfect English; he was in fact a golfing man, and thoroughly well acquainted with St Andrews. Businesslike and authoritative, he arranged for Dr Inglis to receive from the Evacuation Hospital at the docks all patients too badly wounded to move on in ambulance trains. 'It is work we are specially fitted for with our well-equipped theatre and our highly-trained nurses,' she wrote.[5]

Kropensky also established them in a building actually designed as a hospital: one-storeyed, built of wood, light, airy, convenient, new, and *clean.* So new that it was not quite complete, they pointed out to her: there had been no time to instal second panes in all the windows. This she brushed aside as a detail; it was one of the best hospital buildings she had ever had. The women's private quarters were also attractive: a curious, comfortable little folly of a house with a tower, standing on high ground near the hospital and commanding glorious views to the Danube and the hills beyond.[6]

With Austrian prisoners detailed as orderlies, men who compared with Russians seemed models of briskness and hygiene, and who to Dr Inglis's surprise could almost all speak something that passed for Russian (for she never fully understood the ethnic and linguistic complications of Eastern Europe), and with a supply of 'real' beds, mere planks across trestles but a luxury to the nurses after weeks of caring for men on palliasses on the floor, even Dr Inglis admitted herself 'well pleased'[7] with the arrangements.

On January 11th, when Kropensky paid his first visit, Mrs Haverfield also arrived from Odessa. She had been organising the transport on her own initiative since being separated from Dr Inglis in the First Dobruga Retreat in October. 'The work the transport has accomplished is wonderful,' Dr Inglis wrote.[8] It was a characteristic understatement. The Transport had taken over the entire task of evacuating the wounded from the Dobruga, Russian ambulances having proved unreliable. Later it had moved all the Russian hospitals out from Tulcea, the last Dobruga town to fall, on to barges on the Danube. Even after these had been moved to safety, the Transport women went back into the Dobruga, picking up wounded stragglers and helping to move small isolated field dressing stations, their cars overcrowded almost to breakdown point, and always with the consciousness of the enemy hard on their heels.

The cars, however, Mrs Haverfield reported now, had been so badly knocked about that they must go to Odessa for repairs and refitting and would be useless until spring.

The weather in early January turned unexpectedly fine and everyone's spirits rose. The lively girls were youthfully resilient and when the 30th Cossack Regiment invited them all to a concert in the mess, Dr Inglis, though 'much amused and a little amazed' (the front line was only five miles off and the guns booming incessantly), agreed that they might all go, chaperoned by Dr Corbett. The entire party danced till midnight and arrived back just in time to receive the first batch of fifty seriously wounded men, with half as many more arriving within a few hours. 'They invited us to another one the next week, too,' Dr Inglis wrote wonderingly.[9]

That was on January 16th. For days they were exceedingly busy again, with the day staff working on until midnight. For the time being all went well. Ration problems were solved now they were working for the open-handed Russians, although Dr Inglis had all along to provide any special diets for patients out of her own resources; and water was brought from the river. They all knew their Danube too well by now to enjoy drinking it, but everyone agreed that soup made with it looked 'lovely, so rich and thick'.[10]

The patients, Dr Inglis was touched to find, seemed happy; begged her to operate on them rather than pass them over to Russian doctors; and pleaded with her not to move them back to base hospitals. She learned from a Captain Bergman, sent by the man-of-the-world Kropensky to replace the helpful little Sister Marie, that in Petrograd there was only one opinion about the organisation and comfort of a Scottish Women's Hospital; though the language, it was said, was always a drawback.[11]

On January 19th they awoke to find ice thick on the windows. General Winter had resumed command. A biting north wind had already drifted snow deep around the hospital block. The need of those double-glazed windows was brought home to Dr Inglis. She installed extra stoves, distributed more blankets, but she could not keep the patients warm; and 'the poor Russians', she wrote to Eve Simson, 'do mind cold so much'.[12]

Once again things—and people—worked together for her. The chief military inspector chose that moment to pay a visit, and the temperature of the wards blotted out all other considerations for him. 'I have no doubt some [glass] will be found,' she wrote.[13]

The cold was to persist well after the middle of March. The winter of 1917 was the hardest of this century, bringing fighting to a standstill everywhere. The guns above the hospital at Reni were silenced; the snow blotted out other noise. It grew more bitter daily. Ten days after the first snow, two wounded men, brought in the usual open carts to the hospital from the wharf less than half a mile away, arrived frozen to death. When the Unit moved their convalescents out, they too went in open carts. The feckless inhumanity of the Russians to their own men appalled the Scottish Women, who noted that the men would not be given so much as straw or blankets if the Unit did not provide them.[14]

By January 22nd the hospital was running smoothly enough to be left with Dr Corbett and Dr Potter while Elsie went to Odessa. It was in good hands. A few days after her departure there was an inspection by a Russian 'military big wig'[15] who examined everything in portentous silence which kept the women on tenterhooks until he pronounced impressively, 'At last—at last, I see women work.'

The journey of 150 miles to Odessa took Dr Inglis four days. The city, when she arrived, was sparkling despite the prevalent war-weariness. Bells tinkled everywhere on the frosty air from sleighs pulled at a spanking pace by horses in brilliant net blankets which streamed out behind them; snow was piled high in the streets, the waves of an unbelievably blue Black Sea danced in the sun.[16]

Dr Inglis had no time to admire the scenery. She spent her time, as she put it, 'going into details' with Mrs Haverfield and Dr Chesney.[17]

Among the 'details' was the wholesale mutiny of the Transport. With a few exceptions they had resigned, and set out for home. The most enterprising and dashing of all the S.W.H. Units, they had also been the quickest to rebel once the strain was eased. Now, young fillies feeling their oats, they were footloose in Russia, and it was worrying. True, they had performed deeds of great courage, initiative, and mechanical expertise, had done things no man had been found to tackle; but they were still young ladies, and guilty of a damaging breach of convention in travelling about the country unchaperoned. It was all highly irregular; but there was nothing to be done about it, Dr Inglis regretfully concluded—except hope that for the credit of the Unit they all went home quickly, and make regulations for other parties travelling, considerably stricter from now on.[18]

Their defection was no problem in itself for the cars were out of commission anyway. It did, however, call Mrs Haverfield's leadership in question.

Dr Inglis was generous in her praise. 'The success of the transport was due to two things—the pluck and staying power of the girls and [Mrs Haverfield's] splendid power of initiative and indomitable spirit. Very few other women could have put it through.'[19]

Her methods, however, and in particular her total indifference to comfort or even regular meals, for herself and for other people, put a great strain upon the young women. Dr Inglis wrote strongly to her Committee and must have expressed herself similarly to Mrs Haverfield. But, she wrote, 'There isn't a particle of ill-will between us. Mrs Haverfield is as generous and open-minded and as ready to face facts as she always was. All we either of us care about is the success of the Unit, and our ideas differ.'[20]

They must have had a hard-hitting discussion for Mrs Haverfield, who believed that dual control—the fact that the Transport was ultimately responsible to Dr Inglis—had occasioned the difficulties, wanted to wire home giving 'dissatisfaction with the leadership' as the reason for the girls' revolt. 'So like her,' commented Dr Inglis drily,[21] and persuaded Mrs Haverfield to go instead to lay her views personally before the Committee at home, taking with her an open letter from Dr Inglis. Mrs Haverfield, the letter said, wanted the Transport to become autonomous. Dr Inglis disagreed. It would hamper the Hospitals, and she questioned whether Mrs Haverfield 'should be allowed to do this until she has shown that she can manage'.[22]

Another, connected, 'detail' was the future of Dr Chesney's hospital, which had been stationed so far away that it was now virtually a separate Unit. And Dr Lilian Chesney, though hard-working, loyal, thorough and a splendid doctor, was not good, either, at handling her staff.

Dr Inglis had hoped to unite all the groups under her own eye in the large premises at Reni. But this posed another intractable 'detail': Dr Chesney and Mrs Haverfield, though they had 'tried heroically', could not hide their antipathy. Elsie now admitted it had been unwise to expect it. After all, she had seen them in Serbia. But she had been sure that knowing the danger, they would avoid it! She had had long talks with them both! They were both such bricks! Each now assured Dr Inglis that she had been perfectly polite to the other. 'Bless them. But the fact remains that they bring out the very worst in one another'[23] she wrote confidentially to Miss Palliser.

She hated to be beaten. She admired each of the women so much that the difficulty seemed absurd. Finally she decided it would be unfair to sacrifice Dr Chesney who had made a success of her work. Mrs Haverfield might be an old friend, a more congenial spirit, a woman personally deserving of the highest degree of love and devotion, but in the interests of the work, Dr Inglis could still wield a hatchet. She wrote privately to the Committee indicating that she would prefer them to accept Mrs Haverfield's resignation.[24] Mrs Haverfield left for England. The two women never met again. Mrs Haverfield to the end of her days held Elsie Inglis as 'the truest and most faithful friend a woman ever had'.[25]

More important than these personal dissensions was the problem which had principally brought her to Odessa. She had come out to work for the Serbs, and after the first weeks at Megidia, was still doing nothing for them.

Both her own hospital and Dr Chesney's—now in Odessa—were full of Russians, although they knew there were thousands of Serbs needing help. The British Red Cross Unit which had gone out for the 2nd Serbian Division was in like case and had been nursing Roumanians; and all efforts by Dr Clemaud, head of that Unit, had failed to get an explanation.

'I think we must get the question settled,' Dr Inglis had written shortly before. 'I know some Serbs are feeling very sore about it—and I imagine somehow think it is our fault . . . But it would be criminal to refuse such work as we had to do at Braila and Galatz, and now at Reni, when the Serbs don't even use the hospital they have got.

'I get on so well with Serbs that I shall probably find out more easily than anybody what is the matter.'[26]

What in fact was the matter was the complicated and bitter relations between the three nations on this front. Roumania had been induced to join the Allies to keep her natural resources out of German hands, but she was for Russia a detestable liability.[27]

Towards Serbia, Russia was in theory more friendly; they shared a common culture, Serbia's hope of leading a pan-Slav Balkan state suited Russia's book, and at the personal level the Serbian Crown Prince was a protégé of the Emperor and suitor for his daughter. But the Serbian Divisions in Russia were a different matter; former subjects of Austria, they had all along been regarded by Russia as a more doubtful quantity.

Serb officers had said to Dr Inglis that Russia would not mind if Serbia were wiped out; in fact would be glad of it. Their fears for their race were not unfounded; when the nations counted their losses after the war, it was found that Serb casualties amounted to 23% of her population* as compared with 3.7% for Great Britain, 8.5% for France and 9.3% for Germany. No small nation can suffer a loss such as Serbia's, drawn moreover entirely from its able-bodied manhood, without coming somewhere near the risk of extinction. Every single man who could be saved from the débâcle strengthened the hope for the future.

Feeling between the Serbians and the Roumanians was equally bitter. Nobody lightly voiced to Dr Inglis criticisms of Britain or Serbia; at this time Mrs Milne, the Unit's cook, in Odessa for treatment for neuritis, was finding that people were saying England was making too much profit to wish the war to end;[28] but the way Roumanians were putting it to Dr Inglis was that everyone was now trusting to Britain's staying power. Now, however, criticisms of Serbia were made even to her, and she was told more than once, with a sneer, that the Serbs had stated they would fight for their own country but refused to help Roumania. Her retort, predictably, was that she felt sure this did not represent the facts.[29]

The Serbian Commander in Odessa, Colonel Geraitch, when she asked for an explanation, put a more acceptable complexion on things. The authorities, he said, realised that many more fights such as the Serbs had put up in the Dobruga would virtually exterminate their nation. They did not feel it their duty to protect Roumania at so great a cost. 'The duty of defending Roumania is a Russian duty, not ours,' Geraitch affirmed. 'When Roumania has been retaken, and the advance is again properly organised, the Serb Divisions are ready to take their share again.' This point of view, he told her, had been fully laid before the

* *Geographical Statistical Atlas,* Professor Hichmann.

Czar (at this stage still in personal command of his armies) and received his sympathy and approval.[30]

But the Czar was a thousand miles away and the Serbian Divisions were entirely dependent upon local Russian commanders for their rations, equipment, uniforms, transport, everything. Supplies were so short that one unit had to be kept indoors for weeks because they had no boots, and deficiency diseases had begun to affect the men's health.[31]

Dr Inglis had known some of this, and guessed some. Now she found herself deeply touched at the full realisation of how difficult the position of these volunteer Divisions had become, how gloomy the future looked to them, what trust they seemed to repose in the British in general—and in the Scottish Women in particular.

There was no question of either Division going into action yet, Geraitch told her. Indeed, there was the chance that both Divisions would be sent to Salonika later in the year.

After discussion, she asked what he would like her to do. They spent a further hour and a half working out a joint plan. It was clear to them both that the Russians really needed hospitals for the front. Not only had they 'borrowed' the Scottish Women's Hospital and the Red Cross Unit, but they had taken over one of the purely Serbian *lazarettes* for their own, giving the usual undertaking to return them all when needed.

In the meantime an order had been made that Serbian sick or long-term wounded should be treated in Russian hospitals. When Dr Inglis asked if this was indeed a good plan, Geraitch answered promptly, 'No. It would be much better to have a Serbian hospital.'[32]

'Then,' she persisted, 'shall I insist on our two hospitals working for you at once?' She had no doubt that what she insisted upon, she would get. But Geraitch dissuaded her. He believed it would help their cause more in the long run to do what the Russians wanted now. Moreover, he had no means of rationing a hospital; when the Divisions went to the front their hospitals would be rationed as part of the whole operation by the Russians, but until then, the Russians would supply nothing.

Dr Inglis next suggested that she might take her Unit home until it was needed by the Serbians.

'You must not go.' Geraitch was emphatic. Was it purely the usefulness of the hospitals he had in mind? Or had he some premonition that by keeping her where she was, Dr Inglis might some day be in the position to render the Serbian Divisions an even greater service? 'You really help us by doing this for the Russians,' he repeated emphatically several times. It was clear that the Hospitals had become a bargaining counter in the hand of the Serbs; a counter, though neither Geraitch nor Dr Inglis knew it then, which would one day tip the balance against annihilation.

'Is there, then, anything we can do directly for you now?' was her last question. There was. They were very short of certain drugs and she promised to wire home for supplies.

'I know the Committee would have been very touched', she wrote home in confirmation, 'if they could have talked to Colonel Geraitch and realised how difficult the position of these volunteer Divisions is here—and not only that but how gloomy things look to these men—and how they seem to trust us. The money spent on drugs will do a great deal more than merely supply the drugs—it will be one more proof to them that we care.

'Perhaps Dr Potter could bring out the whole consignment,' she added. She had just learned that another huge consignment sent to her by rail with no one in charge had disappeared without trace at Jassy. *'I hope the Committee will make a point of seeing Dr Potter.'*[33]

Dr Lena Potter, going on leave, was to be the first of several emissaries Dr Inglis sent home charged with verbal messages. The situation was more complex than she could explain in any letter likely to pass the censor. She wrote a long confidential report of her talk with Geraitch, decided it was too frank and replaced it with a shorter version, adding, 'Would the Committee think it advisable to allow the Serbian Legation to see this report as it is most important they should understand? Probably also they will be able to explain various points too.'

These problems kept Dr Inglis in Odessa until the second week of February. Just before returning to Reni a small incident cheered her.

She had gone to the station to enquire about her train, and a Russian officer there approached her deferentially. 'You are the Commandant of the automobiles, are you not?'

'Yes,' she replied. 'The cars belong to us.'

'They have done magnificently,' he told her.

Dr Inglis's eyes must have shone with pleasure, and she

murmured that it was very kind of him to say so; she thought they had done pretty well. Noticing a map on the wall, she began to point out to him where the Transport and hospitals had been operating.

A puzzled look spread over his face. After a minute he said, doubtfully, 'Yours are the automobiles that carry cannon—are they not?'

He had believed, and perhaps it was not surprising after what happened at Galatz, that she, a woman, was in command of the Royal Naval Air Service Armoured Cars. She hid her amusement, and explained to him gravely that *her* cars were simply for carrying the wounded.

'I should have said something more than "pretty well" if I had known he was talking about the Armoured Cars,' she wrote to Miss Palliser. 'For they have done "magnificently". And as one was not their Commandant, one could have said so.'[34]

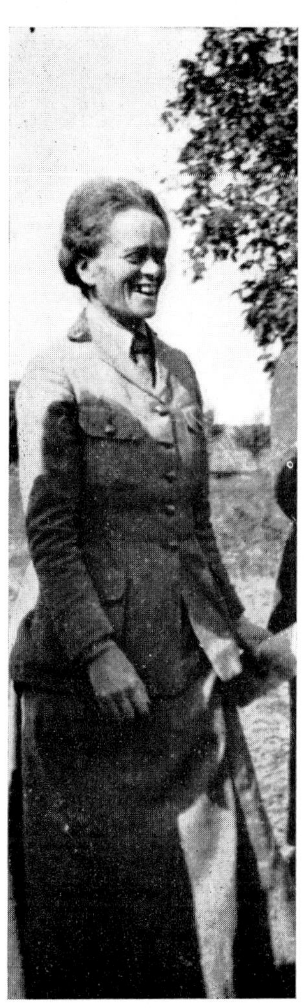

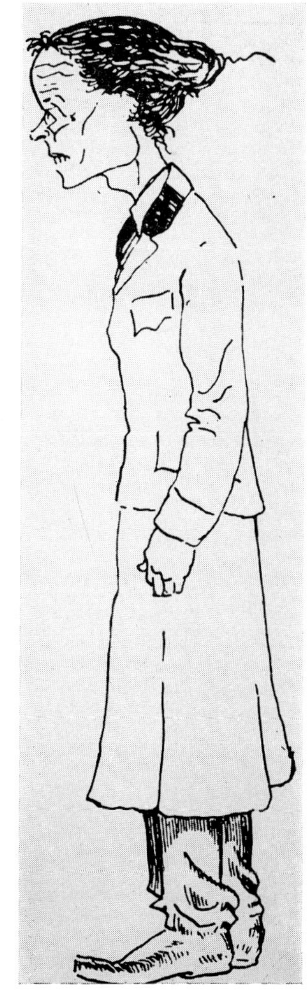

Right Dr Elsie Inglis, drawn in the late summer of 1917, by Sibe Miličića *Left* Dr Elsie Inglis, late summer 1917.

THE DAILY MIRROR, Saturday, December 1, 1917.

GERMANS ON GUNFIRE ON THE WESTERN FRONT

The Daily Mirror

CERTIFIED CIRCULATION LARGER THAN THAT OF ANY OTHER DAILY PICTURE PAPER

No. 4,401. Registered at the G.P.O. as a Newspaper. SATURDAY, DECEMBER 1, 1917. One Penny.

WOUNDED.

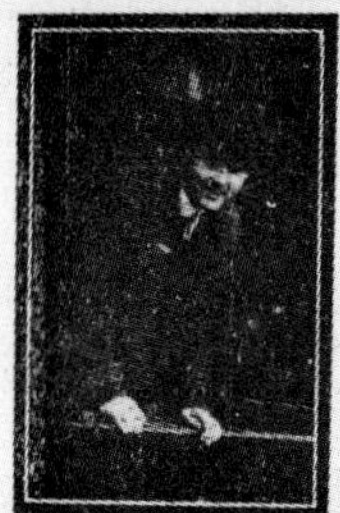

Captain Lord Folkestone, Wiltshire Regiment, son of the Earl of Radnor, who has been wounded in Palestine.

M.P.'s DAUGHTER TO WED

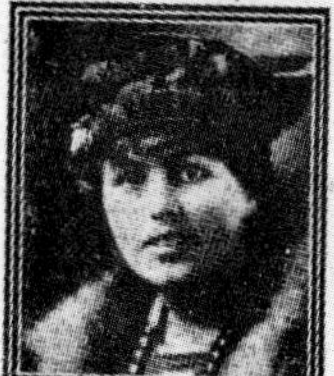

Florence, daughter of Mr. John R. Starkey, M.P., to marry Major B. T. Wilson, R.E., eldest son of Mr. Alexander Wilson, F.R.C.S.

SERBIANS' LAST TRIBUTE TO WOMAN DOCTOR

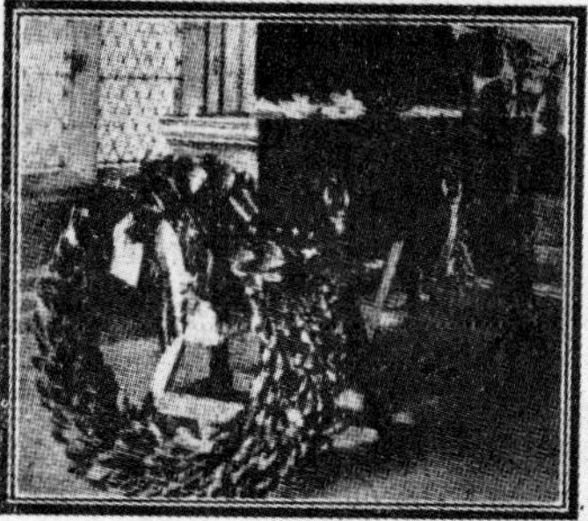

The coffin lying in St. Giles' Cathedral, Edinburgh.

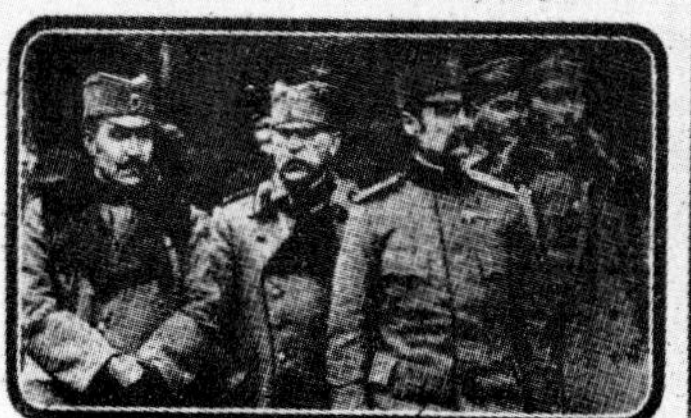

The Serbian Minister and other members of the Legation.

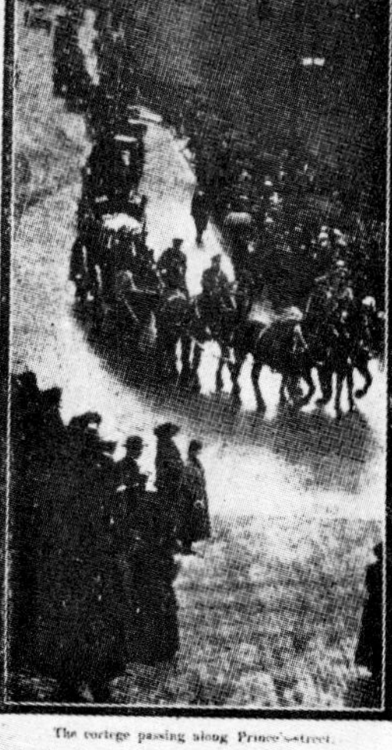

The cortege passing along Prince's-street.

Dr. Elsie Inglis, a pioneer of the Scottish Women's Hospital, was buried at Edinburgh with military honours, the coffin being borne on a gun-carriage drawn by six horses. Dr. Inglis was in the Serbian and Rumanian retreats, and was made prisoner by the Enemy. The Serbian Minister was among the mourners.

NAVAL MEN DECORATED—AN HONOUR CONFERRED BY FRANCE.

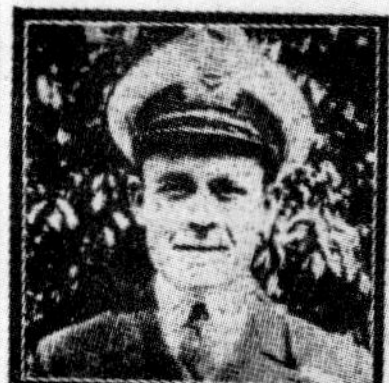

Flight Lieutenant Basil Deacon Hobbs, D.S.O., D.S.C., R.N.A.S., who has now been awarded a bar to his Distinguished Service Cross.

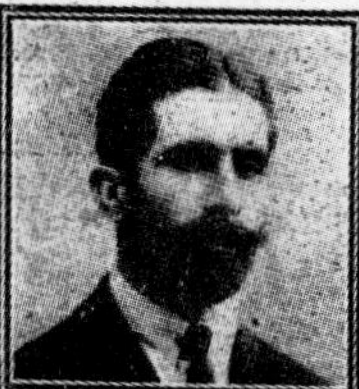

Wing Commander C. L. Courtney, R.N.A.S., awarded the D.S.O. The wing under his command has invariably shown a high standard of efficiency.

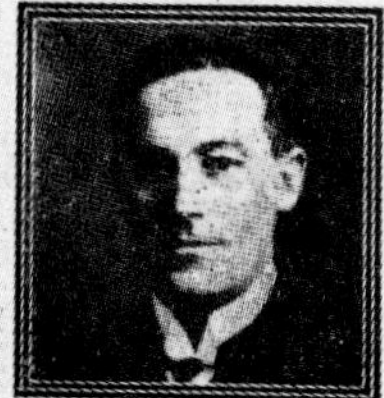

Lieutenant Commander Daniel McDowell, D.S.O., R.N., on whom the President of the French Republic has conferred the Croix de Guerre.

ACT OF SACRIFICE.

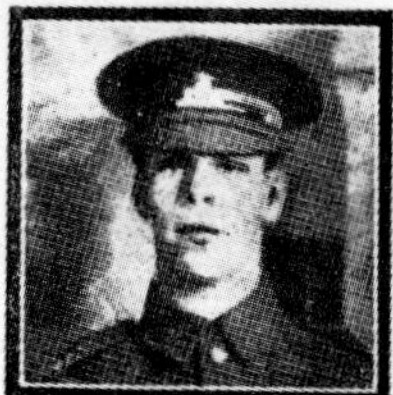

Private W. J. John, Lancashire Fusiliers, who, while lying wounded in a hospital in France, voluntarily gave a pint of his blood to a comrade, thus saving his life.

The front page of the *Daily Mirror*, 1st December, 1917.

CHAPTER 21

When Elsie returned to Reni in mid-February, the hospital on its hill was exposed to biting blizzards and the temperature was minus thirty degrees centigrade. The patients, fortunately few since the frost had stopped hostilities not only here but all over Europe, were moved into one single ward, for fuel for the stoves was almost impossible to come by. Food was equally scarce, and for water they were now drinking melted snow, more palatable than Danube water. Twenty horses were given to Dr Inglis by the Russians, to cart supplies, but nothing whatever on which to feed them, and the women gave their own black bread to the brutes. (Although they did not know it, railway disorganisation with its consequence of lack of fodder was a chief cause of Russia's military failure, and at this time all cavalry units were being reduced.[1]) The incident strengthened Dr Inglis's conviction that she had done the right thing about the Transport; her hospital must never be less than independent in this respect.[2]

By the 25th the Danube was frozen from bank to bank ('so nice of it to do it just when we are here! I would not have missed it for anything'[3]) and now her twenty carts could drive a mile across the ice to collect wood from the Roumanian bank. Bergman developed a gift of solving the ration problem and 'getting things even when he had been told the things did not exist'; while Matron Vizard, hitherto gentle and ineffectual, also suddenly developed a gift of initiative and became a tower of strength.[4]

Elsie badly needed someone of the kind now. Mrs Haverfield and Dr Potter had gone home; Dr Corbett been posted to assist Dr Chesney. At Reni, her only medical colleague was now Dr Laird, who replaced Dr Potter: another veteran of Serbia and a delightful woman, but very young.

Elsie, ill, ageing, and overworked, acutely felt the burden of lonely leadership. When Miss Palliser wrote that she herself might chaperone a party of new orderlies travelling out, Elsie responded warmly. 'Do you really *mean* you could come out?—

Because if you do—do come—and not to look after the orderlies—but after the Unit—as Administrator. I never dared to hope for such luck as getting *you*. It would be such a help ... Dear Miss Palliser, I do hope you will be here soon.'[5] Miss Palliser, however, never came.

The fact of having only one doctor at Reni besides herself had another serious aspect. On March 3rd the Russian Chief of Medical Staff descended on them for an inspection, 'and that was indeed a thorough inspection. The men's pyjama suits were taken off and searched for lice; the sheets were turned up and the mattresses beaten to see if they were dusty; the food was tasted and the orderlies' room raided. The Report eventually ran that the patients were *ochin cheste* (very clean), well cared for medically, and well nursed; but that the condition of the orderlies was disgraceful. This report is absolutely true. But the condition of the orderlies shall no longer remain "disgraceful".'[6]

The orderlies had been lousy. Bergman had always insisted that he was in charge of them, but now the Chief of Medical Staff asked Dr Inglis abruptly, 'Do you hold yourself responsible for the condition of the orderlies?'

'Yes,' she replied briskly. 'And the next time you come you will not find a single louse.' The old gentleman chuckled with pleasure. Not only could women work; here was one who could accept responsibility. But Dr Inglis made a mental note to settle once for all with Kropensky the question of Bergman's duties.[7]

The inspection was almost certainly connected with the typhus then breaking out along the front. In Roumania, Barclay reported secretly to the Foreign Office, the disease reached epidemic proportions in March and April but was hushed up for security reasons.[8] Strangely, Dr Inglis seems to have been unaware of it, and nobody in authority thought fit to enlighten her. If she really did not know of it—and all the evidence is that she did not—it is an indication of how completely the language barrier isolated the Scottish Women.

At all events, at about the same time, a patient with a puzzling fever was admitted. Dr Inglis sat on his bed for twenty minutes examining him. Not till ten days later did the characteristic spotted typhus rash appear. It spoke well for the hospital, she said with mild complacency, that no other case appeared although the man had been in a crowded ward all that time.

She realised with a qualm, however, that she herself might

easily have caught the disease, leaving young Dr Laird in sole charge of dozens of patients whose language she could not speak and of a bunch of women needing much tact to control.[9]

Elsie Inglis was not alarmist; it is accepted that in typhus, medical personnel are at special risk; and her concern was entirely for the future of the hospital. One can also, however, see in this incident an indication that her own health was beginning to turn traitor, and that private anxieties as to how long she could carry on, were perhaps rationalised as a risk of typhus.

By early March the weather was colder than ever. On March 1st Elsie awoke to the memory of one of the happiest days of her life: it was just one year since she had arrived in Scotland from her imprisonment in Serbia, and the memory of 'all you dear people at home', of the little rose-patterned bedroom in her sister's house, and the security of what must have seemed almost another existence, swept over her in a wave of nostalgia.[10]

Next day the worst blizzard of the winter brought deep drifts of snow almost cutting off the staff quarters from the hospital. Day after day the women struggled through it in their top boots, their skirts shortened to mid-calf. Night after night the enemy searchlights played over the hospital; occasionally shelling was heard from Galatz, ten miles away, which had never fallen and where the Armoured Cars still had some men. Over the front as a whole the lull continued.[11]

Dr Inglis opened a small out-patients' department for units of the Reni division; and it was found that the reputation earned there, helped a good deal in handling new in-patients. When work allowed, the girls went in turns to Odessa for leave. At Reni they enjoyed a lively existence, were made much of by the Armoured Car men passing through, and invited to a variety of entertainments by the Russians. Chaperoning her girls to these affairs exhausted the little doctor far more than the clock-round operations at Galatz had done; for Dr Laird, although a veteran of the Serbian typhus epidemic and the Great Retreat, could not chaperone the girls 'as she is so young herself'.[12] Elsie owned she was thankful when Lent put a stop to such amusements, and officers merely came instead to take tea.

One of these in particular impressed her with his command of English, his knowledge of English history, his advocacy of the Commonwealth as undoubtedly the most interesting period of all European history, and his remarkable familiarity with, of all things, the political writings of Milton. When she complimented him, he replied, a little surprisingly, that he had had an English nanny.[13]

Social life might be outwardly urbane, but the physical problems of mere existence became ever more acute. 'Some people will always wash, but others will only do so if it is made easy for them,' said Dr Inglis and ordered buckets of icy water distributed to the rooms of the staff.[14] Occasionally brilliant sunshine would bring an illusion of spring, to be quickly followed by more snow and biting winds. By mid-March, however, it was thawing. Out walking in glorious sunshine during their off-duty on the 17th, some of the women found the road flooded in places with melting snow; two days later the Danube was flowing freely.[15]

Spring, however, had come too late. The Scottish Women had found it hard to struggle through the winter. For the poverty-ridden Russian masses, the economic disorganisation it brought had proved, at last, too heavy to bear. On March 11th massed demonstrations in Petrograd were fired on by soldiers; the next day army units in the city refused to obey their officers. On the 15th the Emperor Nicholas II abdicated. The Revolution was in being.

CHAPTER 22

The first news of the Revolution reached Reni and the Scottish women on March 18th, from soldiers who had just heard it from the enemy radio transmitters beyond the Danube. The women saw that the effect upon the whole army was electric. No one could think or speak of anything else. Everyone was beaming, there was the wildest enthusiasm and confidence everywhere, all were on the side of the change. The Russian officers who came to tea replied to Dr Inglis's questions with beaming smiles and an emphatic '*Harosho*' (good).[1] Defeatism had vanished, there was a renewal of enthusiasm for continuing the war.[2]

A few days later the women splashed through the mud to Reni's first Free Speech Revolutionary Meeting[3] in the old market square, much beflagged in scarlet for the occasion and with frequent mournful Slavic renderings of the 'Marseillaise'. The gist of the speeches was the duty of citizens to continue the war and defend Russian soil; and the women were deeply moved when the mass of men knelt, cap in hand, on the cobbles, and with bowed heads sang the 'Kontakion' for their comrades killed in the Petrograd fighting.[4]

There seemed no reason to believe the change would adversely affect the hospital, and Dr Inglis's comments in letters were characteristic. They had all been 'awfully excited and interested in the news' and it was 'most interesting to see how everybody is on the side of the change'. She had been having second thoughts about the officer so well-versed in the Commonwealth and Milton's writings; had he perhaps meant more than she had understood?[5]

The army authorities in the area had the situation well in hand, and took pains to maintain morale in the face of new regulations relaxing discipline.* All leave was stopped, revolutionary notions from big cities being more infectious than typhus;

* On this front at any rate, the famous decree abolishing the death penalty in the army, was in practice superseded by sentences of flogging of such severity that death in fact resulted. Stanojevitch, p. 137.

and Prince Dolgourokoff, who commanded in the area, made a hastily arranged round of visits to units.

He took Dr Inglis entirely by surprise, arriving on March 20th well in advance of the telegram announcing him. She was thankful she had impressed on the Unit that they had as commandant an old maid who could not stand dirt and muddle; and found, showing the tall and handsome Dolgourokoff and his 'gilded staff' around, that even she could feel *fairly* satisfied with the hospital 'in its ordinary' and that it was *almost* worthy of having the Union Jack over it.

Two or three very severely wounded patients were decorated with the St George's Medal 'for bravery under fire', and one young sergeant got the St George's Cross, the dream of all Russian soldiers. Then the prince had the staff assembled and gave each of the Scottish Women the Medal, and posed good-humouredly for photographs, and complimented the matron. When asked about the Revolution, however, his gilded staff were markedly uncommunicative.[6]

The rapport between the women and their patients was unprecedentedly high. The women already respected the 'brave and patient men', now the men rejoiced at the honour to their 'little sisters from Scotland' and impressed upon them that the Medal carried a pension of one rouble (one and sixpence) a month for life. To the men this meant much. The Russian soldier of 1917 was paid seventy-five kopeks, about one and twopence a month, and had no hope of leave, little or no news of home, and the knowledge that in the event of disablement, he would be turned off with a gratuity of ten roubles (fifteen shillings) and possibly a licence to beg.[7]

Three days later rapport rose even higher. Elsie had come to realise how much religion meant to the Russian soldier in this land where (as the British Military attaché, Knox, personally witnessed) a general could, in a discussion of professional technicalities, quite simply and naturally interject 'You must always remember too the value of prayer—with prayer you can do anything.'[8] She asked Sister Kolesnikoff, the Russian nurse now attached as interpreter, whether they would like ikons in the wards; and was told that it would indeed make a great deal of difference to the men.

So four ikons were bought, and a bearded army priest, a green and gold vestment thrown over his grey greatcoat, came to the main ward. The ikons were there, with candles, a crucifix, a bowl of holy water. Prayers were chanted, the patients crossing themselves and making the responses with great heartiness. Holy water was sprinkled over the ikons and the men. Then the ikons were put in the corners of the wards, with tiny lamps burning always before them. When, in the evening, the men turned to the ikons and sang their evening hymn, Elsie's mind went back eighteen months: she had first heard that hymn sung by Russian prisoners in the barrack yard at Krushevatz. And when Russian officers said to her 'Indeed, Madame, that was a kind thought', she was, she admitted, much touched.[9]

She still felt impelled to justify to her insular, practical, and Protestant Committee the spending of forty-five shillings for the ikons and the priest. 'When I tell the Committee of our next adventure I am sure they will think the money was well spent', she wrote (again the voice of Inglis Sahib), 'for it is a great thing in a foreign country to show the people that one has sympathy for them.'[10]

The next adventure was indeed potentially serious. Dr Inglis, and Miss Agnes Murphy, an orderly, were arrested as spies.

Spy fever was rampant all along the front, for the Central Powers were taking full advantage of the disorganisation brought about by the Revolution.[11] Moreover, fresh troops who knew nothing of the Scottish Women's Hospital were arriving in the area, their lax discipline, boorish manners and unpredictable upsurges of violence and hostility reflecting the new influences at work in Russia as a whole—so much so that some Armoured Car men who visited the hospital at the end of March were markedly pessimistic about the Revolution: the first time the women had heard this note sounded.

One evening while Elsie and three companions were playing bridge, their quaint little folly of a house with its pagoda-like tower was invaded by half a dozen unkempt soldiers who addressed the women brusquely in Russian. Sister Kolesnikoff, summoned to interpret, explained that contrary to appearances, these uncouth men were officers, who had come about some signalling from the tower. Elsie, assuming they wished to use the tower for signalling, began to escort them upstairs, but found her way barred by a soldier with fixed bayonet. After a good deal of altercation she was allowed to go to the first floor and remain there while Sister Kolesnikoff took the men to the tower.

The lower room meanwhile filled with soldiers, undisciplined and rude. And when Sister Kolesnikoff returned, she was distressed. She had got the whole story: coloured lights seen from the tower, a regular morse system, signals to the enemy, it was said. The whole house was surrounded by sentries and it took all Dr Inglis's force to get permission for her routine night visit to the hospital. When she returned, sentries were posted round the house for the night.

Five minutes after Dr Inglis's return, there was another invasion, this time by the Commander of the Expeditionary Force in person. He arrested Miss Murphy, an Irish girl of singular beauty and charm,[12] who slept in the tower room and had charge of some stores there, and she was allowed only time to pull on some clothes over her pyjamas before being taken, under escort, to his office for questioning. Dr Inglis insisted upon going with her.

Even now the implications had not dawned upon them. Cut off by the language barrier, they knew little of the tales circulating in Russia, of the local outbreaks of sudden, irrational violence among those who had been so long oppressed and who now took affairs into their own hands, in response to their own whims. 'This is perfectly intolerable,' Dr Inglis burst out at Murphy's arrest, adding, 'I think we must go back to our Serbs who would never have doubted us.'[13] She had no conception that this could possibly be placed beyond her power to do.

She supposed that a few simple answers to questions would clear up the matter.[14] When the women reached the Commandant's office, however, they were pushed into a small room and the door locked harshly behind them. No one put questions to them, or gave them any chance to clear themselves. Twelve hours passed. They remained in close confinement, and were refused permission to get in touch with Kropensky, or with the British Consul in Odessa.

At last help came. It had taken hours, but Matron Vizard at last discovered their whereabouts. Then she approached their old friend Visolskin, who still commanded the Danube Russian Flotilla at Reni. Even Visolskin had to walk warily in the new Russia, but he suggested a compromise solution—the whole Unit was to sign a guarantee of Murphy's 'fidelity', in effect to go bail for her—and this secured the release of the two women. It was humiliating, when they had been held on no charge but purely on the whim of the revolutionaries. However, Dr Inglis had to accept it; until she was free she could take no steps to establish the Unit's integrity.

Then she hurried to Commander Gregory whose yacht was at Reni, and an Armoured Car despatch rider went post haste to Kropensky. Returning to the house, she found her rooms had been searched and, it was said, incriminating objects had been found. The whole affair was taking a grimmer turn than she had anticipated. It was almost a relief to give way to laughter when the incriminating objects turned out to be some coloured medicines from Miss Murphy's stores; but it pointed up the ignorance and irrationality of the men with whom they had now to deal.

Kropensky's arrival late that evening was the signal for explanations all round. The colonel of the offending regiment also appeared, profuse in apologies and excuses. Dr Inglis, not at once appeased, retorted that if spies existed, naturally no one was more anxious than she for them to be found. She lectured him at length upon the care with which her staff were chosen and dragged him across to ask if the patients had complaints. The patients and orderlies, more in awe of Dr Inglis than of anyone else, declared they had never heard anything so ridiculous as suspecting the little sisters from Scotland of spying.

The colonel was a kindly man, fatherly in the way of so many Imperial Russian officers, and annoyed at the behaviour of his subordinates; but now he was no longer certain of his control over them. He intended, he said, to address the regiment on the subject that afternoon; but if he should make no impression, it would be a favour if Dr Inglis and Kropensky would put in an appearance.

The meeting went well, however, and Kropensky departed. Even while he was taking his leave, Miss Broadbent, another of the women, who had gone out for a walk, was placed under arrest by two private soldiers and marched before the town commandant. She managed to signal to two friends, and Dr Inglis was summoned. The town commandant turned out to be an old acquaintance from that disastrous journey to Ciulnitza in December. He too was profuse in apologies and explanations. He kept, however, two books belonging to Broadbent.

'As you can imagine, this last incident simply added fuel to the dying flames of our wrath and the whole thing blazed up again', wrote Dr Inglis to her Committee. 'I must say I think the Unit would hardly have been British if they had not been angry ... However during the night I realised that we might do a great deal of harm by simply throwing up our work and going away leaving so false an impression of British subjects behind us. I also realised as a result of the long talks I had had with General Kropensky and the Colonel of the Regiment that in common fairness we must look at the other side—a country in revolution with all the disorganisation which must inevitably accompany so great a change, even if that change be beneficial. The undoubted presence of spies all along the Front and the fact that foreigners by the ordinary people in any country are always regarded with suspicion ... Taking all these things into consideration and realising that we should make these men understand that Great Britain is absolutely loyal and intends to carry this war through, I spoke to the Unit next morning. I think everybody saw the point for several said to me that it would never do to go away leaving the thing uncleared.'[15]

It hardly occurred to her that it might not be within her power to take her Unit away and leave the thing uncleared; that in other parts of Russia incidents were occurring of inoffensive people being shot out of hand on mere suspicion. Jivkovitch himself and his chief of staff were at about this time placed under close arrest by a Soldiers' and Workmen's Committee, and only released on the intervention of the British Ambassador in Petrograd.[16] As much now as at any time before, Dr Inglis was conscious of 'the whole might of the British Empire' at her back.

From then on, however, things improved. Men crowding the out-patients' clinic were punctilious with salutes. A telegram of 'heartiest regret' was received from General Zourikoff commanding the 6th Army, to which she responded with the cordiality she could feel for an opponent wise enough to climb down. Two sergeants arrived on their own initiative—representing the new Free Speech Revolution spirit of the army, she said—to express personal regrets over the business. Kropensky congratulated her upon her English *sang-froid* and *savoir faire* which had saved the situation. 'I am afraid', she commented tartly, 'there was not much *sang-froid* among us, but some of us managed to keep hold of our common sense.' Visolskin was reported to her to have said, 'I told these fools they were going about it the wrong way. You can give orders to Russians—but the English are not in the habit of obeying orders.' 'What a libel on the most law-abiding nation in Europe,' Dr Inglis indignantly wrote to Miss Palliser. 'I told them we always obeyed orders if we recognised the authority.'[17]

And when, on April 15th, the Orthodox Easter, Dr Inglis was presented with a letter from all her patients, who, like the two sergeants, clearly did not consider that demonstrations from generals and admirals fully met the case, she was able to feel the spy incident had even strengthened her position.

To the much-honoured Elsie Maud Ivanovna the letter, written for the Patients' Committee by Sister Kolesnikoff,[18] began: and the Russian patronymic must have delighted her who never forgot that she was 'the daughter of John'. She sent a translation* to her committee.

> We, all the patients, sick and wounded, belonging to the Army and Navy and coming from different parts of the Great Free Russia, who are at present in your hospital, are filled with feelings of the truest respect for you. We think it our duty as Citizens on this beautiful day of Holy Easter to express to you, highly respected and much beloved Doctor, as well as to your whole Unit, our best thanks for all the care and attention you have bestowed upon us. We bow low and very respectfully before the constant and useful work which we have seen daily and which we know to be for the well-being of our allied countries.
>
> We are quite sure that, thanks to the complete unity of action of all the allied countries, the hour of gladness and the triumph of the allied arms in the cause of humanity and the honour of nations is near.
>
> Vive l'Angleterre.
> Russian Soldiers, Citizens, and the
> Russian Sister, Vera V. de Kolesnikoff.

After producing their letter, the patients shared the traditional Easter food of white bread, painted eggs, Easter cake and wine. The women had their evensong in the afternoon, beautifully read as usual by their Dr I., with three Easter hymns and a sung

* The original has not survived. Two slightly different translations exist. That given here was made on the spot at the time, probably by Sister Kolesnikoff. A different version in *A History of the Scottish Women's Hospitals*, ed. Mrs McLaren, seems to indicate that Elsie Inglis kept the original until her death.

Magnificat she had got them to rehearse; an Armoured Car man was present and, she wrote with a certain wistfulness, 'it was nice to have a man's voice in the singing'.[19]

Later there was a party in the wards, with tossing for the doctors, cheers for the Russian dead, and even an attempt to get dancing going; it was unsuccessful either because the men were shy or unversed in the polka,[20] or perhaps just because, as one of them was overheard to say a few days later, 'The Russian sisters are pretty but they are not good—the English sisters are good but they are not pretty.'[21] In the evening however, the girls were invited to a more formal dance, by the officers of the 195th. The period of festivities and chaperonage had begun again for their Dr I.

CHAPTER 23

By the Orthodox Easter, spring had transformed the steppe around Reni with irises, soft grey willows, carpets of violets and scarlet windflowers, cherry trees in bloom. Wild geese were flying north, storks nesting or balancing in blue, reed-fringed pools. Fairy-tale villages of quaint whitewashed houses were seen hidden among acacia trees or set in orchards of apricot and almond blossom; between were vineyards and streams and flocks of sheep watched by tiny shepherd boys.[1]

Just to feel warm was delicious, and Dr Inglis had tents pitched for their sleeping quarters. By day it was even hot enough for her to worry about sun hats and summer uniforms; soon the sun became so strong as to bleach every scrap of colour from the year-old medal ribbons she wore.[2]

Riding was the women's newest off-duty pastime. Their twenty horses were not now overworked and with strange padded Cossack saddles they ranged far and wide. Dr Inglis joined in. A photograph[3] shows her beaming delightedly like a child having its first seaside donkey ride when, at the decorous age of fifty-two, she flung to the winds the conventions of her youth, and rode astride for the very first time; she even childishly enjoyed careering across the vast expanse of the steppe when a single shot from an anti-aircraft gun set the horses off: 'we just sat tight and *went*'.[4]

They were beginning now—like the Armoured Car men—to revise their ideas about the beneficial effect of the Revolution. Among the local soldiers' committees, support for the Scottish Women's Hospital was still strong. Matron Vizard, coming from arranging for supplies at the commandant's office, was greeted by a crowd of soldiers who asked if she had got what she needed. She replied that it was in the commandant's hands. The men retorted, shouting, 'The commandant must be told that the *Schottlandsche bolnitza* is the best hospital on this front and must have whatever it wants. That is the opinion of the Russian soldier.'[5]

As early as April 9th, however, there were rumours of mutiny and desertion at Galatz.[6] Odessa had been a hotbed ever since the *Potemkin* affair. And elsewhere in Russia the unrest which was showing itself among the troops spread also to hospitals, where patients' committees dictated hours for doctors' visits, times of meals, and other matters of organisation, making established routines unworkable. The Anglo-Russian Hospital in Petrograd, for instance, actually had to close because of the intractability of the patients.[7]

Dr Inglis had one, and only one, manifestation of this kind. 'There is a sailor in the hospital from the Expedition, who plays the violin and sings beautifully. But he is rather a troublesome patient in that he thinks he can go out whenever he likes to visit the Regiments round about,' she wrote on May 27th. She may have guessed, though she did not say so, that the man was engaged in spreading propaganda and disaffection—sailors were always more active revolutionaries than were soldiers. 'However, I have put a stop to that with a firm hand. There is no good trying to keep the hospital clean if the men go out and stay for hours in dirty barracks.'[8] Just what kind of firm hand she used, is not clear; but it seems to have held the Russian Revolution in check in the area under her personal command. We hear no more of trouble along these lines, and one is tempted to speculate, tantalisingly, on what might have happened to the course of history if her sphere of influence had been larger!

Soon after Easter Lenin arrived in Petrograd from Germany; but as yet Kerensky, urging discipline and a continuance of the war, spoke with the more persuasive voice. On April 21st the Scottish Women learned from two Armoured Car men that enemy aeroplanes had dropped leaflets in Russian in the trenches,[9] abusing the English and saying England was responsible for the deposition of the Emperor; the first recorded instance, and the possible source, of that curious *canard* which has ever since been current, to the effect that Kerensky's Revolution was first hatched in the British Embassy. On the following day came the first rumour that Russia intended a separate peace.

It was only a rumour. The signs were of an impending offensive and Dr Chesney's hospital had been ordered to another sector of the front in readiness. 'She wrote me a very cheerful letter,' reported Dr Inglis. 'She went up to the Serb headquarters to say goodbye. They expect we shall have to join them soon. She added the startling remark "I was kissed by everybody" but added "fortunately only on the hand". She is a most amusing person.'[10]

By now the girls noticed that their Dr I. was getting distinctly restless for news of a transfer back to the Serbs.[11] Work in the hospital was slack and there was an average of only forty in the wards. Two of them were Vaughn and Eckroyd, men of the Armoured Cars, wounded near Galatz in April. 'It is very nice having one's own countrymen to look after,'[12] Dr Inglis wrote, and got herself into a complicated muddle trying to spoil them with special delicacies at meals without risking a charge of favouritism from the Russian patients; coming at last to the conclusion that she was not born to be a conspirator.

On May 8th there was a welcome break in the sense of isolation. Miss Henderson arrived from England, having been two months on the journey, with a large consignment of equipment and a quantity of letters and news. Some of it was excellent. Money was rolling in for the S.W.H. and the other Units were all doing valuable work. Elsie learned that her old friend Mrs Harley, who had been administering civilian relief in the recaptured front-line town of Monastir, in Serbia, had been killed by a shell splinter just after finishing a distribution of bread. 'How terribly sad,' wrote Elsie to Miss Palliser. 'And yet I don't know. There was something just right about it. It was what you would have expected of her, to die in harness.'[13]

With Miss Henderson had come from Petrograd a chaplain of the English colony, Mr French, who was spending his leave visiting scattered British groups. This was a joy to Elsie.[14] The daily services read by herself from the Euchologion were all very well; but only a priest could administer the Holy Communion which touched the sacramental essence of her life. A little tent was put up, an altar improvised of packing cases draped with sheets. At the service she knelt in deep meditation from which she had to be roused to receive the sacrament. It was in fact to be the last time she did so. To those with her (writing with hindsight, it must be said) it seemed that 'her soul was reaching out beyond this present consciousness and that her spirit was already dwelling in "the secret place of the most High".'[15]

Mr French was also a practical man. He had helped Miss Henderson bring all the equipment through safely, for constant supervision was needed to defeat the established system whereby railway officials customarily listed and passed on only 75% of goods, retaining the rest for private speculation.[16] Some consignments sent to Dr Inglis had entirely vanished; and of blankets, drugs, needles and food stores she was now seriously short and was having to buy in Odessa at inflated prices.[17]

Miss Henderson also brought news of six more orderlies and an administrator on the way, for which Dr Inglis was thankful. She had been harrying the Committee constantly for more staff of which she was now very short. The fact was that the position of women had entirely changed since 1914; any woman who could do useful work was in great demand. As early as October 1914 Dr Inglis had foreseen this and forecast that the S.W.H. would eventually have to pay the same salaries as the R.A.M.C.* As far as the doctors were concerned she now partly won her point. On May 11th she wrote, 'Your telegrams about the salaries have arrived ... Many thanks from myself for the doctors. Personally I am more than content but I cannot help thinking that if you want to keep the supply you would be wiser to put the remuneration on the War Office basis,'[18] and in August she was hammering away in the same vein: 'Girls *must* think of these things ... And we are a women's organisation which has always stood for equal pay.'[19]

Pay, however, was not the whole difficulty. Although Dr Inglis was unaware of it, a movement was on foot to prevent any Englishwomen travelling to Russia after the Revolution.

In April, after the S.W.H. in London enquired about travel permits, the Foreign Office had consulted the War Office who refused consent for doctors and nurses proceeding abroad.[20] The War Office, it is true, no longer asked women to go home and sit still. It now expected them to join the R.A.M.C. or the Q.A.I.M.N.C. as nurses or, if doctors, to remain at their civilian duties to release men; it was still commissioning women not in the R.A.M.C.

When the War Office refusal was told to Dr Inglis's Committee, they pointed out that they did not propose sending extra staff, merely replacements. But the War Office remained adamant in refusing even this.[21]

The Red Cross was also opposed to women going out. In May, Mr Kimens, the British Red Cross representative in Petrograd, with the support of the ambassador, Sir George Buchanan, wrote

* The pay of a medical man holding a temporary commission was twenty-four shillings a day and allowances.

to the Hon. Arthur Stanley, chairman of the Red Cross in London, with special reference to the Scottish Women's Hospitals. Conditions in Russia since the Revolution, he wrote, were quite unfit for Englishwomen; if they insisted upon coming they must do it on their own responsibility.[22]

Mr Stanley, whose brother Lord Derby was of course Secretary of State for War, could only reply that he had no jurisdiction whatever over the Scottish Women's Hospitals.

On May 21st the Serbian Legation in London begged the Foreign Office to allow Dr Inglis replacements; the British Minister in Roumania was consulted and declared himself in favour. The Foreign Office now proposed that an exception might be made, in favour of the Scottish Women's Hospitals, to the general ruling that no Englishwoman might have a travel permit. It would be politically serious if the Scottish Women were prevented from helping the Serbs.[23]

And on June 8th, with the face-saving compromise that they would allow medical replacements to go, but not women drivers, the War Office climbed down.[24]

Dr Inglis had won another victory by remote control.

CHAPTER 24

In spite of the qualms of Mr Kimens and Sir George Buchanan, most of southern Russia was fairly quiet in the early summer, although there were sporadic outbreaks of violence like that at Yalta in May when sailors ransacked villas of the aristocracy.[1] It was however an open question whether Russia would continue the war.

In a report on June 5th Dr Inglis wrote, 'We cannot give you any idea of what our future movements will be just yet, for we must wait and see how things develop. In any case we must stand by until the Serbs know definitely what they are going to do, as we and the British Red Cross are the only hospitals they have got.'[2] In a private letter to Miss Palliser of the same date she wrote, 'It is rather trying work—waiting and wondering where we will go next.'[3] Even Dr Chesney, so reliable and sturdy, was having doubts, and told Dr Inglis she could sign on for only another three months.[4]

If Dr Inglis had doubts about Russian intentions, she did not voice them, except, guardedly, to her Committee. In public she was confident and encouraging. On June 5th in the ward a man remarked to her that the Sister was going home soon, and asked, 'When are you going home?'

'I am not going home,' Dr Inglis replied sturdily. 'I am going to Sofia with the Russian Army.' The shout from all over the ward at the mention of the Bulgarian capital showed that she had scored a direct hit.[5]

Early in June Miss Genge, the new administrator, arrived with the six replacement orderlies. 'I cannot tell you how glad we are to have them. They have all picked up their different bits of work splendidly ... I think they seem a very nice set of girls.' But Elsie was scathing about their equipment. 'The necessaries for this Unit were very carefully thought out and the list left ... in both offices at home. Yet these girls have been sent out without ground sheets, without canvas basins and pails, without plates and mugs ... without summer hats and with cheap rubber boots that the Committee have been told over and over again do not wear ... the original cheap boots that will prove useless in a month.'[6]

Muddle and inefficiency roused Dr Inglis to fury and she was surrounded by them. Hunter in Serbia two years before had found her gentle-hearted and lovable.[7] But Serbia in 1915 had been a bed of roses compared with Russia in 1917 and Hunter might hardly have recognised the wiry little martinet she had of necessity become. War is anyway 'the most muddled of all human activities'[8] and the Russia of 1917 possibly the most muddled of all human societies. There was also the muddle which sprang from the fear she inspired in the weaker of the Unit's members. Few were so efficient as never to fail her and only the strongest could endure submissively the stinging rebukes they occasionally received. The girl who had run the office for months pending the new administrator's arrival had already been dismissed once for insubordination; then worked so hard that the dismissal was withdrawn; then made important mistakes she could not bring herself to own to; and finally 'lost' part of the telegram announcing her successor's arrival. A clear, and typical, example of difficulties created by those who attempted to live up to Dr Inglis's enormous expectations without being quite big enough to do so.[9]

Miss Genge, however, was not exactly Dr Inglis's idea of an administrator either. Ladylike and well-intentioned, with prudish notions of women's role in a hospital of men, she lacked method and was not a woman of the world. 'She sticks tightly to the office —and does that all right—but as to any idea of being Administrational! She never can put anything through and then is annoyed because I do it myself or give it to someone else to do,' Dr Inglis wrote in August. 'And she is head of the Unit when I am away! I am really rather sorry for her for she has undertaken a piece of work she cannot do. She hasn't the remotest idea of how to do it, in fact, she hasn't it in her ...'[10]

Simultaneously there was trouble with Miss Marx, who had replaced Mrs Haverfield in charge of Transport. The cars had been repaired in Odessa with the help of two male mechanics sent out from England, but no drivers arrived and as an interim measure Serb drivers were being used.[11] As we have seen, efforts were being made in London to prevent women from travelling out; and the same thing was going on in Odessa.

The first Dr Inglis heard of it was when Miss Marx proposed

that no more women drivers be recruited. Dr Inglis commented in evident excitement to Miss Palliser on June 5th:

'Miss Marx seems to have got very panicy about the condition of things in Russia—but if she were right (which she isn't!) it would be a reason for giving up the hospitals, not for having men drivers for the cars!'[12]

'I wrote to her,' she elaborated a week later, 'saying that the first object of the Scottish Women's Hospitals was to care for the wounded, and the second was to do it through a women's organisation.'[13] (To Mrs Fawcett, about the same time, she wrote, 'Before the war, I had only two thoughts—surgery and suffrage; and now I feel that I am working for suffrage still.'[14])

Miss Marx, however, wired her resignation; and when asked to 'come down and talk it over' did not come. 'Some paltry excuse about not being able to leave the cars,' commented Dr Inglis crossly to Miss Palliser.[15]

It was no wonder Miss Marx did not care to face her. At the end of April she and Miss Henderson had persuaded Mr Bagge,* British Consul in Odessa, to telegraph to the Foreign Office that it was inadvisable to send out more women drivers. On May 30th he had sent a stronger telegram to the S.W.H. in London that it would be 'criminal' to do so.[16] When Dr Inglis found out, she was wrathful indeed. Her letter to Miss Palliser betrays in style and spelling the indignation and haste in which it was written.

'We should never have had any Scottish Women's Hospitals at all if they and their sort—dear things—had been listened to. How they would have disapproved of Florence Nightingale's little band! Miss Henderson solemnly talked to me for an hour the other day about the wickedness of risking young lives (in the middle of this terrible, terrible war, remember) and what was and what was not woman's work! ...

'And worse still the Consul, without even seeing me ... has wired to you ...

'Now I cannot manage these hospitals if that sort of thing is done, can I?—and what is more he never would have done it if a man had been head of these hospitals. Imagine him wiring home about the Armoured Cars without consulting Commander Gregory. Or wiring to the Red Cross about the personnel of the British Red Cross without talking it over with Dr Clemo—unless indeed he thought Commander Gregory or Dr Clemo were doing

* Later Sir John Picton Bagge, (1881-1967).

their job so badly that they ought to be superceded.—And apparently he does not think that of me.—But he think because I am a woman it does not matter interfering!—

'Now, dear Miss Palliser, will the Committee realise that they cannot have it both ways. They cannot expect me to be always ready and always on the spot and to take no risks. The B.R.C. units ran away from Galatz.* We held on—and apparently you were pleased—Certainly we managed to do a big bit of work.'

(There is no evidence that the Committee 'expected' anything. This was Dr Inglis's way of putting it; the targets for the hospitals were set by her alone.)

'Now—if you want me to stay here—will you back me up by helping me to be always ready—with personnel and with material?—And will you help me to keep the hospitals what they were originally intended to be—viz, women's organisations?—I am quite willing to have Serb orderlies ... but I want women doctors, sisters, cooks, women orderlies under the sisters, and women drivers for the cars. We all run exactly the same risk, no more and no less in Red Cross Hospitals and Red Cross Transports. The point is whether what we are fighting for is worth the risk. I say it is.

'And don't think I am the sort of fool who takes unnecessary risks. I haven't lost one bit of your equipment, through the enemy, except one Ludgate boiler! And I cleared the whole personnel out *in front of me* from the Dobruga, except the Field Hospital which made its own way with the Serbs and I knew was safe. Whenever there is a question of evacuating I always get my orders clearly *in writing* and I always make sure of being able to get out. These it appears to me, are the elementary duties of a leader. There is no sense in losing equipment and getting taken prisoner unnecessarily. We *had* to stay behind in Serbia—because there was no one else to look after the wounded. But only volunteers stayed. The rest all got out through Montenegro.

'I am going up to Odessa in a few days to see Miss Marx and the Consul and the Serbs at Headquarters. The uncertainty or rather I fear the *certainty* on this front is very trying, and I must find out what the Serbs intend to do. There is no good them and us sitting here indefinitely while the war needs us in other places. Could the Committee do anything about getting the British

* See page 208. The B.R.C. left Galatz on December 22nd when ordered to do so by the head of the Russian Red Cross.

Government to take over the financing and management of these divisions and get us on to the Western or Salonika Front—or to Mesopotamia!—They are *first rate* fighting men, worth their weight in gold . . .

'We have got twenty-five Serb orderlies here now. I wrote and asked for them as I wanted a nucleus of trained men whom we could take with us when we leave the Russian Red Cross. They are nice!

'Is this letter quite clear. It is so difficult to know how a written thing will strike the reader—isn't it? But I have written it very carefully. Read it several times.'[17]

She was hampered by the censorship, but it is clear that now she had no expectation that Russia would continue the war, and supposed that in the event of a separate peace the Serb divisions would simply be abandoned to sell their lives as dearly as they could in Roumania.

About now—a question was put down in the House of Commons on June 28th[18]—terms were published in Russia of a Secret Treaty said to have been signed with Roumania the year before and promising Roumania a large tract of territory to which Serbia also laid claim. This, again, convinced the Serbs that their allies had abandoned them. The Serb Government in Corfu, seeing they had nothing more to hope for from Russia, were already engaged in the talks with the Yugo-Slav Committee which were to culminate on July 20th in the Corfu Declaration, proclaiming a federal state, the Kingdom of the Serbs, Croats and Slovenes, with Alexander as its King; which in 1929 would be re-named Yugoslavia.

It was against this background that Dr Inglis went to see the Serbian Command in Odessa. The conversations she had threw a different light on the problems that worried her.

'I am very glad I came up to Odessa', she wrote to Miss Palliser on June 24th. 'Not only because of the Transport but because of the very satisfactory talk I have had at the Serbian headquarters. I *do* wish I could write it all now, but you must wait for news.

'We had lunch there—at the Serbian headquarters one day. Miss Henderson will tell you all about it. She starts for home tonight . . . I am bursting with news but I particularly want this letter to reach you so I am not going to risk any censor stopping it.'[19]

The news was—it seems clear—that the Serbian divisions were to be transferred to the Salonika front. Her letter to Miss Palliser is full of dark hints which the latter was clearly intended to interpret, with the help of Miss Henderson, the bearer.

'I agree with the Consul about chauffeurs not coming out just now—but for reasons entirely different to his!—Also I have had a long talk to Miss Marx and she has quite come back to her bearings.

'So

'1st. I am keeping her as Transport Officer

'& 2nd. I have sent a telegram through the Consul to you asking the Committee immediately to engage women chauffeurs and *to begin to train them on Ford cars* but not to send them out till I wire. Lots of girls are quite good chauffeurs but cannot manage Fords. We need *someone who has driven and managed them for some time.*

'Then I have also had a long talk with Day [one of the two mechanics sent from London]. And he says the Fords are the only possible kind of car on the roads we shall have to drive on—but the Committee must understand that it is *essential* to supply a very large amount of "spare parts"—many more than you would have to supply with any other kind of car—but—of course—on the other hand Fords are cheaper than any other car—just as a car. I have asked Miss Marx to make out a complete list of what she will need for *hard* work for six months and to send it home by Miss Henderson, who starts tonight.

'Day especially asked me to say that after all the knocking about the cars got in the Dobruga—they are really secondhand cars now but that "on the Bath Road he would guarantee them for two years". *On the roads we shall have to use and for hard work he gives them four months. And he thinks we ought gradually* [to] *begin to add new cars—he suggests two more ambulances at once.*'[20] (E.I.'s emphasis)

The references to bad roads, hard work and the need for Fords seem intended to convey that they would be used in Serbia. It had already been found from experience that the high wheel base of the Ford made it the only practicable vehicle for the rough mountain roads there.[21]

Miss Henderson had been returning to England in any event.

She now became the second of the messengers charged with information Dr Inglis would not risk in a letter.

On June 25th Dr Inglis returned to Reni. Just before leaving Odessa she learned that her favourite nephew, Major James Simson, had been wounded in the eye at the Battle of Gaza while commanding the 5th King's Own Scottish Borderers.

Observers who saw her dealing with wounded men were always impressed by her compassion and humanity; there was nothing of the case-hardened doctor in her. That she had even deeper feelings which she seldom allowed to show, is revealed by the letter she sat up late on June 24th to write.

> 'Dearest, dearest Amy,
>
> 'Eve's letter came yesterday about Jim, and though I start at seven tomorrow morning for Reni, I must write to you, dear, before I go. Though what one can say I don't know. One sees these awful doings all round one, but it strikes right home when one thinks of Jim. Thank God he is still with us, the dear, dear boy! ...'

Even in so personal a letter she could not resist a side-glance at her overriding preoccupation, the fate of the small nations. 'Whatever we suffer and whatever we lose, it is for the right we are standing. I wish you could realise how the little nations—Serbs and Roumanians and Poles—count on us ...

'Miss Henderson is taking home with her today a Serb officer, quite blind, shot right through behind his eyes, to place him somewhere where he can be trained. I heard of him just after I had read Eve's letter, and I nearly cried. He wasn't just a case at that minute, with my thoughts full of Jim.'[22]

At Reni she found waiting a telegram, with the news she had been hoping for thirty years to hear. On June 19th the House of Commons had passed by 385 votes to 55 the first and second readings of the Bill which would extend the franchise to women over thirty.

'So the vote has come! And for our work! Fancy its having taken the war to show them how ready we were to work!' she wrote. 'Or even to show them that work was necessary. Where do they think the world would have been without women's work all these ages?'[23]

All that had taken her to Russia had been accomplished, with the winning of the vote. For her, a larger loyalty had supervened. What did the risk to the Unit count, in a situation of steadily increasing danger, compared with the absolute certainty that if she abandoned her efforts on their behalf, thousands of men might be uselessly, inevitably, sacrificed? Little now stood between them and their fate, save for her own will-power. Could her will prove strong enough?

At Reni, she fell ill with German measles. She wrote in amusement, 'The consul asked me what I meant by that at my time of life! The majority of people say how unpatriotic and Hunnish of you! Well, a few days off did not do me any harm. I had a very luxurious time lying in my tent.'[24]

If she enjoyed the rest, it was because her health was definitely worsening. It may not have been apparent to the newly-arrived, who had not known her long. Mrs Milne however was an old hand; she read the signs and saw that only the little doctor's will-power was preventing the others from knowing how ill she was.[25] If she was unwell occasionally, it was common to most of them; bouts of dysentery or food poisoning were almost impossible to prevent, so oppressive was the heat, so ubiquitous the flies; few of them, probably, believed Dr Inglis to be suffering from anything worse than afflicted them all; for the symptoms which in her meant mortal illness were also the accompaniment of the milder infections from which they all suffered.

For the moment, work was slack. The trained nurses who had stayed on to help when they were needed, were going home. Reliefs were said to be coming. They never came. The Foreign Office, while recognising that one nurse there would be worth more than ten in England, had now reluctantly applied to the Scottish Women's Hospital a general ruling that ladies must not be allowed to travel to Russia.[26]

On July 15th a large party, including many of the best nurses, left. Dr Inglis accompanied them to Odessa, summoned by a telegram from Jivkovitch. The letter she wrote to Miss Palliser afterwards was cheerful and, once more, full of mysterious hints and dark allusions. The Serb Command seem to have confidently expected a transfer to Salonika soon. In the first week of July the Serbian Minister in Petrograd asked for this, the Russians had agreed and the British had signified approval.[27]

At Odessa Dr Inglis found waiting a letter saying that her

Committee would leave her to do what she thought wisest in the chaotic circumstances. She also found the able and tactful Miss Onslow, who had returned from leave bringing with her the young Dr G. Ward, to replace Dr Laird, who was going home to be married.

'Many many thanks for your awfully nice kind letter ...' she wrote on July 15th to Miss Palliser. 'Miss Onslow and Dr Ward have arrived and Miss Onslow and I have had a most satisfactory talk. But for numerous reasons you'll have to wait for particulars! She is taking on the cars because Miss Marx has been recalled by the W.V.R.* for some special work at home. I want you to know that Marx has worked well and faithfully with the cars. (She quite lost her bearings at one point but that was all right after she and I had had a talk) ...

'I came up here on a telegram from Serbian Headquarters ... Wait for particulars as to all that too.

'As the sisters haven't come and 13 of the present staff are going home I have closed the Hospital at Tecuci. Dr Chesney may form a dressing station with a staff of four or five. It is a pity, just at this psychological moment.

'Well, I hope to write or wire soon.

'Ever, dear Miss Palliser, with many thanks for yours and the Committee's expression of trust repeated in this letter, believe me, yours affectionately, Elsie Maud Inglis.'

And in a P.S. she wrote, 'This letter is mysterious but I cannot help it! Wait and see.'[28]

At this moment in fact Dr Chesney's small remaining party, sent forward to the Carpathian foothills to be ready for the attack known to history as the Kornilov Offensive, was busy, and was even moved forward some miles in the middle of July. But the advance petered out;[29] it became clear that the Russians would not fight, and by August Dr Chesney's group were on their way back to Reni.[29]

Demoralisation in Russia was growing fast. In mid-July the Bolsheviks, protagonists of a negotiated peace, made their first bid for power and Kerensky lost for ever the chance to crush them absolutely. The number of Russian deserters was estimated at one million, one in fourteen of the men on the strength.[30] The Kerensky Offensive began at the end of July but petered

* Women's Volunteer Reserve, the central registry for qualified women doing war work.

out. At Tarnopol, Stanislau and Kaluz, 'the freest army in the world' committed atrocities against civilians which rang round the globe.[31] The Assistant War Minister remarked to the British attaché, General Knox, that the Russian soldier was 'good natured at ordinary times but a wild beast when drunk or in panic', on which Knox privately commented, 'the worst of it is that he is now generally drunk or in panic'.[32]

Roumania still wished to fight and her army had been reorganised by the French, but without support could not withstand the attacks which began on July 19th. Roumania more than Russia now had reason to wish the help of the Serbs who, with the abdication of the Czar, had lost a powerful friend.

The Serbian divisions had been told they would go to Salonika, but orders to move never came. After waiting a week after his interview with Dr Inglis, Jivkovitch approached Sir George Buchanan to ask England to put pressure on the Russians to let them go.[33]

To Buchanan's enquiries the Russians pleaded lack of transport, and proposed that the divisions went to the Roumanian front in the meantime. Buchanan telegraphed the Foreign Office for instructions on July 22nd.[34] In London, there was delay in reaching a decision. The Admiralty had some transports available, but so many panic-stricken requests for help in getting out of Russia had now been received that it was necessary to call a conference to settle priorities; the date was fixed for August 9th.[35]

In the meantime, on July 26th, the Russian 6th Army H.Q. ordered the Serbs to the Roumanian front.

This was communicated by a deeply distressed Jivkovitch to Dr Inglis the next day. The Iron General was moved almost to tears.

'The men want to fight. They are not cowards,' he said. 'But it goes to my heart to send them like this to their death for nothing.'[36]

Earlier, the Serbs had said Dr Inglis would be 'helping them by helping the Russians'.[37] Now was the moment for the Russian debt to be paid. Perhaps her influence could tip the scales. Anyway it was worth trying. The Serb staff itself was powerless, entirely dependent on England to effect their release. And the only Englishman unequivocally on their side seemed to be a woman: Dr Inglis. Could she work the miracle?

She telegraphed home next day, using the Foreign Office

cypher, via the Consul in Odessa, to several people she thought might help: Seton Watson, Lady Selborne, sister of Lord Robert Cecil the Under Secretary at the Foreign Office, and Mrs Kinnell of the N.U.W.S.S. who as the sister of Lady Cowdray* had influence.[38]

> Serbian Division has been ordered to front. After 7 months intimate acquaintance with and personal observation of officers and men it is clear to me that Russian Army cannot fight now. Fear repetition of what took place in Dobruga. It is waste of splendid men to leave Serbian Division in Russia. It is imperative to get them removed to France or Salonika as quickly as possible but action must be taken immediately as they are ordered at once to Roumanian front. Do not think it will meet point to recall hospitals. If Serbian Division goes to Roumanian front hospitals should go also and do their best. But if possible division should be prevented from going and being probably wiped out as in Dobruga. Could not transports be sent to Archangel immediately? Ends.

The telegram never reached those for whom it was intended. When it arrived, as it dealt with military matters, the Foreign Office referred it to the Director of Military Intelligence before passing it on. The D.M.I. tartly remarked that he did not regard the removal of these troops to another theatre of war as being the proper concern of Dr Inglis, and was therefore opposed to the message being passed to the addressees. The D.M.I. would suggest that Dr Inglis should be told that he (sic) could rest assured that the question had not escaped the attention of the military authorities.[39]

Even while the Military Intelligence department were composing this message, however, another reached them from their own representative in Petrograd, General Barter, who had just heard (August 6th, ten days after Dr Inglis's telegram) that it had been decided to send the 1st Serbian Division to the Roumanian front;[40] and transfer to Salonika only the 2nd Division, which had been reduced to a strength of just over 3000 in order to make up the 1st Division. The War Office passed this information to the Foreign Office along with their comments about Dr Inglis;

* Lord Cowdray was at this time President of the Air Board, forerunner of the Air Ministry.

adding that Barter was making representations on the matter to the Russian General Staff.[41]

Unaware that her telegram was to be stopped in this way, Dr Inglis next day sent off Miss Marx, whom she had briefed thoroughly on the situation and armed with several letters of introduction.

'Dear Mrs Kinnell,' the first of them read.

'This is to introduce Miss Marx to you ... I have asked her specially to see you about the question of the Serb Division ...

'I sent you a telegram yesterday. You once said to me that if I wanted anything, to come straight to you, and I have taken you literally at your word. You'll know who to go to and what to do—so I shifted the trouble on to you! For I am miserable about it. You know how the Serb Divisions were left high and dry in the Dobruga—held out for 24 hours without support and came out of action having lost 11,000 out of 15,000. Well, that will simply happen again now. Miss Marx will tell you why ...

'We have orders to go in three days—but there'll be some delays I have no doubt. What we want is orders to go to Archangel to be ready for the Transports ...'

She described her interview with Jivkovitch and went on, 'They are such a splendid body of men. It is such a wicked wicked *waste* from every point of view.

'We are still at Reni, with tents pitched to make more beds to be ready for this so-called offensive ... I am up here [Odessa] to see what I can do to get this miserable tangle about this Division, undone. They want the Division to go on to the Front to "encourage" the Russians! Miss Marx will tell you.

'Goodbye, dear Mrs Kinnell. It is such a comfort to know you are there.'[42]

To Miss Palliser she wrote similarly, ending on a note that was, for her, unusually downcast. 'If the Serbs go to Roumania we shall probably not have to come up to Odessa, but join them on the way there. And the Field Hospital will, of course, join up too.

'In the meantime the work goes on at Reni as it has in the past, but it seems to get less and less. What a lot of interesting things I might write to you—but I don't suppose this letter would ever reach you then.

'Goodbye for the present. Tell the Committee we are doing our best in difficult circumstances—all of us!'[43]

CHAPTER 25

Miss Marx also bore with her a letter and a memorandum from Dr Inglis which when she arrived in London were sent, on August 23rd, to the Prime Minister and the Foreign Secretary. The Memorandum read:[1]

Dr Elsie Inglis, Chief Medical Officer of the Scottish Women's Hospitals attached to the Serbian Army in South Russia begs to draw the attention of all who may have the power to approach the British Government to the urgent need of removing the army of the Serbs, Croats and Slovenes from Russia to the Salonika or French fronts.

This Army was composed (July 28, 1917) of approximately 20,000 fighting men with 10,000 others including invalids. All ranks were insistently begging to be taken out of Russia. The tradition amongst the Yugoslavs was that Russia was as their big brother on whom they could always rely, that faith is now destroyed both by the events of the last year and by the demoralisation of the Russian Army consequent on the Revolution.

Last year the 1st Division went to the Roumanian front and fought heroically, the Russians on the one side and the Roumanians on the other failed to support them and at one time they held on for 24 hours alone. They went into action 14,000 men and lost 9000.

The remnant withdrew to Russia with headquarters at Odessa.

At that time the Treaty by which Russia promised the Banat to the Roumanians was still a secret, it is now known to the Serbs and because of it, too, the Officers and men of the 1st Division, which includes those surviving from the Dobruga last year, unanimously refuse to fight on the Roumanian front.

A telegram was received in Odessa from Russian headquarters on or about July 21 saying that the situation in Russia and Berlin* required the presence of the Serbian divisions on the Roumanian Front as the Bulgarian-German forces were weak and it was advisable to make an offensive and the Serbs were needed to encourage the unwilling Russians to advance; a few thousand Serbs to lead on the millions of Russians!

The Divisions are recruited from the Serbs, Croats and Slovenes who were Austrian subjects and as such were forced to fight in the Austrian Army and who after being made prisoners of war by the Russians were given their liberty to enable them to join as volunteers the Divisions of the Serbian Army in South Russia.

The General Commanding and some officers and a few of the men are Serbians from Serbia.

General Jivkovitch told Dr Inglis that the men were ready and keen to fight but demand to be placed where they can trust the troops on either side of them. (End).

Miss Marx left with this memorandum on July 29th but did not reach England until the third week of August. In the meantime, Dr Inglis, having done what she could for the moment, returned to Reni, where on August 10th a rush of work had again begun, the result of the Kerensky Offensive. The hospital soon had well over its nominal capacity of two hundred and had so many urgent operations that although they began at five in the morning to avoid the intense heat of the day, they often had anyway to continue till late afternoon.

'A great many of these cases are very severely wounded, but on the other hand at first before the authorities began to use this hospital as it should be used, namely for serious cases only, a great proportion of the men had very slight wounds, and a very great proportion of these were wounded in the left hand,'[2] Dr Inglis wrote in her official report, amplifying it in a private letter, 'if you know what that *means*. I don't think the British Army does know!'[3]

The work was more difficult because all the trained Sisters had now gone, and none of the new nurses coming out had had surgical training or understood the uses of antiseptics. 'These so-called sisters' was how Dr Inglis described them.[4] Miss (later Professor) E. M. Butler, who as a Russian linguist had been accepted as an orderly principally so that she could escort the

* This refers to reports of unrest in Berlin in July 1917.

last four of them out to Reni, was franker, when she came to write her memoirs nearly forty years later: of her four, one was a tower of strength, one lanky and limp, one incompetent, raddled and rouged, and the fourth 'almost a nympho'.[5]

Even on her journey Miss Butler had come to believe firmly in the power Dr Inglis could exercise from a distance. Mr Kimens in Petrograd had tried to prevent her party from travelling on, but crumpled completely when she quoted Dr Inglis's orders, 'being obviously far more frightened of what Dr Inglis would say to him than of anything the Russians could do to us'. And later, when her own resolution was wavering, there had been an inexplicable encounter with a gypsy who had seemed to be seeking her, told her the names of her six brothers and sisters, and finally said 'Elsie? Go where you are waited for. You are wanted there. Go.'[6]

Their arrival was indeed timely, for it coincided with the Kerensky Offensive and they were plunged into the rush before Dr Inglis could even instruct the Sisters in elementary surgical nursing. Miss Butler, put straight on to night duty as a ward orderly, noticed that out of doors in the stillness of the night, a strange sound could be heard, a sound never heard by day, as if the steppe were sighing, gently, hopelessly. It was the subdued moaning of hundreds of wounded men.

Professor Butler has left a picture of Dr Inglis as she was at this time.

'She was both lovable and fierce in the highest degree. The standards she set and the demands she made on us were as nothing to what she performed herself, but they were severe, and her wrath was great at any failure to come up to the mark. I for one went in mortal terror of attracting it, and never shall I forget my sensations when after a particularly gruelling night I was aroused from my afternoon sleep to interpret between Dr Inglis and some outpatients ... I dressed in a panic, seized my dictionary and rushed to the consulting tent where I found a handful of peasants all of them, as far as I could see, smitten with different and (to me) mysterious diseases. Lightning swift at diagnosis, Dr Inglis had already examined them and identified their complaints. It now devolved on me to pass on her instructions. Why, oh why, had I ever boasted of knowing Russian? and would I even understand Dr Inglis's medical terms? I should have known her better. She used none but the basic words and they summoned up as if by magic the equivalent Russian root ... I heard the redeeming word *Panimayu* (understood) from one illiterate peasant after another. "You know more Russian than I gave you credit for," said Dr Inglis when it was over.'[7]

Meanwhile, in London, as we have seen, on August 9th a conference had been called to decide whether the Serbians could be removed from Russia.

On the morning of this conference, *The Times* carried a report from its Russian correspondent that a belief was gaining ground that Odessa was to be the main target of enemy attack; a number of people in London must have been extremely worried about the safety of individual members of the Scottish Women's Hospitals; and some, Lady Selborne and Lady Cowdray for instance, were undoubtedly in a position to exercise both official and unofficial influence. Their exact weight cannot be estimated, but the outcome of the conference was an agreement that the Serbian divisions should have first priority, and that about 4000 could certainly be moved from Archangel on about September 9th, with possibly a further 15,000 then or later.[8]

On the same day the Foreign Office asked the War Office to have the Scottish Women, at least, withdrawn from Russia; and wrote to the same effect to the British Red Cross Society. The War Office replied that they quite concurred in the suggestion, but had no power whatever to carry it out.[9]

Dr Inglis knew nothing of all this. In mid-August she was in Odessa again, still nagging anyone she thought would help the Serbs. Nagging, and not without result. She had created enough indecision in the minds of the authorities to prevent the Serbs from being sent to Roumania, and by now the offensive was petering out.

On the day before her fifty-third birthday, still unaware of the decisions taken in London, she wrote in a private letter, 'The work at Reni is coming to an end, and we are to go to the front with the Serbian Division. I cannot write about it owing to censors and people. But I am going to risk this: the Serbs ought to be most awfully proud. The Russian General on the front is going to insist on having them "to stiffen up his Russian troops". I think you people at home ought to know what magnificent fighting men these Serbs are, and so splendidly disciplined, simply worth their weight in gold. There are only two divisions of them after all.'[10]

At about this time she also telegraphed direct to the Foreign Office, through Buchanan. Her message is reproduced as it was received on August 24th:

> As my telegrams could not be delivered, might I submit to you facts within my knowledge. First Serbian Division which was under orders for Archangel is now ordered to Roumanian front at special request of Russian General who requires them to stiffen his Russian troops (? wounded) of which troops are now coming into (? our) hospital. 40% to 50% of wounds are self-inflicted in left hand. His troops are completely disorganised. Perhaps several Army Corps might stiffen them. One division of Serbians will only be sacrificed. Russian Government are sheltering behind hope that Transports cannot be given but if you think it right to remove them that would (undecipherable) a minor difficulty. They are needed for a (undecipherable) rather than fighting division not for refugees. Extraordinary Russian compliment to their quality proves this. The coming winter is a further question. It was difficult last winter when there was plenty, to get food and fuel for Serbians. This winter condition of Serbians will be miserable as there is a shortage. They should leave before Archangel closes if there is not a disaster before then.
>
> Our hospitals accompany division and will stand by and save as many as possible. We shall be safe having (? troops) transport. Ends.[11]

A note attached in the Foreign Office files reads 'Lord Robert Cecil would like this telegram dealt with officially but whatever decision is taken a nice reply should be sent to Mrs Inglis.' Two days later a telegram went to Buchanan: 'Please convey following message to Dr Inglis. Your telegram received I will do what I can but decision must rest with the military authorities.'

On August 20th she arrived back at Reni; and it is worth remarking on the toll this constant travelling in arduous conditions and the heat of summer must have taken of her health. Even the previous year the journey was taking four days and now in August 1917 one-quarter of all Russian locomotives were out of service.[12] Dr Inglis must sometimes have longed for rest. She kept in her travelling wallet, with her writing materials and a copy of the 'Suffrage Hymn', a printed picture postcard adorned with sentimental flowery patterns around a quotation attributed to Goethe but actually from John S. Dwight's very free translation; 'Rest', it read, 'is not quitting this busy career. Rest is the fitting of self to one's sphere.'[13]

She arrived at Reni, and, keyed up as she was, almost burst into tears on being handed a telegram saying simply 'Many happy returns of the day' which had arrived from Mrs Simson. When she recovered, she felt, she wrote a week later, 'happy for days'. 'You don't know how nice it was to get it and to feel you were thinking of me.'[14]

Immediately on her return she despatched a long report. She had, she said, now received firm orders to rejoin the Serbians (at, though this she did not mention in the report, Hadji Abdul, a small village about fifteen miles to the rear), there to wait till the Serbians received orders and then to go with them. 'I am sorry that it is impossible to give details of the conversations I had with people in authority there in this report. The final result however is that we are going back to our original work and I greatly fear that the work will take on its original intensity ... Dr Chesney, who always said she could not have another winter out here, now tells me that she meant she must be home in England by the winter.* She will therefore leave us when the hospitals leave Reni ... We shall therefore be left with three doctors, only two of us surgeons ...

'Miss Robinson and Miss Holme, whose agreement ended some time ago and who stayed on to help us, are now going home and I hope the Committee will make a special point of seeing them ...'[15]

Not only was Dr Inglis's communication with home hindered by the censorship (Miss Robinson and Miss Holme were in fact being sent by her with a special message) but the timelag in communication was such that this report was not received in London until September 17th; and two days after it was written, i.e. on August 22nd, the appeals she had sent as early as July by Miss Marx, were read to the Committee of the S.W.H. At the same meeting the Committee was shown a telegram from Mr Kimens in Petrograd, who, with the support of Buchanan, was now urging the withdrawal of Dr Inglis even if this should leave

* Dr Chesney served again with the S.W.H. in Serbia in 1918.

the Serbians in the lurch. Immediately *after* the meeting, too, the Red Cross in London approached several Committee members privately, urging the Foreign Office view that the Unit be brought home. All were agreed that *of course* the Foreign Office's wishes should be met. The Red Cross, however, like the War Office, had to own that they really had no jurisdiction over Dr Inglis: she was entirely independent of any other body.[16]

This same meeting heard the verbal messages brought home by Miss Marx and next day, as we have seen, they were passed to 10 Downing Street and to the Foreign Office. The latter, which may have had the sensation of receiving from all directions a bombardment which nice replies were inadequate to avert, replied to the Committee that Lord Robert Cecil had already been in touch with Dr Inglis and that the Government was aware of the situation and making an effort to secure the Serbs' removal.[17]

In any event, before the meeting at which all agreed that Dr Inglis must certainly come home, Mrs Kinnell and Miss Palliser had, on their own account, telegraphed her encouraging and reassuring messages with just the opposite sense; and on August 27th she wrote acknowledging them. The shaky handwriting betrays her health and, perhaps, emotion.

'Your telegram asking if Miss Hedges and Miss Arbuthnot should come on cheered me very much because it showed that Miss Marx had got home.

'We are closing this hospital today after nearly eight months work here. On Friday we join the Serbian Division ...

'I wonder how long we shall be at this special place! And what will happen next—I have had a long talk with Colonel Milotinovitch who is in command of the Division ... It will be very nice being back among our dear Serbs again ...

'I do long for a good talk with you about the whole organisation of these Units. And perhaps that will come about before long ... I confess I am quite sorry to say "Goodbye" to this little hospital here. It has done some quite good work ...'[18]

While she was actually writing this, another telegram was brought to her. It had been sent after the Committee's deliberations. It advised her to leave the Serbs and to withdraw from Russia; but left the final decision in her hands. She broke off her letter to telegraph a brief reply: 'I am grateful to you for leaving decision in my hands. I will come with the Division.'

And in a postscript to the letter upon which she was engaged she wrote, 'Your telegram has just come about going home and I am answering that we shall stay on here. If there was a disaster we should none of us ever forgive ourselves if we had left. We must stand by. If you want us home—get *them* out!'[19]

This letter was read to the Committee in London on October 8th. In the meantime, however, Miss Frances Robinson and Miss Vera Holme had arrived in England. Elsie had taken the drastic step of sending these two of her best people, whom she could ill spare, as bearers of the third message she dared not trust to the mails.

It was a report of the political situation as it affected the divisions and had been drawn up for Dr Inglis by Dr Jambrishak, a member of the Yugo-Slav Committee who was at that time in Odessa.

It was clearly dangerous to carry so confidential a document through Russia. Miss Robinson, who was a schoolteacher in peace time, therefore committed the whole thing, some 2,500 rather turgid words, to memory. On a tiny scrap of paper no bigger than a postage stamp[20] Dr Inglis noted the headings of the report:

Formation 1 Div & 2nd
Croats and Slovenes forced to enter
3 Causes discontent with R. Situat;
Austrian spies in corpus
Soldiers & Workmens Committees
Intervention B. Em.
Emigrant Officers
Italian Propaganda
Desire to leave Russia
Ordered to Roumanian Front.

This was concealed in a humble little packet of needles from the Army and Navy Stores; and carried on her person by Miss Holme, the girl from the D'Oyly Carte company, who had spirit enough for anything but said she could never remember words unless they were set to music.

They left Reni some time after August 27th and reached London on October 9th; and soon after laid the missive, re-typed to Miss Robinson's dictation, before Lord Robert Cecil of the Foreign Office and Lord Derby, the Secretary of State for War, in person. Miss Robinson told Miss Curwen, secretary of the London

Committee, that after this experience she would never again force her pupils to commit anything to memory by heart.[21]

The full text of the missive appears in the Appendix. Its gist was as follows:

> The 1st Serbian Division consists of only 12,000 rifles, could depend on no support, and had no reserves. The Serbian Division had suffered in the previous winter from lack of food and equipment; far greater shortages were now expected and sickness and malnutrition would take their toll. The 2nd Division had left Russia.
>
> The Serbian troops had proved their quality in the Dobruga, but would be thrown away in Roumania. Many were conscripts, for the Yugoslavs had, like the British, adopted conscription rather than simply sacrificing the nation's better elements. Efforts were being made to educate these conscripts in the conception of a Yugoslav nation, but were hindered because the circumstances inside Russia made it seem improbable that a Yugoslav state would ever be achieved.
>
> Furthermore Austrian agents had infiltrated among the Division and used the Soldiers' and Workmen's Committee to foment trouble so that many men deserted and at one stage General Jivkovitch and his Chief of Staff had actually been prisoners of the Soldiers' and Workmen's Committees and had only been liberated through the intervention of the British Ambassador.
>
> Simultaneously there was an outbreak of anti-Serb feeling among younger officers of Croatian descent, a number of whom had to be transferred to the Russian Army.*
>
> The Italians meanwhile conducted their own anti-Serb propaganda. The Serbian Divisions were thus threatened by disintegration through the work of interested parties and also by annihilation if sent without support to the Roumanian front.
>
> The Divisions now looked to England as their principal protector and guardian.[22]

It will be noted that this memorandum brought by Robinson and Holme speaks of the 2nd Division as having already left.

* When Kerensky finally escaped from Russia in 1918 it was in the disguise of a Serbian officer.

What had happened was that in response to British pressure the Russians had agreed to release one division, which was all that transport could be found for at the time. It was not practicable to keep thousands of men hanging around for transports at Archangel, which itself had expanded to the very limits, until ships arrived. Rail and sea movements needed careful co-ordination.

Before the 2nd Division left, however, men were withdrawn from it to bring the 1st Division, which was being retained, up to strength. Approximately 3,000 men, therefore, comprised the entire Serbian 2nd Division which left Archangel in early September, passed through Britain, and arrived at Salonika on December 5th.[23]

There is no record to show whether Elsie Inglis ever knew that Miss Robinson and Miss Holme had got through to deliver their message.

CHAPTER 26

On August 31st, one year to the day after they had sailed from Liverpool, the Scottish Women's Hospital Unit rejoined the 1st Serbian Division at its new headquarters.

Hadji Abdul, straggling over a wooded hillside where a windmill stood like a sentinel, was an old village which had once been within the Turkish empire and now was full of Roumanian refugees. On the lower outskirts, among the trees of an apricot orchard, were pitched the tents of the Hospital, now completely under canvas for the first time. Its once immaculate white tents, camouflaged a dirty brown (for German reconnaissance planes were probing in this rear area) looked from the far hillside like a village among the trees and the mess tent stood in an old vineyard.[1]

The hospital soon filled with sick, for there was a good deal of malaria among the Serbians and a number of long-term wounded. But for the overriding anxiety about the future, however, life during September at Hadji Abdul must have been pleasant enough for the Scottish Women's Hospital, with useful work but no terrible rushes of wounded. In off-duty hours there were picnics, riding, a variety of entertainments, and nearly every afternoon Dr Inglis would sit under an enormous walnut tree at one side of the camp, holding court in the dappled sunshine, beaming genially at her girls and at the officers who came to pay their respects.[2]

At Hadji Abdul, however, she began to be very ill. Miss Hedges, who had been with her in the early days in the Dobruga but been home on leave since March, now arrived with Miss Arbuthnot, the grandchild of Elsie's old friends the Muirs. Miss Hedges was shocked at the change in Dr Inglis and even Miss Arbuthnot, who had not met her before, saw that she looked very ill. Her eyes, quite grey now, seemed enormous in the thin face whose pallor emphasised every freckle. Reduced almost to a skeleton by sickness and anxiety she was still strict and forceful on duty; straightbacked and well-groomed, her wispy hair tightly combed; sterner even with herself than with others, she could not often be persuaded to so much as breakfast in bed. She still worked in the theatre, mostly on minor operations, though she performed at this time a gastro-enterotomy lasting three hours on one of the Serb chauffeurs, a man they all knew as Joe, of whom she was especially fond.[3]

Nothing, however, could now convince the Unit that she was fit; they had all been asked not to refer, in letters home, to her illness. Whether they realised she was dying is another matter. In the light of hindsight, some claimed they did. Others, including some in a particularly good position to judge, believed almost to the end that she would recover.[4] She herself seems by now to have believed she could hold death off by the force of her will alone. She *meant* to live.

The future looked dark. A day or two after arriving at Hadji Abdul, Elsie sent Miss Onslow at Odessa instructions to send the Transport to join the Hospital. 'No one really knows,' she explained, 'what the Russian Government means or will do. I don't think the last explanation of how the last order for Archangel came to be altered* improves things at all. It shows there is no settled policy but that they are swayed by the last opinion. Such a wave may carry us right into Roumania and I want this Hospital at any rate to be ready, and then one often gets a chance of helping one would otherwise lose. It is awfully nice being back with the Serbs.'[6]

During these early days of September the last chance of restoring order in Russia was slipping away. On September 2nd martial law was proclaimed in Petrograd and on September 8th Kerensky quarrelled with Kornilov, who had stood for continuing the war with the Allies; after Kornilov fell, Britain was unprepared to make any further efforts on Russia's behalf.[7]

The state of indecision was reflected in the Serbians' orders. On September 1st General Barter in Petrograd telegraphed the C.I.G.S. to say the 1st Division was not going; on September 5th he telegraphed that they had orders for Archangel;[8] on the same day Sir George Barclay, British Minister in Roumania, intervened to try to get the division moved to that country.[9]

On the 11th, the Scottish Women's Hospitals office in London

* On September 1st the Russian C.I.G.S. informed Knox in Petrograd that at the request of the Russian C.-in-C. Roumania, the 1st Serbian Division would be retained, and would not be available for embarkation before November.[5]

asked the Foreign Office if they could confirm or deny a rumour that the Serbian Division was already in action. The Foreign Office replied by letting them know of Barter's secret telegrams and Mr (later Sir) Lancelot Oliphant, himself an expert on Eastern Europe at the F.O., noted that there could be no possible harm in this as 'much of our information on this subject is itself derived from members of the Scottish Women's Hospitals'.[10]

Meanwhile disorganisation in Russia was having inevitable economic effects. Not only had transport broken down, but the lack of manufactures and the devaluation of currency were causing the peasants to withhold their produce.[11] The country was on the verge of famine.

Dr Inglis, it would seem, had some anxiety about her own sinking condition and began to ask herself who could take charge in an emergency. Miss Genge, nominally her deputy, 'hadn't it in her'. The Committee had sent out someone else they had fondly hoped was the competent woman of the world Dr Inglis so much needed. But Gertrude, Lady Decies, was more useless than Miss Genge; over-made-up and of eccentric gaiety, the widow of a man whose only claim to fame was that the same pack of foxhounds had been in his family since the early eighteenth century; speculation was rife among the junior members of the Unit as to what on earth the Serbs made of her.[12]

Miss Onslow was reliable, but an admirable second-in-command only. Dr Chesney had gone home, Dr Corbett was more doctor than leader, and Dr Ward was newly arrived and very young.

On September 24th Dr Inglis sent for the cook, Mrs Milne, and raised her to the rank of officer, cutting, because there was no spare insignia, the tabs from one of her own uniforms for Mrs Milne to wear. Mary Milne wrote later that she had been perfectly happy as 'only the cook' but that what pleased her was Dr Inglis's approval and trust. The loss of the four steriliser drums had at last been completely redeemed.[13]

Two days later Dr Inglis collapsed. She was unable to leave her tent, and from then onwards was never well and more often really ill. With a puritanical independence she refused being waited upon and was quick to see through any attempt to prepare for her special delicacies or comforts. She continued to read the church service on Sundays and to direct the Unit from her sick bed, or, on better days, from a chair in the sun outside her tent.[14]

Two days after her first collapse the news came that the division was to leave in three days for Archangel, there to be picked up by French transports. This time there was every reason to believe the matter settled. She rallied and wrote home: something she had not had strength to do since leaving Reni. Only certain inaccuracies betray her weakness

'Dear Miss Palliser', she wrote on October 1st. 'I must sent you a line from this lovely place—even though we may be home ourselves before you get this letter. Think of it! Isn't it joyful!'

She gave a detailed account of the camp arrangements, a side glance at the shortcomings of her administrators and ended, 'I won't plan new things at the moment—as so soon I hope to talk everything over with the Committee. We shall have about six weeks at home—I hope—to refit.'[15]

The competition for the services of the Serbs, if it had delayed their departure, had at least convinced even the War Office that they must be very useful troops, since so many people wanted them. Only, where could they best be used? By mid-September the War Office was swinging to the view that, as transport before ice closed Archangel for the winter was so difficult to arrange, it would be best to send them to back up the re-formed Roumanian Army.[16] The French, whose General Berthelot had reorganised the Roumanians, were saying the same, and on October 9th, the Foreign Office learned that the Roumanian king was, contrary to all protocol, making a personal plea to the same effect.[17]

It was on this day that Miss Robinson and Miss Holme arrived in London with the long memorised report. They saw Lord Robert Cecil and Lord Derby on the 16th,[18] but of this Dr Inglis knew nothing. She became sick at heart as hope was deferred. Days passed, the hospital was cleared of patients, equipment was packed; still no orders came to move.

On October 17th she wrote to a niece, 'I wonder if this is my last letter from Russia! We hope to be off in a very few days now ... The question was whether we were going to Roumania or elsewhere. It is nice being back with these nice people. They have been most kind and friendly ... Now we are packed up and ready to go, and I mean to walk in on you one morning. It does not stand thinking of!

'We shall have about two months to refit, but one of those is my due as a holiday, *which I am going to take.* I'll see you all soon.—Your loving aunt, Elsie.'[19]

By now the weather was extremely cold, especially at night. In her emaciated condition, Dr Inglis felt it acutely. The Unit were worried, but could not help her, for a reason which in other circumstances might have been comic. The Scottish Women always had an eye for the attractive peasant markets of Eastern Europe; now they had placed unwise reliance on going home and had bartered almost all their warm clothing, and their stout boots, for the handwoven rugs of the Roumanian refugees.[20] They were not the only ones: most Russian soldiers had gambled away their boots by now.[21]

On October 22nd, Dr Inglis heard from the Serbian H.Q. that their orders were again altered: they were to proceed to Ackermann on the Black Sea and thence to Roumania.

To Mrs Milne, summoned that afternoon to the tent where she was confined to bed, Elsie Inglis admitted that for the first time in her life she felt homesick. She did not however spend long on that. Quietly, methodically, she outlined to her newest officer her plans for the winter. While things were quiet, Matron Vizard, who had also been ill, would go home on leave, as would Dr Corbett; only when they returned would she, Dr Inglis, go home for a rest. Ill as she was, all the details were clear in her mind and now she had made sure that a reliable deputy knew them too. 'I was very miserable when I left her,' wrote Mary Milne. 'She was so obviously unfit to stay on, yet she would not give in.'[22]

Next morning, Dr Inglis received a letter from Miss Onslow in Odessa. Was it true that the Serbian division was to go after all to Roumania? Dr Inglis replied at once:

Dear Onslow,

Thanks for your letter about the Roumanian rumour. I am afraid it is more than a rumour and that there is a determined effort on the part of the Roumanian [British?] Minister at Jassy and various other people, naturally the Roumanians among them, to keep the Serbs here. The day before yesterday a telegram came saying our departure was again postponed. Colonel Milotinovitch has gone to Michaeloff, the Russian General Headquarters, to see about it all.

Now it may end all right, but what I am writing about is this. Would it be worth while for you to go at once to Petrograd and see the Ambassador? If I were not tied by the leg to bed, I should certainly go myself, and, though I should like you to have a talk with the Consul about it, I cannot help feeling that you might do the trick by going up now. Explain to him that these men have not got their winter clothing, have had all their ammunition except 6 rounds taken away from them, that last winter they were short of fuel and clothing and food, that he will have one difficulty after another if he lets them stay in this country and that the only thing is to get them out. And impress upon him that the whole Division must go together, the idea of sending one brigade and the General Staff and then the second brigade simply means that the second brigade would never go.

Now if this plan is worth carrying out it must be done at once so that the Ambassador can wire to the authorities at Russian General Headquarters immediately. I cannot imagine how they imagine that England is going to send transports to Archangel while they play these irresponsible games at this end, but if the Transports have been sent and are there, it seems to me the Ambassador is in a very strong position.

If you think it necessary take Hedges with you and send the other girls back here, or if Hedges's back is still bad, take Butler. I do wish I could go with you, it is just like our luck that I should be laid on my back at this point. I believe you and I together might do something with the Ambassador.

Will you send the man I am sending up with this straight back, telling me what you are going to do?

I have not said anything to the Serbs here about your going up to Petrograd, because I think that had better just be our own business and we must take the full responsibility but you need not say that to the Consul. Of course, if the Consul thinks telegrams will do, well and good, but personally I feel sure that if you went up and saw the Ambassador it would be far more effective.

Yours ever, Elsie Inglis.[23]

It would, of course, be overstating the case to assert that in the general confusion Elsie Inglis was alone and entirely responsible for the eventual transfer of the Serbian Division. Yet that is what it comes to in the end. The Foreign Office, and the Serbians in London and Petrograd, were requesting the transfer. They were opposed by the Russian military authorities, the Roumanians, and the French; who, as the Serbians were already approximately where they wanted them to be, had all the force of inertia on their side. The War Office had an open mind, and the Kerensky Government, whatever its views, had at this stage no ability to enforce them.

When opposing forces are evenly balanced, as were the forces for and against moving the Serbians, even the lightest weight, if hurled with sufficient conviction, can effect a change. This was the weight and, more importantly, this the sufficient conviction, which Elsie Inglis threw into the scales to save thirteen thousand men from useless death and in some degree to change the course of history.

For another six days matters hung in the balance. The cold was becoming intense. The Unit begged Dr Inglis to move to a room in the village, but she refused unless all the rest could do so too. The search for quarters was still going on when on October 27th a Serbian officer arrived in the camp,[24] his delighted face telling his news even before he could get the words out: orders had come and they were for England. The first troop train was leaving that very night; the Scottish Women's Hospital would travel with the Staff in three days' time.

It was by now a question whether Dr Inglis was fit to make the journey.

The sun shone, matching their mood as they dismantled and packed their tents, cooking equipment, everything. Food had to be procured for the journey. Dr Inglis, determined to be better for the moment, sat in the sunshine directing operations, and even inspected a row of excessively bulky kit bags and bed rolls, turning an indulgent eye on their untidy dimensions.[25] She wrote on October 29th a final report for her Committee; even now she hardly dared credit that they would go. 'There really seems a prospect of getting away soon. The Foreign Office knows us only too well. Only 6000 of the Division go in this lot, the rest (15,000)* to follow.'[26]

* These figures seem not perfectly accurate, but accurate figures are hard to arrive at. In early September there were said to be 16,000 Serbian troops in Russia. The 1st Division was made up to strength before the 2nd Division, reduced to 3000, left; leaving just under 13,000 in the 1st Division. Nearly 7000 of these went at the same time as the S.W.H. In view of Dr Inglis's gloomy prophecy (p. 269) the fate of the rest is of interest. They could not go via Archangel, but Britain had realised the importance of getting them away and refused a further request for them by Roumania. They eventually left via the Manchurian Railway and Dairen, with the help of the Japanese, and rejoined their Division in Salonika.[27]

Early that evening the Scottish Women's Hospital left Hadji Abdul. Never had it looked more charming than in the evening sunlight as they slowly pulled away, in the longest train they had ever seen, across the vast dreaming steppe with its little pink and blue villages set amid the sunflower fields,[28] in the direction of Odessa and on to Archangel for home.

CHAPTER 27

The journey took four weeks all but a day. While the Unit divided themselves between two fourth-class wagons, Dr Inglis had the second-class compartment due to an officer of high rank. She had with difficulty been persuaded to accept it, and shared it with Matron Vizard.

With no proper bed, no comfort of any kind, a strictly limited amount of linen which her Unit knew better than to try to increase (there had once before been an awful row when they tried to smuggle extra bedding into her kit), with makeshift meals which anyway she could hardly share for she now needed a liquid diet, with no suitable drugs and almost no privacy, the journey must have been a nightmare.[1]

For much of the time, weakness forced her to lie down. Every day she insisted upon dressing; on the very worst days, Miss Arbuthnot was permitted to tie her bootlaces. Now that there was no work and little responsibility, her autocratic manner was seldom seen. She was all kindness, charm and fortitude, and even hugged Miss Arbuthnot, saying 'Dear child, it was your duty' when the latter was almost left behind through going to say goodbye to the chauffeur Joe who was still too ill to travel.[2]

It was an anxious journey. Before they were out of the Ukraine they had seen real revolution, passed through a town where twenty people had been shot that morning and mutinous troops were in control. Mostly the train crawled so that the young women found running alongside the engine a healthy exercise. At other times it would stop for hours, sometimes at a village miraculously untouched by revolution where white bread, poultry, fruit, fresh eggs and good milk could be bought, but equally often in the midst of forests where the wood-burning engine could be replenished, and sometimes in the trackless wastes of the tundra while the driver made repairs to the ludicrously dilapidated engine.[3]

Dr Ward, who attended Dr Inglis during the journey, wrote

almost fifty years later, 'My most vivid recollection of that journey is of rushing to the local chemist wherever we stopped, only to find that there was nothing with which we could alleviate Dr Inglis's sufferings. When told she generally made a joke of this. There can never have been anyone who made more light of pain and discomfort. Her main care seemed to be for the rest of the Unit and their very minor discomforts ... Next to her courage I think her affection for her Unit was her most striking characteristic, and I think she knew how deeply this was felt and reciprocated.'[4]

As they went north, the extreme cold added to Dr Inglis's sufferings. Worse than the present privations, however, must have been the knowledge that some time before November 15th ice would close the port of Archangel.[5] The meandering progress of the train became a race against winter.

Moscow they did not enter but skirted by and slipped away from, contrary to the pre-arranged plan, in the dead of night. Though they did not know it at the time, Moscow was in the hands of a drunken mob and thousands had been killed in street fighting. On November 7th, while the train creaked its way across the tundra, the Petrograd garrison went over to the Bolsheviks, Kerensky fled and the entire body of ministers was placed under arrest.

The train arrived at Archangel late in the evening of November 9th so that they spent the night in a siding. Next day Mrs Milne went to enlist the help of their old friend Bevan, now a Commodore.[6] English sailors she met were not reassuring; the last convoy which left for England had been lost and all outward bound vessels might expect to be torpedoed. They were not exaggerating. The final months of 1917 were the blackest of the war from the North Sea submarine menace.[7]

Bevan was kind, helpful, and so far as he could be, reassuring. Their ship, the S.S. *Porto*, was located; she would sail on the 13th, giving ample time to transfer their forty tons of equipment (the cars having been sold in Odessa). With three Russian ships, the *Czar*, *Czaritza* and *Dwinsk*, the *Porto* comprised the third set of transports provided for the Serbs. One set had gone out with the 2nd Division in September; another sent for the 1st Division in mid-October had found no Serbians ready to sail and had filled up instead with a Czech labour corps destined for France and with refugees from the Revolution.*[8] Mrs Milne arranged with Bevan that the women would take with them a sick naval officer and nurse him.

In the thirteen days they spent in the train, Dr Inglis had twice found the will to walk on the station platform, during waits, for five minutes. Each time the effort exhausted her completely. Now, since there was no other way aboard, she managed with help to climb twenty feet of rope ladder to the deck of the *Porto*.[9]

They found her a comfortable cabin. As she had known ever since those strong head winds in the Indian Ocean forty years earlier, she was a good sailor and did not fear the sea. Now her condition even improved a little.

It was bitterly cold, snow covered everything in the almost Arctic twilight of the short days. Late on the evening of the 11th there came to Dr Inglis as she lay in her bunk, her eyes closed with exhaustion and pain, the stores orderly, Butler, who had spent the whole day hanging around a locked and deserted station, trying to locate the stationmaster and have the equipment vans, which had been uncoupled a good mile away, moved to the quayside.

She had just found him; he had been attending revolutionary meetings all day and now told her that a general strike had been called and he could do nothing for her.[10] We know now, what the Scottish Women did not, that on the previous day the Bolsheviks had formed their government, that almost their first action was to call a general strike, and that Trotsky had at once given orders that no British subjects were to leave Russia, pending the release by Britain of the interned Russians Petroff and Chicherin. Even the British Ambassador, who had been planning a visit to England, was forced to stay in Russia.[11]

Butler reported on the situation as she knew it, and Dr Inglis opened her eyes. In her small white face they appeared enormous. In a voice so weak that she could hardly raise it above a whisper, she said, 'You must either get the equipment on board before we sail or stay behind to guard it. Your duty is to the equipment,' and shut her eyes again.

Butler, convinced she had been ordered to achieve the impossible, determined on one last appeal to the stationmaster. Early

*Among those applying for passage to Britain was Sister Vera Kolesnikoff who had of course left the S.W.H. when it joined the Serbians. She was granted a Foreign Office permit to travel as an English nurse in this party.

next morning as she confronted him, the whistle of an engine was heard. '*He's* working.' 'No—he's putting the engine away. Ask him yourself if you like.'

She did so, and met another refusal. Then, as she later described, a will stronger than her own took charge. In more fluent Russian than she had believed she knew, she begged and pleaded with him; and felt a British horror, even, when she found herself pulling the *vox humana* stop.

She stopped, exhausted. Without a word, the driver ran his locomotive to the Scottish Women's vans, coupled them on, and drove them to the quay, where Serbian soldiers unloaded and handed the precious equipment to the lascars of S.S. *Porto.* With a single sentence, the dying woman, exhausted in her bunk, had broken the nation-wide revolutionary strike and eluded Trotsky's ban. 'I knew I could trust you to do it,' was all she said when Butler reported to her.[12]

Ice breakers cleared a path for them as they left Archangel to assemble with the rest of their convoy which, on the morning of the 15th, finally steamed away from Russia under the escort of H.M.S. *Vindictive.*[13]

Five days later the Edinburgh Committee of the Scottish Women's Hospitals received a telegram Dr Inglis had sent before sailing. 'On our way home, everything satisfactory and all well except me, please do not arrange any meetings for me, the others will see reporters if you wish am going myself direct to London to report to Committee inform headquarters and relations. Inglis.'[14]

It was the first intimation they had had that she was even slightly unwell, and they did not take it too seriously.[15]

The *Porto* was old and unseaworthy. The crew was lascar, the captain and officers English. It was a relief to the women to be in the company of those Englishmen. Unlike the fatalistic Russians or the stoical Serbs, they diffused that security which only one's compatriots can give. The more introspective women realised now that while none of them had seriously felt frightened in Russia, neither had they ever felt safe.

The feeling, now, was an illusion. They were in as great danger as they had ever been. The second night out, a tremendous storm separated them from the rest of the convoy, with whom they never re-established contact, and drove them within the Arctic Circle. The *Porto* took on the look of a ghost ship, with icicles hanging from every point. The captain admitted he had no idea where he was within a hundred miles; in twenty years he had made no voyage which caused him such anxiety. Besides the threat of submarine and iceberg, the lascars were almost ready to mutiny and the pumps broke down so that seven feet of water flooded the engine room. Only unceasing work by the two engineer officers, who merely remarked in a reassuringly un-Slav understatement that they did not intend to let the women drown so near home after all they had been through, kept the ship afloat.[16]

Dr Inglis was a good deal better during the early part of the voyage. She was delighted; she joined the others in the saloon; found energy to play patience; read *The Old Dominion* and a volume of Browning, comprising *Sordello, Paracelsus* and *Pauline*;[17] attended and prescribed for the sick naval officer whose condition was serious; and said to Mrs Milne, 'After each time that I go down, I rise higher and higher. I shall soon be quite well again.'[18]

But soon she had to return to bed in great pain. Now she spent her time checking accounts and preparing lists of needed equipment, making fresh plans to take the Unit to Salonika. She interviewed each woman to ask if she would sign on again, and many did. She could hardly speak above a whisper; but told them that she expected to be ready to start for Salonika in six weeks' time.[19]

After they passed Orkney, the passage became even worse. The naval officer they were nursing, died as they tossed in a storm.

Then a strange feeling began to take possession of those on board: that only the will to live of the indomitable woman who had somehow brought them all together here to plough through the grey wastes of the North Sea, was keeping the *Porto* afloat. They were by no means sure that she must die. But they were convinced that if she did, not one of them would see land again. Only the Serbs, of course, spoke of it. But when they did, the English knew what they meant.[20]

On November 22nd they were within sight of land all day, that evening they were escorted through the narrow mine-swept path to the Tyne entrance, and at night they anchored off Newcastle and sent telegrams to their families.

The soldiers disembarked in the morning,* their homesick bewilderment contrasting miserably with the excitement of the women, who were to go ashore later. But towards noon the wind got up and no launch could come alongside. All day and through the night the *Porto* tossed in a blizzard that raged across the whole country. It was one of the wildest and most dangerous nights since they had left Archangel and more than one ship in the Tyne went adrift.[21]

At one moment a great liner was seen to be out of control and bearing down upon the *Porto*. She was within a few feet of ramming her when the *Porto*'s own moorings gave way and she swung out of danger. An orderly went to tell Dr Inglis. 'Who cut our moorings?' she asked. 'No one cut them. They broke,' was the reply. The two women looked at one another, and an unspoken question was in the air between them.[22]

On November 24th the Serb staff landed. Ill as she was, and having slept not at all the night before, Dr Inglis insisted upon dressing, and, wearing all her decorations, stood for nearly twenty minutes on deck, quite unsupported, to bid them goodbye. With her quiet air of gentle dignity, her face ashy pale and drawn, her worn uniform and faded medal ribbons, she was a figure that none who saw her could forget, as she stood there extending her hand to each officer to kiss and flashed at each of them the smile which still spoke of an unquenchable spirit.

When it was over she telegraphed to Seton Watson: 'Serbian headquarters staff with the brigade left here for Winchester, hope to be in London next week myself to see you. Inglis.'[24] Then she collapsed from weakness but refused to return to bed. Even now, nobody who saw her could accept that her illness was mortal. She did not accept it herself, and next day insisted upon

* In the absence of any announcement as to their identity, then or later, some at least of those who watched them marching from Newcastle Quayside and past Close Power Station, have believed up to the present day that these were the legendary 'snow on the boots' Russians whose arrival in England was persistently rumoured throughout the First World War. One witness, Arthur Johnson of Newcastle, then a power-station apprentice, wrote in *The Guardian* (10.12.69), 'They sang as they marched along the road ... By our own forces' standards at the time these marching men were badly clothed. Some wore greatcoats frayed out at the bottom without a hem. There was no snow on their boots and most of the marching feet were bound in a sort of hessian puttee or bandage. By comparison their officers were immaculately dressed and all wearing knee-length leather boots. Many of the men were carrying balalaikas slung over a shoulder.'

walking from her cabin and down the gangplank to the tug waiting to take her ashore. Dr Ward, who had attended her all through the past weeks, still believed she could be saved.[25]

She was taken to the Station Hotel where some of the Unit were putting up for the night, and wired to her family who had for forty-eight hours been trying to get into communication: 'I am in bed, do not telephone for a few days.'[26]

Eve Simson, with whom Elsie had a close bond of affection, set off on receipt of this and reached Newcastle in the small hours of Monday morning. They were unalarmed, but merely thought one of them should be with Elsie if she was unwell.[27]

When Miss Simson saw Dr Inglis—who had characteristically sent away the night nurse—early next morning, she was shocked at her wasted state; but was clasped in such a strong embrace that she was convinced good food and rest might soon restore her aunt. Dr Ward, however, arriving soon after, saw so much deterioration that she arranged to call in a second doctor. Dr Ethel Williams, who came, diagnosed peritonitis and privately held out little hope; but various treatments were tried. 'Now don't think we didn't think of all these things before,' said Elsie 'But on board ship nothing was possible.'[28]

The morning was given to goodbyes with the women who had stayed at Newcastle overnight. 'Goodbye, thank you for what you've done. We shall all meet again and we'll all go out to Serbia,' Miss Arbuthnot was told.[29] Mrs Milne was asked to see the Scots girls as far as Edinburgh and to report to the Committee. 'In a few days, come and see me in Edinburgh,' Dr Inglis added.[30] To Miss Onslow she said, 'I shall be up in London in a few days' time and we will talk the matter of a new Unit over.' Miss Onslow turned away to hide her tears.[31]

Later, Dr Williams returned. Now something in the faces of those about her made Elsie ask if this was the end. Miss Simson could not dissemble. Without hesitation Elsie said, 'Eve, it will be grand starting a new job over there.' She paused, then with her old dry humour added, 'Although there are two or three jobs here I would like to have finished.'[32]

Then she began to dictate final messages to her committees, her Units, her family. Her serenity made Dr Williams believe she had not grasped the fact of her condition; but she soon saw that Elsie was simply meeting a new challenge with her customary courage and adaptability.

To Miss Palliser she dictated a message (quoted here as it was received): 'So sorry I cannot come to London. Dr Williams and Dr Ward are agreed and quite rightly. Will send Gwynne in a day or two with explanations and suggestions. Colonel Miliantinovitch and Colonel Tcholah Antitch were to make appointment this week or next from Winchester; do see them, and also as many of the Committee as possible, and show them every hospitality. They have been very kind to us. And whatever happens, dear Miss Palliser, do beg the Committee to make sure that they (the Serbs) have their hospitals and transport, for they do need them.

'Many thanks to the Committee for their kindness to me and their support of me. Elsie Inglis.'[33]

To each of those who had been with her in Russia she sent the same message. It read simply 'My dear Unit—Goodbye.' Some of them have kept that faded slip of paper for fifty years.[34]

The storm which had been raging all day was blowing itself out when Mrs Simson and Mrs McLaren, summoned by telephone, arrived late in the afternoon. They were both in mourning for Mrs Simson's son James who had died of his wound on November 9th.

Elsie's first words to them were, 'So I am going over to the other side,' and then, with a smile, 'For a long time I meant to live, but now I know I am going.'

Her lucid intervals grew shorter. During one, Mrs McLaren said encouragingly, 'You have done magnificent work.' The answer was ready, and delivered with a flash of the old spirit: 'Not I but my Unit.'[35]

No more than she had shown fear in life did she now shrink from dying. There was just time for a few gentle sisterly exchanges of Christian courage and comfort, a short reading from the scriptures—characteristically, not specially chosen passages but those prescribed for that and the following days, in her little book of daily devotions.[36]

Then, with as little expense of time and fuss as she had ever in life given to her own personal affairs, she died.

Her old friend Dr Wallace Williamson made the first public announcement of her death next afternoon, and now the furore over her work knew no bounds.[37]

The Queen wrote to Mrs McLaren; William Hunter wrote to *The Times.* Columns upon columns of press eulogy ranged from the dignified and long obituaries in *The Times, Morning Post* and *Scotsman,* to the sober professional assessment of *The Lancet* and leading articles of the *Manchester Guardian* and *Glasgow Bulletin.* The *Aberdeen Free Press* perhaps predictably reported a War Office spokesman as having said that Dr Inglis's organisation got twice as much for their money as he did. The *Westminster Gazette* revealed that she had been on the point of receiving the very highest decorations from Russia and Serbia, the Gold St George medal and the White Eagle with Swords;* and the *Daily Sketch* summed up in a single headline what the ordinary man and woman in the street were thinking: 'Why Not V.C.s for Women?'[38]

There was a lying-in-state in St Giles' Cathedral in the district which had seen all the devoted years of unspectacular work. Royalty of England and Serbia were represented at the funeral; so was the Scottish Military Command which had once told her to sit still. Medical and suffrage colleagues were there, old friends and young from all periods of her life; doctors and nurses of her Units, Serbian soldiers who had known her in Kragujevatz, others who had been in Russia; and there were present twenty-five Serb boys who had made the Great Retreat and were now at school in Edinburgh.

The tattered banners of Scotland's heroes hung above where the small coffin lay, draped in a Union flag. The Hallelujah Chorus was played, the Last Post sounded. When the coffin was taken on a gun carriage drawn by six black horses at the head of a long procession down the winding miles to the Dean Cemetery, crowds eight deep lined Princes Street under their umbrellas in the dripping murk of the November afternoon;[39] and in the meaner streets women in shawls lifted shoulder-high small children she had brought into the world, so that they would always remember they had seen her coffin pass.

Then, a few days later, the memorial service at St Margaret's Westminster, with royalty again represented, and the diplomatic corps and government departments turning out in full force. There were more columns upon columns of press tributes. They all, for reasons of censorship and security, kept completely silent

* This was in fact bestowed posthumously on the representation of Gen. Jivkovitch. It had not before been given to a woman.

about her final and greatest achievement, the return of the Serbian divisions.[40] The *Scots Pictorial* summed up in two sentences the gist of them all: 'Not often has a death excited such profound and general regret as that of Dr Elsie Inglis. She was a supreme heroine in a time that has produced many heroines and she laid down her life for her fellow beings as truly as though she had given it on the battlefield.'[41]

'If she were a Serbian,' remarked an Orthodox priest to Dr Curcin, 'we would declare her a saint. In Scotland, she is only a doctor.'[42]

In the half century spanned by Elsie Inglis's life it is possible to see, in an extraordinarily compact pattern, the interwoven threads of the causes which inspired her.

She was born only months before the first M.P. supporting women's suffrage was elected to Westminster and the first woman qualified in medicine in England. When she died, women had that same year won the vote; women doctors had also at last won full recognition as competent to treat any patients who needed them. Both these things owed much to the work of herself and a handful of others of similar calibre.

At her birth, the Kingdom of Serbia for which she was to sacrifice herself did not yet exist; almost conterminously with her own life, it ceased, and became part of the greater unity now called Yugoslavia.

When she was born, the British Raj in India was in its infancy; the very name of Empire and its greatest days lay ahead, the implications of empire had still to be worked out. When she died, although the Empire still survived, everyone knew things would never be the same again. The guns of the Great War had shattered for ever the old sanguine confidence. Would anyone, ever again, be able to be totally unafraid simply because 'Britain was there'?

In a less easily defined way, it is possible to see that woman, in this half century, achieved a nobility unimagined for her before. At the beginning of it, she was still legally a slave, an idiot, a nothing. Individual kindness, individual strength, might mitigate this hard fact. But the hard fact was there.

Among the many who raised woman's stature, Elsie Inglis was of the greatest. In any single sphere, in politics, medicine, education, there were others who outpaced her. Many were more intellectually gifted, others more brilliant professionally, still others more politically adept or better rabble-rousers. None was more compassionate, more selfless or more determined. In all-round service therefore she matched the best of them; in heroism outdid them all.

When the Great War brought out among the often quite ordinary men in the trenches that upsurge of selflessness, endurance, idealism amid the pain and squalor, which dignified those years, the women too, *ordinary* women, were capable of sharing it all and, most of them, of still upholding also the gentleness of an older tradition. It was a peak of womanhood which may not recur again, and though many, to their honour, shared in it, it was outstandingly personified in Elsie Inglis. If to be splendidly identified with all that one holds valuable in life is to be happy, she must be accounted among the happiest of women.

APPENDIX

DOCUMENT BROUGHT TO ENGLAND BY MISS ROBINSON AND MISS HOLME MEMORISED BY MISS ROBINSON AND RETYPED TO HER DICTATION

The following is a short statement by Dr Jambrishak of Odessa to illustrate the difficult and dangerous position of the Serb Army on the Roumanian Front.

The Division consists of only 12,000 rifles and if it goes into action cannot depend at all on the support of the Russian troops.

It has *no reserves*, since the 2nd Division has already left Russia, and the Russian Government is now preventing the leaders from carrying on their propaganda and obtaining recruits from Yugoslav prisoners.

The Serbian Army suffered terribly last winter from shortage of food and equipment, e.g. at Berezovka the men had to be kept indoors for weeks because they had no boots, and the food supplies obtained from the Russians were often most unsatisfactory. There will be a far greater shortage of everything this winter and many men will be lost through sickness. Many even now are not at all fit, some of them suffer from night-blindness brought on by insufficient nourishment. Owing to the disorganisation and lack of transport there is already a serious shortage of fuel in South Russia. Difficulties of transport will also grow greater, owing to depreciation of rolling stock, permanent way, etc; except in Bessarabia where there is a rather mysterious activity in railway building and road repairing.

The Serbian troops are exceedingly good, as is shown by the magnificent work they did in the Dobruga in spite of terribly bad equipment; on the Roumanian Front they are being thrown away.

Many of these men were not willing to join our corpus but they were forced to do so because it was the opinion of the leaders that not only the best of our compatriots should die for the Yugoslav idea. This opinion was based on the opinion of the British Government, which has seen in the large number of the British volunteers the plebiscite of the English people, and not being willing that only the best of the English elements should perish in this way, has proclaimed military service as a duty for every Englishman.

For these so-called volunteers a special school was opened in the corpus, where they were educated in the Yugoslav idea. Many inconveniences must be noted here, because the higher military command misunderstood the character of this institution and regarded it as a purely military and not a political institution.

Many of these men were politically ripe but they did not join our corpus, because they could not see in the circumstances of Russia, any guarantee for the carrying out of the Yugoslav programme.

The great difference between the Austrian and the Russian military equipment also affected our men. In Austria the Yugoslavs were always very well treated at the Front and the commissariat arrangements were more than satisfactory. Food arrangements in Russia could not satisfy our men and there was added at the same time a cause of intellectual discontent.

Under Nicholas II Austrian spies conquered all Russia and they entered our corpus too. They began a disastrous campaign not only in our corpus but in the big Slav prison camps in Russia. It was obviously to Austria's interest to annihilate our corpus and these spies did everything in their power to accomplish that end. They applied the Austrian principle of *divide et impera* and tried to separate the Serbs from the Croats. They told our men that as foes of Austria they would never be able to return to their homes and families and said that Yugoslavia would never be formed. There were rumours too that Serbia was not fighting to liberate Croatia and Slovenia but to conquer them and create a greater Serbia, etc.

These spies were helped by Sturmer's Government.

Under these circumstances in our corpus, there broke out the Russian Revolution and the general trouble in Russia gave the spies an opportunity to work at full speed. They used the principle of revolution—Freedom—to destroy our corpus, which at the same time came under the influence of the soldiers' and workmen's committees. Our enemies entered these committees and under the pretence of defending the principle of freedom they pointed at our corpus as an institution composed not of volunteers but of men who were forced to join it. These committees became tools in the hands of the Austrian spies and they employed against our corpus all the means justifiable in the annihilation of an enemy but disastrous when applied to an allied army. A member of these Committees—a Bulgar by origin but a Russian subject—said in the presence of the Serbian Colonel Geraitch that our corpus must be destroyed and that he would use all his knowledge and influence to bring about this end.

If the higher military authorities were not willing to introduce into the Serbian division reforms in correspondence with the Russian army, they demanded that soldiers' committees should be introduced into our corpus too. In consequence of this request the committees were formed, but they were of a purely formal character. This did not satisfy the soldiers' and workmen's committees and they demanded the appointment of a commission whose duty it should be to ask every man whether he wished to remain as a volunteer in the Serbian corpus or not. The military authorities in Odessa and the Ambassador in Petrograd appealed to the Russian Government to interdict the carrying out of this resolution but it was not able to do anything, having no rights and no powers. The government replied always that it was not able to give any help, being in need of help itself to get power into its own hands. No obstacles were to be placed in the way of the committees' will, but if the corpus were disbanded the government would reform it as soon as it should be able to do so. So the committees entered on their disastrous work. Not content with asking every man whether he wished to remain in the corpus or not, they used every argument to persuade our men to leave the corpus. They told them that Russia would make a separate peace, that as foes of Austria they would never be able to return to their homes, that if they did they would be hanged, whereas if they left the corpus they would be free Russian citizens, and the committee guaranteed that they would be able to get four or five roubles a day as earned money—no small inducement to men who were earning less than three roubles a month.

This first commission was immediately followed by a second and the result was that 8000 men left the Serbian Division. These results did not satisfy the committees and the soldiers' and workmen's committee at Alexandrovsk arrested the Commandant of the 2nd Division and his Chief of 2nd Division Headquarters Staff. It was only owing to the presence of mind of the Commandant that a great bloodshed was prevented. The General commanding the Division was forced to ask for the intervention of the British consul at Odessa and the British Embassy at Petrograd. In consequence of this intervention and the protection and help of the British Embassy, the arrested Commandant and his Chief of Staff were liberated. This intervention had as a further result the issue of an order by the Russian military headquarters forbidding the formation of a third commission to enquire of every man whether he wished to remain in the corpus or not.

The results of this intervention communicated to our men, raised cheers and thanks for England and the feeling of sympathy for England was increased in the souls of our men. We speak with pride of the intervention for with English help we were able to save some 17,000 brave Yugoslav volunteers.

The outbreak of the Russian Revolution coincided with the outbreak of discontent among some Serb, Croat and Slovene officers. They were dissatisfied with the severe discipline of the corpus, with its denomination and finally with the really low pay. They demanded especially that the denomination should be changed from 'Serbian Volunteer Corpus' to 'Yugoslav Volunteer Corpus' and wished also to have some control over some of the acts of the higher command.

These officers were under the influence of some men who were for some time suspected of being Austrian agents in Russia.

We cannot deny that these officers were right in many points but we cannot understand why their actions bore such a hostile character.

Many of these young officers were unable to understand how pernicious their actions could be to our Serbian national affairs, they regarded the matter as being an affair of students, whereas those who led them were acting on very good plans. They still today, misled by some ideas and principles of the Russian Revolution, try to prove themselves to be better patriots than their comrades in the corpus.

We cannot doubt that there are among these emigrant officers many good and patriotic men, but we could not permit them to introduce a Russian disorder into our army and we therefore determined to get rid of them.

Those officers joined the Russian Army.

We believe that affairs like this can produce only Russia of today, and we are sure that if our corpus had been located in any other Allied country such things could not happen, or if they did, the Allied government would know how to deal with them more quickly and more efficiently.

We have nothing against these emigrant officers from the national political standpoint for they still emphasise their Yugoslav feelings, i.e. they long for the liberation and union of all Yugoslavs and it is of no importance that they represent the Serbian element as being chauvinist and aggressive because all men who are politically ripe, the Yugoslav organisations in America, and the common representative of all Yugoslavs—the Yugoslav Committee in London—look at our problem correctly and practically and not at all from the point of view of these emigrant officers, many of whom are young and inexperienced in politics, fantastic and naïve and who do not realise that they are being led by men whose only aim is to annihilate our corpus and destroy the credit of the Serbian Government and the Yugoslav Committee.

We must mention here also that the Italian Consul in Odessa began a propaganda among our officers and men, especially those from Istria and Dalmatia, with the object of persuading them to join the Italian army, but the movement was so entirely unsuccessful that the consul was forced to stop.

Having seen that our corpus was in continual danger of being disbanded and that no further prosperity could be guaranteed for it in Russia, we determined to send it to the Anglo-French or Salonika Front. But the opposite happened. After having made all this trouble and difficulty for us, the Russian government and military authorities realised the importance of our army for the Russian Front and on the repeated request of the Russian general commanding, our 1st Division left for the Roumanian Front. Thus our purpose of putting an end to the grave and bad position of our corpus in Russia was frustrated.

We tried to inform English political circles of the state of affairs in our corpus and we feel that it is only with English help that we can hope to leave this unhappy land and join our compatriots on the Salonika Front. Before the war we looked always toward the great eastern Slav state but all that has happened during the war, and especially the treatment of our element in Russia has completely changed the opinion of our men, and they now look towards the west. We hope to find in England our chief protector and assistant in guarding Serbia and the Near East from the Germans. England has now a unique opportunity of gaining the sympathies of all Yugoslavs.

This information was obtained from Croat sources.

Copy of paper dictated by Dr Jambrishak of Odessa, translated by Lieutenant Lipovschak. Transcribed from memory in London, October 9th, 1917.

signed. E. Frances Robinson

BIBLIOGRAPHY

UNPUBLISHED SOURCES

Admiralty Papers, at the Public Record Office.
Elizabeth Garrett Anderson Hospital Archives, London.
Foreign Office Papers, at the Public Record Office.
Hospice and Bruntsfield Hospital Minute Books, Edinburgh.
Inglis, Dr Elsie, Reports and Letters to Scottish Women's Hospitals Committees, at the Fawcett Library.
Inglis Family Papers, belonging to Mrs Maddox and the Rev. Roy MacNicol.
Medical Women's Federation records of early medical women, London.
Scottish Women's Hospital Records, at the Fawcett Library and the Imperial War Museum.
Serbian Relief Fund Archives, at the School of Slavonic Studies.
Seton Watson Papers, belonging to Professor H. Seton Watson.

PRIVATELY PUBLISHED SOURCES

CORBETT, DR C., *Diary of Serbia.*
HANSON, DR H., *Address to the Royal Society of Arts*, 23.2.1916.
HUNTER, WILLIAM, *The Serbian Epidemics of Typhus and Relapsing Fever, 1915* (Royal Society of Medicine).
PAGET, LADY, *With Our Serbian Allies.*
TAIT, DR H. P., *Dr Elsie Maud Inglis.*
WHITCHURCH, HOWELL, B., *Typhus Fever Epidemic in Serbia, 1915.*
Serbian Outpost (*Predstrezhe Srbski*) (Scottish Women's Hospital Records, Imperial War Museum).

PUBLISHED SOURCES

ANDERSON, L. G., *Life of Elizabeth Garrett Anderson*, Faber, 1939.
BALFOUR, LADY FRANCES, *Dr Elsie Inglis*, Hodder & Stoughton, 1918.
BELL, E. MOBERLY, *Storming the Citadel*, Constable, 1953.
BERRY, JAMES (and others), *The Story of a Red Cross Unit in Serbia*, J. & A. Churchill, 1916.
BUCHANAN, MERIEL, *Ambassador's Daughter*, Cassell, 1958.
BUTLER, E. M., *Daylight in a Dream*, Hogarth Press, 1951; *Paper Boats*, Collins, 1959.
CLARKE-KENNEDY, A. E., *Edith Cavell*, Faber, 1965.
CRUTTWELL, C. R. M. F., *A History of the Great War, 1914-1918*, O.U.P., 1934.

EDMONDS, BRIGADIER-GENERAL SIR J., *A Short History of World War I*, O.U.P., 1951.

FALKENHAYN, F. H., *General Headquarters 1914-15 and Its Critical Decisions*, Hutchinson, 1919.

FALLS, CYRIL, *History of the Great War, Macedonia, Vol. II*, H.M.S.O. 1933; *The First World War*, Longmans, 1960.

FAWCETT, MILLICENT, *What I Remember*, Fisher Unwin, 1925.

FEDDEN, MARGUERITE, *Sisters Quarters Salonika*, Grant Richards, 1921.

FITZROY, YVONNE, *With the Scottish Nurses in Roumania*, John Murray, 1918.

FULFORD, ROGER (ed.), *Dearest Child*, Evans Bros., 1964.

GRIFFITHS, P. J., *The British in India*, Robert Hale Ltd, 1946.

HANAK, HARRY, *Great Britain and Austria-Hungary During the First World War*, O.U.P., 1962.

HAY, IAN, *One Hundred Years of Army Nursing*, Cassells.

HOBMAN, D., *Go Spin, You Jade*, Watts, 1957.

HUTTON, I. EMSLIE, *Memories of a Doctor in War and Peace*, Heinemann, 1960; *With a Women's Unit in Serbia, Salonika and Sebastopol*, Williams and Norgate, 1928.

INGLIS, E. and others, *Study of the Diet of the Labouring Classes in Edinburgh*, Otto Schultz & Co.

JENKINS, ROY, *Asquith*, Collins, 1964.

JEX-BLAKE, SOPHIA, *Medical Women*, Hamilton Adams & Co., 1886.

JONES, FORTIER, *With Serbia into Exile*, Andrew Melrose, 1916.

KAMM, JOSEPHINE, *How Different From Us*, Bodley Head, 1958; *Rapiers and Battleaxes*, Allen and Unwin, 1966.

KNOX, MAJOR-GENERAL SIR A., *With the Russian Army 1914-17*, Hutchinson, 1921.

KRUGER, RAYNE, *Goodbye Dolly Gray*, Cassells, 1959.

MCLAREN, BARBARA, *Women of the War*, Hodder & Stoughton, 1917.

MCLAREN, E. SHAW (ed.), *A History of the Scottish Women's Hospitals*, Hodder & Stoughton, 1919; *Elsie Inglis*, S.P.C.K., 1919.

MANDIC, ANTE, *Fragmenti za Historiju Ujedinjenje*, Zagreb, 1956.

MANSON, C. and C., *Dr Agnes Bennett*, Michael Joseph, 1960.

MANTON, JO, *Life of Elizabeth Garrett Anderson*, Methuen, 1965.

MATTHEWS, CAROLINE, *Experiences of a Woman Doctor in Serbia*, Mills & Boon, 1916.

MURRAY, F., *Women as Army Surgeons*, Hodder & Stoughton, 1916.

NOWELL-SMITH, S. (ed.), *Edwardian England*, O.U.P., 1964.

POPE-HENNESSY, J., *Queen Mary*, Allen & Unwin, 1959.

SACKVILLE-WEST, V., *Saint Joan of Arc*, Cobden Sanderson, 1936.

SCHARLIEB, DAME MARY, *Reminiscences*, Williams & Norgate, 1924.

SCOTT, SIR E., *A Short History of Australia*, O.U.P., 1947.

STANOJEVITCH, DR V., *Moje Ratne Veleske i Slike*, Ljubljana, 1934.

TODD, MARGARET, *Life of Sophia Jex-Blake*, Macmillan, 1919.

WEST, REBECCA, *Black Lamb and Grey Falcon*, Macmillan, 1944.

WOODHAM-SMITH, C., *Florence Nightingale*, Penguin Edn.

PRIVATE INFORMATION

Inglis Family: Miss V. Inglis, Mr Moray McLaren, Miss Amy MacNicol, Rev. R. MacNicol, Mrs Maddox, the late Miss May Simson. Others: Miss E. Arbuthnot, Mrs Carlile, Mrs Cochrane-Shanks, Dame May Curwen, the late Miss G. Hedges, Miss G. Herzfeld MRCS, Miss V. Holme, Mrs Sherry, Mr K. St. Pavlowitch, Rev. Edward Vernon, Dr G. Ward, the late Sir Frederick Whyte.

NOTES

Chapter 1

1. *Serbian Outpost,* June-September 1915, S.W.H. Papers, Imperial War Museum.
2. Falls, *The First World War,* p. 371 et seq.
3. Stanojevitch, *Moje Ratne Veleske i Slike,* p. 92, Falls, *History of the Great War, Macedonia,* Vol. II p. 69, and Mandic, *Fragmenti za Historiju Udejinjenje,* pp. 33-49.
4. Butler, *Daylight in a Dream.*
5. *Englishwoman,* April 1916.
6. E. I. to May Simson 5 March 1917.
7. Private information, Mrs Sherry and Miss Hedges.
8. E.I., Report, III.
9. Cruttwell, *A History of the Great War, 1914-18,* p. 295.
10. *New Europe,* 6 December 1917, p. 249.
11. E.I., Report III.
12. *Daily Telegraph,* 14 December 1916.
13. E.I., Report III.
14. Fitzroy, *With the Scottish Nurses in Roumania,* pp. 30-3.
15. E.I., Report III.
16. Fitzroy, p. 33 et seq.
17. Ibid., p. 43.
18. E.I., Report III.
19. *Englishwoman,* November 1916.
20. E.I., Report III.
21. Ibid.
22. Fitzroy, op. cit., pp. 45-50.
23. Stanojevitch, op. cit., p. 110.
24. E.I., Report III.
25. Ibid.
26. E.I. to Lady Ashmore, 9 January 1917.
27. *Common Cause,* 24 June 1909.
28. Private information, Miss Holme.
29. Fitzroy, op. cit., p. 56, and E.I., Report III.
30. E.I., Report III.
31. Ibid.
32. Fitzroy, op. cit., pp. 50-1.
33. Ibid., p. 51.
34. E.I., Report III.
35. Ibid.
36. *Blackwood's Magazine,* April 1918.
37. E.I., Report III.

Chapter 2

1. Falls, *The First World War*, p. 371 et seq.
2. Mr Thomasen, Lieutenant-Governor of United Provinces, to Sir Henry Hardinge, quoted in Balfour, *Dr Elsie Inglis*, p. 12.
3. Balfour, op. cit., pp. 10-11.
4. Griffiths, *The British in India*, p. 105.
5. *Encyclopaedia Britannica*, 11th Edition, 'John Lawrence'.
6. Balfour, op. cit., pp. 14-15.
7. Private information, Miss V. Inglis.
8. Harriet Inglis to Amy Inglis, 21 December 1864.
9. Balfour, op. cit., p. 15.
10. John Inglis to E.I., 27 August 1876
11. E.I. to Amy Inglis, undated.
12. John Inglis to E.I., 8 September 1876.
13. Napier of Magdala to E.I., 17 February 1875.
14. Notes of Mrs McLaren, Inglis Papers, undated.
15. Harriet Inglis to Amy Inglis, January 1865.
16. Private information, Mrs Maddox.
17. E.I. to Amy Inglis, 20 June 1871.
18. McLaren, *Elsie Inglis*, pp. 7-8.
19. *Encyclopaedia Britannica*, 11th Edition, 'John Lawrence'.
20. Harriet Inglis to Amy Inglis, 3 January 1865.
21. Harriet Inglis, fragment, April 1873.
22. Harriet Inglis to Amy Inglis, 3 January 1865.
23. Jex-Blake, *Medical Women*, p. 235.
24. Fulford, *Dearest Child*.
25. Jex-Blake, op. cit., generally.
26. Balfour, op. cit., p. 27.
27. Private information, Mrs Maddox.
28. Inglis Papers.
29. *Encyclopaedia Britannica*, 11th Edition, 'John Lawrence'.
30. Balfour, op. cit., p. 28.

Chapter 3

1. John Inglis to Amy Inglis, 16 August 1864.
2. Manton, *Life of Elizabeth Garrett Anderson*.
3. Eva Inglis to Amy Inglis, 2 July, (no year).
4. Eva Inglis to Mrs Simson, 25 September 1878.
5. Horace Inglis to Mrs Simson, 1 October 1877.
6. Eva Inglis to Mrs Simson, 20 December 1877.
7. E.I. to Henry Simson, 24 December 1877.
8. Eva Inglis to Mrs Simson, 25 September 1878.
9. Balfour, op. cit., p. 28.
10. Kamm, *How Different From Us*, p. 36.
11. Ibid., p. 82.
12. John Inglis to Mrs Simson, 14 February 1879.
13. Eva Inglis to Mrs Simson, 20 December 1877.
14. Balfour, op. cit., p. 29.
15. *The Scotsman*, 15 July 1889

16. Scott, *A Short History of Australia*, p. 225.
17. Hugh Inglis to Herbert Inglis, 1895.
18. Cecil Inglis to E.I., 8 December 1895.
19. Private information, Miss V. Inglis.
20. Notes of Mrs McLaren, Inglis Papers, undated.

Chapter 4

1. Advertisement in *The Scotsman*, 27 August 1879.
2. Isabella Thornton to Mrs Simson, 2 December 1917.
3. Balfour, op. cit., p. 30.
4. Jex-Blake, op. cit., p. 230.
5. E. Moberly Bell, *Storming The Citadel*, p. 134.
6. Todd, *Life of Sophia Jex-Blake*, p. 477.
7. Ibid., p. 457.
8. Balfour, op. cit., p. 30.
9. E.I., Report III.
10. Mrs E. G. Osborne in Inglis Papers, 20 January 1918.
11. Balfour, op. cit., p. 31.
12. Mrs E. G. Osborne in Inglis Papers, 20 January 1918.
13. Balfour, op. cit., p. 37.
14. John Inglis to E.I., 20 November 1882.
15. Harriet Inglis to E.I., 10 January 1883.
16. Undated fragment from E.I., Inglis Papers.
17. Balfour, op. cit., p. 38.
18. Private information, Miss Hedges.
19. Private information, Mrs Cochrane Shanks.
20. Butler, *Paper Boats*, pp. 66-9.
21. John Inglis to E.I., 13 November 1882.
22. John Inglis to E.I., 20 November 1882.
23. Harriet Inglis to E.I., 6 February 1883.
24. Balfour, op. cit., p. 38.

Chapter 5

1. Woodham-Smith, *Florence Nightingale*, p. 62.
2. Kamm, *How Different From Us*, p. 39.
3. Inglis Papers.
4. *The Lancet*, 8 December 1917.
5. E.I. to 'Aunt Dorry', 6 October 1898.
6. *Glasgow Herald*, 16 August 1964.
7. Balfour, op. cit., p. 33.
8. Ibid., p. 32.
9. Jex-Blake, op. cit., p. 227.
10. Balfour, op. cit., p. 40.
11. Todd, op. cit., pp. 70-1.
12. MS. note in Inglis Papers.
13. *The Scotsman*, 19 July 1889.
14. E.I. to Ernest Inglis, 15 March 1894.
15. Jex-Blake, op. cit., pp. 157, 160.
16. Todd, op. cit., pp. 479-80.

17. Jex-Blake, op. cit., pp. 177-81.
18. Anderson, *Life of Elizabeth Garrett Anderson*, p. 104.
19. Moberly Bell, *Storming The Citadel*, p. 105.
20. *The Scotsman*, 19 July 1889.
21. Reports in *The Scotsman*, 19 and 20 July, 24 October, 4 November, 1889, of the Action of Lady Medical Students.
22. Todd, op. cit., p. 417.
23. Jex-Blake, op. cit., p. 181.
24. Tait, *Dr Elsie Maud Inglis*, p. 23.
25. Balfour, op. cit., p. 47.
26. Manson, *Dr Agnes Bennett*, p. 30.
27. Balfour, op. cit., p. 57.
28. E.I. to John Inglis, 9 February 1891.
29. Balfour, op. cit., p. 50.
30. Ibid., p. 53.
31. Private information, Miss May Simson.
32. Balfour, op. cit., p. 51.
33. Ibid., pp. 56-7.
34. Ibid., p. 51.
35. Ibid., pp. 53-7.
36. Ibid., p. 58.
37. Dr B Russell, note in Inglis Papers, undated.
38. Hutton, *With A Women's Unit in Serbia, Salonika and Sebastopol*, p. 191.

Chapter 6

1. Elizabeth Garrett Anderson Hospital Archives.
2. Moberly Bell, *Storming The Citadel*, p. 111 et seq.
3. Scharlieb, *Reminiscences*, pp. 203-4.
4. Balfour, op. cit., p. 72.
5. Ibid., pp. 88-9.
6. Ibid., p. 88.
7. Records of early medical women at Medical Women's Federation.
8. Balfour, op. cit., pp. 90-2.
9. Ibid., p. 95.
10. Photograph in Fawcett Library.
11. Kamm, *Rapiers and Battleaxes*, p. 117
12. Balfour, op. cit., pp. 92-3.
13. Ibid., p. 66.
14. Ibid., p. 69.
15. Ibid., p. 73.
16. Ibid., p. 67-8.
17. E.I. to John Inglis, December 1892.
18. Balfour, op. cit., p. 54.
19. Ibid., p. 68.
20. Ibid., p. 73.
21. Ibid., p. 77.
22. Ibid., p. 75. See also British Medical Register, 1893.
23. Ibid., p. 77.

24. Ibid, p. 78.
25. E.I. to John Inglis, 10 February 1894.
26. Minute Book 1 of Bruntsfield Hospital.
27. E.I. to John Inglis, 10 February 1894.
28. Balfour, op. cit., p. 80.
29. E.I. to Ernest Inglis, 15 March 1894.

Chapter 7

1. Private information, Mrs Maddox.
2. Private information, Mrs Carlile.
3. Balfour, op. cit., p. 68.
4. See Lloyd Osborne's introduction to *New Arabian Nights* (Tusitala edition), p. xv.
5. *The Scotsman*, 23 October 1889.
6. A. J. P. Taylor in *Edwardian England*, ed. S. Nowell-Smith.
7. *The Scotsman*, 20 July 1889.
8. Hobman, *Go Spin, You Jade*, p. 126.
9. McLaren, op. cit., pp. 17-18.
10. Typescript 'Stories from Patients', Inglis Papers.
11. Balfour, op. cit., pp. 127-8.
12. Typescript 'Political Work', Inglis Papers.
13. Dr B. Russell in *Edinburgh Medical Journal*, January 1918.
14. Minute Book 2 of Bruntsfield Hospital, 29 January 1899.
15. Ibid., 24 March 1899.
16. Ibid., 27 March 1899.
17. Private information, Mrs Maddox.
18. Balfour, op. cit., p. 119.
19. Minute Book 2 of Bruntsfield Hospital, June 1899.
20. Balfour, op. cit., p. 113.
21. Minute Book 3 of Bruntsfield Hospital, 22 June 1901.
22. Ibid., 6 July 1901.
23. Minute Book of The Hospice and Bruntsfield Hospital, no date.
24. Minute Book of The Hospice.
25. Typescript 'Stories from Patients', Inglis Papers.
26. Typescript 'Stories from Patients', Inglis Papers.
27. Inglis E. and others, *Study of the Diet of the Labouring Classes in Edinburgh.*

Chapter 8

1. Minute Book 3 of Bruntsfield Hospital, 12 and 20 April, 1905.
2. Ibid., 11 April 1906.
3. Ibid., 6 July 1905.
4. Ibid., November 1905.
5. Hobman, op. cit., p. 96.
6. For this period, see files of *Common Cause*, especially July 1909.
7. *British Weekly*, 6 December 1917.
8. Mary Bury to Mrs Simson, 19 January 1918, Inglis Papers.
9. Private information, Mrs Carlile.
10. Letters from Mrs Snowden etc., Inglis Papers.

11. Typescript 'Political Work', Inglis Papers.
12. Private information, Miss May Simson.
13. E.I. to Mrs Simson, 6 November 1915.
14. Balfour, op. cit., p. 135.
15. Notes of Mrs McLaren, Inglis Papers.
16. *Nineteenth Century*, June 1889.
17. *The Lancet*, 8 December 1917.
18. Minute Book 3 of Bruntsfield Hospital, October 1907.
19. Tait, op. cit., pp. 6-7.
20. Balfour, op. cit., p. 132.
21. Private information, Miss May Simson.
22. Typescript 'Stories of Patients', Inglis Papers.
23. Private information, Mrs Maddox, Miss V. Inglis, Miss May Simson.
24. Balfour, op. cit., p. 133.
25. Entries in Minute Book 3 of the Bruntsfield Hospital, October-December 1909.
26. *The Scotsman*, 19 July, 1911.
27. Private information, Mrs Maddox.
28. Private information, Miss A. MacNicol.
29. Jenkins, *Asquith*, p. 246.
30. *Common Cause*, 1 July 1909.
31. *Glasgow Herald*, 1 December 1917.
32. McLaren, *Elsie Inglis*, pp. 38-40.
33. Hobman, op. cit., p. 113.
34. Shaw, *Prefaces*, p. 745.
35. McLaren, op. cit., pp. 38-39.
36. Typescript, Inglis Papers.
37. McLaren, *Elsie Inglis*, p. 20.
38. Notes of Mrs McLaren, Inglis Papers.
39. Stevenson, *An Inland Voyage* (Tusitala edition), p. 80.
40. Wells, *First and Last Things*.
41. Private information, Miss V. Inglis.
42. Jex-Blake, op. cit., p. 211.
43. Notes of Mrs McLaren, Inglis Papers.
44. Ibid.
45. Private information, Miss May Simson.
46. Hobman, op. cit., p. 114.
47. Jenkins, op. cit., pp. 246-7.
48. McLaren, *Elsie Inglis*, p. 34.
49. Typescript 'Stories of Patients', Inglis Papers.
50. McLaren, *Elsie Inglis*, p. 30.

Chapter 9

1. *Common Cause*, 11 May 1917.
2. Private information, Miss May Simson.
3. Murray, *Women as Army Surgeons*, p. 69.
4. Hutton, *With a Women's Unit in Serbia, Salonika and Sebastopol*, p. 16.

5. Kruger, *Goodbye Dolly Gray*, p. 510.
6. Ibid., pp. 392, 462.
7. Fawcett, *What I Remember*, pp. 170-1.
8. Kruger, op. cit., p. 392.
9. Ibid., p. 215.
10. McLaren, *A History of the Scottish Women's Hospitals*, p. 4.
11. Balfour, op. cit., p. 148.
12. *Sheffield Telegraph*, 30 November 1917.
13. Note by Miss M. Henderson in Inglis Papers.
14. Note by Dame Sarah Mair in Inglis Papers.
15. *Common Cause*, 30 October 1914.
16. E.I. to Mrs Fawcett, 9 October 1914.
17. Private information, Miss V. Inglis; and McLaren, *A History of the Scottish Women's Hospitals*, p. 6.
18. *Central Somerset Gazette*, 6 November 1914.
19. E.I. to Mrs Fawcett, 9 October 1914.
20. McLaren, *A History of the Scottish Women's Hospitals*, p. 8.
21. Scottish Women's Hospitals Records, Imperial War Museum.
22. Hutton, *With A Women's Unit in Serbia, Salonika and Sebastopol*, pp. 19-21.
23. Ibid., p. 21.
24. Fedden, *Sisters Quarters Salonika.*
25. S.W.H. Records, Box 1915, Fawcett Library.
26. *Common Cause*, 16 October 1914.
27. Murray, op. cit.
28. *Evesham Journal*, 2 June 1916.
29. Hutton, *Memories of a Doctor in War and Peace*, p. 93.
30. Clark-Kennedy, *Edith Cavell*, pp. 61-70.
31. McLaren, *A History of the Scottish Women's Hospitals*, p. 12.
32. Ibid., p. 18.
33. S.W.H. Records, Imperial War Museum.
34. McLaren, *A History of the Scottish Women's Hospitals*, pp. 19-21.
35. E.I. to Mrs Simson, 22 December 1914.
36. Ibid.
37. *Aberdeen Free Press*, 30 November 1914.
38. E.I. to Mrs Simson, 22 December 1914.
39. Holograph note by Mrs McLaren, Inglis Papers.
40. B.W.W. in *The Scotsman*, 26 October 1957.
41. Balfour, op. cit., p. 156.
42. Sackville-West, *Saint Joan of Arc*, p. 373.
43. Private information, Mrs Cochrane Shanks.
44. Minute book of N.U.W.S.S., 17 February 1915.
45. Private information, Mrs Cochrane Shanks.
46. Note by Dame Sarah Mair in Inglis Papers.
47. E.I., 'The Tragedy of Serbia', *Englishwoman*, April 1916.

Chapter 10

1. See contemporary newspapers.
2. West, *Black Lamb and Grey Falcon*, Vol. I, pp. 553-5, 575-90.

3. Pope-Hennessy, *Queen Mary*, p. 486.
4. Falls, *The First World War*, pp. 18-19.
5. Edmonds, *A Short History of World War I*, p. 9.
6. A number of translations of this passage exist. I have used that given by E.I. to a public meeting at the Criterion Theatre, London, April 1916. Inglis Papers.
7. Falls, *The First World War*, p. 35.
8. Trevelyan and Watson, *Serbian Relief Fund Archives*, 20 January 1915.
9. Bertram Christian, Serbian Relief Fund Archives.
10. Reports from S.W.H. members, *Ladies' Field*, 3 April 1915, and *Common Cause*, 12 November 1915.
11. Helen Hanson M.D., Address to the Royal Society of Arts, 23 February 1916. Fawcett Library.
12. William Hunter, *The Serbian Epidemics of Typhus and Relapsing Fever in 1915*, Royal Society of Medicine Library.
13. *Common Cause*, 12 February 1915.
14. E.I. to Dr Soltau, 9 March 1915.
15. H. D. Irvine, *Common Cause*, 12 November 1915.
16. S.W.H. Records, Imperial War Museum. See also *Evesham Journal*, 2 June 1916.
17. Hanson, op. cit.
18. Hunter, op. cit.
19. Hanson, op. cit.
20. Minute book of The Hospice, 7 January 1915.
21. E.I. to Miss Crompton, Inglis Papers.
22. Balfour, op. cit., p. 152.
23. Hunter, op. cit.
24. Unidentified cutting, 12 December 1917, S.W.H. Records, Imperial War Museum.
25. Rev. S. Baring-Gould to Miss Burke, Box 1915, S.W.H. Records, Fawcett Library.
26. Box 1916, S.W.H. Records, Fawcett Library.
27. Private information, Miss Hedges.
28. E.I. to Miss McLaren, 2 May 1915.
29. Ibid.
30. Ibid.
31. Ibid.
32. McLaren, *A History of the Scottish Women's Hospitals*, p. 97 et seq.
33. Lady Paget to Lady Brassey, 15 August 1915, S.W.H. Records, Fawcett Library.
34. McLaren, *A History of the Scottish Women's Hospitals*, p. 31.
35. *Serbian Outpost*, June-September 1915, S.W.H. Records, Imperial War Museum.
36. McLaren, *A History of the Scottish Women's Hospitals*, p. 132.
37. Ibid, p. 133.
38. Ibid. p. 134.

Chapter 11

1. Hanson, op. cit.
2. *Common Cause*, 12 November 1915.
3. Hutton, *With A Women's Unit in Serbia, Salonika and Sebastopol*, p. 188.
4. Hanson, op. cit.
5. E.I. to Mrs Simson, Inglis Papers.
6. *Daily Mail*, 23 February 1915.
7. Balfour, op. cit., p. 178.
8. Major Claude Askew, *Englishwoman*, October 1916.
9. Hanson, op. cit.
10. Hunter, op. cit.
11. Ibid.
12. Berry, *The Story of a Red Cross Unit in Serbia*, p. 131.
13. McLaren, *A History of the Scottish Women's Hospitals*, p. 107.
14. Hutton, *With A Women's Unit in Serbia, Salonika and Sebastopol*, p. 101.
15. McLaren, *A History of the Scottish Women's Hospitals*, p. 107.
16. Ibid, p. 106.
17. William Hunter to Mrs McLaren, 1 December 1919, Inglis Papers.
18. See E.I. to Miss Palliser, 5 March 1917, S.W.H. Records, Fawcett Library.
19. E.I. to Mrs McLaren, 16 June 1915, Inglis Papers.
20. McLaren, *Elsie Inglis*, p. 54.
21. Ibid., p. 49.
22. *The Times*, 29 November 1917.
23. Hunter, op. cit.
24. McLaren, *A History of the Scottish Women's Hospitals*, p. 111.
25. Hutton, *With A Women's Unit in Serbia, Salonika and Sebastopol*, p. 101.

Chapter 12

1. *Morning Post*, 20 April 1915.
2. *Serbian Outpost*, June-September 1915.
3. Askew, *Englishwoman*, October 1916.
4. *Englishwoman*, November 1916.
5. Ibid., June 1916.
6. Matthews, *Experiences of a Woman Doctor in Serbia*, p. 40.
7. Hutton, *With A Women's Unit in Serbia, Salonika and Sebastopol*, p. 87.
8. McLaren, *A History of the Scottish Women's Hospitals*, p. 117.
9. *Common Cause*, 10 September 1915.
10. E.I. to Mrs McLaren, 19 December 1916, Inglis Papers.
11. Box 1915, S.W.H. Records, Fawcett Library.
12. Ibid.
13. McLaren, *A History of the Scottish Women's Hospitals*, p. 129.
14. Ibid., p. 114.
15. E.I., *Englishwoman*, April 1916.
16. Note by Miss Holme, Inglis Papers.

17. Hunter, op. cit.
18. McLaren, *A History of the Scottish Women's Hospitals*, pp 115-16.
19. Ibid., p. 120.
20. Private information, Mr K. St. Pavlowitch.
21. McLaren, *A History of the Scottish Women's Hospitals*, p. 128.
22. Falls, *The First World War*, p. 122.
23. Hanson, op. cit.
24. E.I., 'The Tragedy of Serbia', *Englishwoman*, April 1916.
25. Fr Nikolai Velimiroviz, Inglis Papers.
26. McLaren, *A History of the Scottish Women's Hospitals*, pp. 121-4.
27. *Common Cause*, 12 November 1915.
28. Ibid., 7 April 1916.
29. McLaren, *A History of the Scottish Women's Hospitals*, p. 126.
30. Ibid., p. 126.
31. G. Pares, 'With the Serbian Retreat', *Englishwoman*, March 1916.
32. McLaren, *A History of the Scottish Women's Hospitals*, p. 127.
33. E.I., 'The Tragedy of Serbia', *Englishwoman*, April 1916.
34. McLaren, *A History of the Scottish Women's Hospitals*, p. 127.
35. Lady Paget, *With Our Serbian Allies*.
36. Hanson, op. cit.
37. Berry, op. cit., p. 176.
38. Lady Paget, op. cit.
39. McLaren, *A History of the Scottish Women's Hospitals*, p. 207.
40. E.I. at the Criterion Theatre public meeting, 4 April 1916, Inglis Papers.

Chapter 13

1. Falkenhayn, *General Headquarters 1914-15 and its Critical Decisions*, p. 175.
2. Jones, *With Serbia Into Exile*.
3. *Englishwoman*, September 1916.
4. Ibid., April 1916.
5. Photograph in Inglis Papers.
6. Corbett, *Diary of Serbia*, pp. 2-3.
7. Berry, op. cit.
8. E.I., *Englishwoman*, April 1916.
9. Ibid.
10. Curcin, 'British Women in Serbia', *Englishwoman*, September 1916.
11. Lady Paget, op. cit., p. 21.
12. Ibid.
13. Hutton, *With A Women's Unit in Serbia, Salonika and Sebastopol*, p. 97.
14. Hanson, op. cit.
15. Lady Paget, op. cit., p. 36.
16. Hay, *One Hundred Years of Army Nursing*, p. 168.
17. E.I., 'The Tragedy of Serbia', *Englishwoman*, April 1916.

18. Corbett, op. cit., p. 6.
19. E.I. to Miss Mair, 5 November 1915, S.W.H. Records, Imperial War Museum.
20. Corbett, op. cit., p. 8.
21. McLaren, *Elsie Inglis*, p. 51.
22. Jones, op. cit.
23. Corbett, op. cit., p. 12.
24. McLaren, *A History of the Scottish Women's Hospitals*, p. 144.
25. Curcin, 'British Women in Serbia', *Englishwoman*, September 1916.
26. E.I. to Miss Mair, 5 November 1915, S.W.H. Records, Imperial War Museum.
27. McLaren, *A History of the Scottish Women's Hospitals*, pp. 143-4.
28. E.I. to Mrs Simson, 6 November 1916, Inglis Papers.
29. Corbett, op. cit., p. 17.
30. *Northern Whig*, 29 November 1915.
31. Corbett, op. cit., p. 7.
32. McLaren, *Elsie Inglis*, pp. 51-2.
33. Corbett, op. cit., p. 15.
34. Ibid., p. 16.
35. *Common Cause*, 3 March 1916.
36. Corbett, op. cit., p. 19.
37. *Common Cause*, 3 March 1916.
38. *Englishwoman*, June 1916.
39. Ibid.

Chapter 14

1. E.I., 'The Tragedy of Serbia', *Englishwoman*, June 1916.
2. Ibid.
3. E.I., Report XII, 16 April 1917, Fawcett Library.
4. E.I., 'The Tragedy of Serbia', *Englishwoman*, June 1916.
5. Ibid.
6. Ibid.
7. Corbett, op. cit., p. 23.
8. E.I., 'The Tragedy of Serbia', *Englishwoman*, June 1916.
9. I am indebted to Miss Holme for the name of Miss Whitehead, who appears in the writings of Elsie Inglis and Catherine Corbett simply as 'W'.
10. E.I., 'The Tragedy of Serbia', *Englishwoman*, June 1916.
11. Berry, op. cit. Also Foreign Office Papers, F.O. 372/1037/180014.
12. Corbett, op. cit., pp. 31-2.
13. Ibid., pp. 30-49.
14. Holograph note by Mrs McLaren, Inglis Papers.
15. Corbett, op. cit., p. 26.
16. Holograph note by Mrs McLaren, Inglis Papers.
17. Folder marked '1915. S.W.H. Laurie' in Fawcett Library.
18. *Common Cause*, 12 November 1915.
19. McLaren, *A History of the Scottish Women's Hospitals*, pp. 161-2.
20. Corbett, op. cit., p. 27.

21. Pares, 'With the Serbian Retreat', *Englishwoman,* March 1916.
22. McLaren, *A History of the Scottish Women's Hospitals,* p. 150.
23. Pares, 'With the Serbian Retreat', *Englishwoman,* March 1916.
24. Ibid.
25. Minute book of Bruntsfield Hospital.
26. Curcin, 'British Women in Serbia', *Englishwoman,* September 1916.
27. Hutton, *With A Women's Unit in Serbia, Salonika and Sebastopol,* p. 44.
28. Personal Information the Rev. Edward Vernon.

Chapter 15

1. E.I., 'The Tragedy of Serbia', *Englishwoman,* June 1916.
2. Corbett, op. cit., p. 62.
3. Berry, op. cit., p. 51.
4. E.I., 'The Tragedy of Serbia', *Englishwoman,* June 1916.
5. Corbett, op. cit., pp. 19, 35, 41, 56.
6. Ibid., pp. 23-4.
7. E.I., 'The Tragedy of Serbia', *Englishwoman,* June 1916.
8. Seton Watson, notes in box-file marked 'S.R.F. Letters', School of Slavonic Studies.
9. Balfour, op. cit., pp. 160-1.
10. Corbett, op. cit., p. 29.
11. Ibid., p. 164.
12. Ibid., p. 30.
13. Ibid., pp. 21, 28.
14. Ibid., pp. 25-7.
15. Ibid., p. 28.
16. E.I., 'The Tragedy of Serbia', *Englishwoman,* June 1916.
17. McLaren, *Elsie Inglis,* p. 56.
18. E.I., 'The Tragedy of Serbia', *Englishwoman,* June 1916.
19. Ibid., and Corbett, op. cit., pp. 40-3.
20. Corbett, op. cit., pp. 44-5.
21. Pares, 'With the Serbian Retreat', *Englishwoman,* March 1916.
22. *Common Cause,* 21 January 1916.
23. Hutton, *With A Women's Unit in Serbia, Salonika and Sebastopol,* pp. 53-5.
24. Corbett, op. cit., p. 46.
25. Ibid., pp. 47, 50.
26. E.I., 'The Tragedy of Serbia', *Englishwoman,* June 1916.
27. Corbett, op. cit., p. 58.
28. *Common Cause,* 3 March 1916.
29. Typescript, 'Stories about Dr Inglis, by One of Her Colleagues', Inglis Papers. The colleague was Miss Holme.
30. Ibid.
31. Corbett, op. cit., p. 63.
32. E.I., 'The Tragedy of Serbia', *Englishwoman,* June 1916.
33. Ibid.
34. Balfour, op. cit., p. 188.

35. Holograph note by Mrs McLaren, Inglis Papers.

Chapter 16

1. Miss M. Henderson, *Dundee Advertiser,* 28 November 1917.
2. Emerson, 'On Heroism'.
3. Mrs Carrington Wild to Mrs Simson, Inglis Papers (undated).
4. *Glasgow Bulletin,* 28 November 1917.
5. Box 1916 S.W.H. Records, Fawcett Library.
6. *The Times,* 4 April 1916.
7. McLaren, *A History of the Scottish Women's Hospitals,* p. 94.
8. West, op. cit., vol. 1, p. 604.
9. *The Lancet,* 8 December 1917.
10. Undated and unidentified cutting, Inglis Papers.
11. Box 1916, S.W.H. Records, Fawcett Library.
12. *The Times,* various dates, June 1917.
13. Falls, *History of the First World War,* p. 137.
14. Hutton, *Memories of a Doctor in War and Peace,* p. 93.
15. *The Times,* 12 July 1917.
16. Typescript report on these negotiations, S.W.H. files, Fawcett Library.
17. *The Times,* 3 April 1916.
18. *The Times,* 19 July 1916.
19. Miss Stoney, letter quoted in *Women of the War* by Barbara McLaren, p. 46.
20. Manson, op. cit., p. 78.
21. McLaren, *Elsie Inglis,* p. 40.
22. Curcin, *Englishwoman,* January 1918; Serbian Relief Fund minute books, School of Slavonic Studies; report of Kossovo Day Committee, Inglis Papers; appeal of Kossovo Day Committee in Box 1916, S.W.H. Records, Fawcett Library.
23. *New Europe,* 6 December 1917.
24. Private information, Sir Frederick Whyte.
25. Reports in S.W.H. Papers, Fawcett Library.
26. Private information from Miss Hedges, Mrs Sherry, Miss Arbuthnot.
27. *Ladies' Pictorial,* 9 September 1916.
28. E.I. to Mrs Simson, 6 September 1916, Inglis Papers.
29. McLaren, *Elsie Inglis,* p. 36.
30. Interview with Mrs McLaren and Mrs Simson, 8 June 1918. Typescript in S.W.H. Records, Imperial War Museum.
31. Holograph note by Mrs McLaren, Inglis Papers.
32. Minute Book 3, Bruntsfield Hospital.
33. Private information, Dame May Curwen.
34. Box 1916, S.W.H. Records, Fawcett Library.
35. *Common Cause,* 30 November 1917.

Chapter 17

1. See contemporary newspaper denials of these rumours.

2. Fitzroy, op. cit., p. 10; and E.I., Report II, 24 September 1916.
3. Fitzroy, op. cit., p. 10 et seq.
4. E.I. Report II, 24 September 1916.
5. E.I. to Mrs Simpson, 14 September 1916, Inglis Papers.
6. E.I. Report II, 24 September 1916.
7. Miss Mair, typewritten note, Inglis papers.
8. E.I. Report II, 24 September 1916.
9. E.I. to Lady Ashmore, 25 September 1916, S.W.H. Records, Fawcett Library.
10. E.I. to Mrs Simson, 20 September 1916, Inglis Papers.
11. Stanojevitch, op. cit., p. 92.
12. E.I. Report II, 24 September 1916.
13. E.I. to Lady Ashmore, 25 September 1916, Fawcett Library.
14. E.I. to Eve Simson, 24 January 1917, Inglis papers.
15. E.I. 'Three Months On The Eastern Front', *Englishwoman*, February 1917.
16. Fitzroy, op. cit., p. 29.
17. E.I., 'Three Months on the Eastern Front', *Englishwoman*, February 1917.
18. E.I., Report III.
19. See *History of The Times, 1912-1920*, p. 247.
20. Knox, *With the Russian Army, 1914-17*, p. 483 et seq.
21. E.I., Report III.
22. Ibid.
23. Stanojevitch, op. cit., p. 110.
24. E.I., Report III.
25. Ibid.
26. Personal information, Miss Hedges.
27. E.I., Report III, Fawcett Library.
28. E.I., 'Three Months On The Eastern Front', *Englishwoman*, February 1917.
29. E.I., Report III, Fawcett Library.
30. Ibid.
31. Personal information, Miss Hedges.
32. E.I., Report III, Fawcett Library.

Chapter 18

1. Photograph in the possession of Miss Hedges.
2. E.I., Report III, Fawcett Library.
3. Ibid.
4. Ibid.
5. E.I. to Mrs Simson, 11 November 1916, Inglis Papers.
6. E.I., Report III, Fawcett Library.
7. Ibid.
8. Ibid.
9. Fitzroy, op. cit., pp. 58-9.
10. E.I. to Mrs Simson, 11 November 1916, Inglis Papers.
11. E.I. to Eve Simson, 27 November 1916, Inglis Papers.
12. E.I., Report V, 27 November 1916, Fawcett Library.

13. E.I., note in Box 1915, S.W.H. Records, Fawcett Library.
14. Falls, *The First World War*, p. 197 et seq.
15. E.I. to Lady Ashmore, 4 December 1916, Fawcett Library.
16. Stanojevitch, op. cit., pp. 110 et seq.
17. E.I. to Lady Ashmore, 14 November 1916, Fawcett Library.
18. E.I., Report VI, 18 December 1916, Fawcett Library.
19. E.I. to Mrs McLaren, 19 December 1916, Inglis Papers.
20. Corbett, op. cit., p. 37.
21. E.I. to Lady Ashmore, 3 November 1916, Fawcett Library.
22. Foreign Office Papers, F.O. 371/2993/118452.
23. E.I. to Lady Ashmore, 3 November 1916, Fawcett Library.
24. Foreign Office Papers, F.O. 371/2993/18601.
25. E.I., Report IV, 20 November 1916, Fawcett Library.
26. E.I. to Lady Ashmore, 4 December 1916, Fawcett Library.
27. E.I. to Lady Ashmore, 19 December 1916, Fawcett Library.
28. Foreign Office Papers, F.O. 371/2993/197059.
29. E.I. to Lady Ashmore, 14 November 1916, Fawcett Library.
30. E.I., Report IV, 20 November 1916, Fawcett Library.
31. Fitzroy, op. cit., p. 57 et seq.
32. E.I., Report V, 27 November 1916, Fawcett Library.
33. Ibid.
34. E.I., Report VI, 19 December 1916, Fawcett Library.
35. Falls, *The First World War*, p. 197 et seq.
36. E.I., Report VI, 19 December 1916, Fawcett Library.
37. Fitzroy, op. cit., pp. 77-8.
38. Fitzroy, op. cit., p. 79 et seq.; E.I., Report VI.
39. E.I., Report VI, 19 December 1916, Fawcett Library.
40. Cruttwell, op. cit., p. 295 et seq.
41. E.I., Report VI, 19 December 1916.
42. Ibid.

Chapter 19

1. Fitzroy, op. cit., p. 86 et seq.
2. E.I. to Eve Simson, 8 January 1917, Inglis Papers.
3. E.I., Report VII, 8 January 1917, Fawcett Library.
4. Fitzroy, op. cit., p. 86 et seq.
5. E.I., Report VII, 8 January 1917, Fawcett Library.
6. Fitzroy, op. cit., pp. 93-6.
7. Commander Gregory to Mrs McLaren, 28 November 1917, Inglis Papers.
8. McLaren, *A History of the Scottish Women's Hospitals*, pp. 199-200.
9. E.I., Report VII, 8 January 1917, Fawcett Library.
10. Ibid.
11. E.I. to Lady Ashmore, 9 January 1917, Fawcett Library.
12. Fitzroy, op. cit., p. 96.
13. E.I. to Mrs McLaren, 9 January 1917, Inglis Papers.
14. E.I. to Lady Ashmore, 9 January 1917, Fawcett Library.
15. E.I., Report VII, 8 January 1917, Fawcett Library.

16. E.I. to Mrs McLaren, 19 December 1916, Inglis Papers.
17. Armoured Car Reports, ADM 116/1626.
18. Ibid.
19. Ibid.
20. E.I., Report VII, 8 January 1917, Fawcett Library.
21. Fitzroy, op. cit., p. 94.
22. Ibid., op. cit., p. 136.
23. Commander Gregory to Mrs McLaren, 28 November 1917, Inglis Papers.
24. Armoured Car Reports, ADM 116/1626.
25. E.I. to Miss Palliser, 12 June 1917, Fawcett Library.
26. E.I. to Lady Ashmore, 9 January 1917, Fawcett Library.

Chapter 20

1. *Blackwood's Magazine*, May 1918.
2. E.I. to Lady Ashmore, 9 January 1917, Fawcett Library.
3. E.I., Report VIII, 24 January 1917, Fawcett Library.
4. Ibid.
5. Ibid.
6. Fitzroy, op. cit., p. 101.
7. E.I. to Lady Ashmore, 24 January 1917, Fawcett Library.
8. E.I. to Miss Palliser, 7 February 1917, Fawcett Library.
9. E.I., Report VIII, 24 January 1917, Fawcett Library.
10. Fitzroy, op. cit., p. 102.
11. E.I. to Lady Ashmore, 24 January 1917, Fawcett Library.
12. E.I. to Eve Simson, 24 January 1917, Inglis Papers.
13. E.I., Report VIII, 24 January 1917, Fawcett Library.
14. Fitzroy, op. cit., p. 110.
15. Ibid., p. 109.
16. *Blackwood's Magazine*, May 1918.
17. E.I., Report X, 28 January 1917, Fawcett Library.
18. E.I., Report IX, 29 January 1917, Fawcett Library. Dr Inglis's reports were numbered at the London headquarters of the S.W.H. according to the order in which they were received. Report IX is in fact a later one than Report X.
19. E.I. to Miss Palliser, 5 March 1917, Fawcett Library.
20. E.I. to Miss Palliser, 7 February 1917, Fawcett Library.
21. E.I. to Miss Palliser, 5 March 1917, Fawcett Library.
22. Ibid.
23. Ibid.
24. Ibid.
25. *Evening News*, 28 November 1917.
26. E.I., Report VIII, 24 January 1917, Fawcett Library.
27. Cruttwell, op. cit., p. 418.
28. *Blackwood's Magazine*, May 1918.
29. E.I., Report at Fawcett Library, marked 'Strictly Private and Confidential'. This was not sent, but was condensed and re-written as the first part of Report IX.
30. Ibid.

31. See Appendix.
32. E.I., Report at Fawcett Library, marked 'Strictly Private and Confidential'.
33. E.I., Report IX, 29 January 1917, Fawcett Library.
34. E.I. to Miss Palliser, 5 March 1917, Fawcett Library.

Chapter 21

1. Knox, op. cit., pp. 537-66.
2. E.I., Report X, 6 March 1917, Fawcett Library.
3. E.I. to Dr Mary MacNicol, 5 March 1917, Inglis Papers.
4. E.I. to Miss Palliser, 27 March 1917, Fawcett Library.
5. E.I. to Miss Palliser, 5 March 1917, Fawcett Library.
6. E.I., Report XI, 6 March 1917, Fawcett Library.
7. Ibid.
8. Foreign Office Papers, F.O. 371/2993/98075/17.
9. E.I., Report XI, 6 March 1917, Fawcett Library.
10. E.I. to Dr Mary MacNicol, 5 March 1917, Inglis Papers.
11. Fitzroy, op. cit., p. 119.
12. E.I. to Mrs Simson, 11 May 1917, Inglis Papers.
13. E.I. to Mrs Simson, 23 March 1917, Inglis Papers.
14. Fitzroy, op. cit., p. 121.
15. Ibid., p. 125.

Chapter 22

1. E.I. to Mrs Simson, 23 March 1917, Inglis Papers.
2. Fitzroy, op. cit., p. 125.
3. *Blackwood's Magazine*, May 1918.
4. Fitzroy, op. cit., p. 128.
5. E.I. to Mrs Simson, 23 March 1917, Inglis Papers.
6. E.I. to Miss Palliser, 20 March 1917, Fawcett Library; Fitzroy, op. cit., p. 125; *Blackwood's Magazine*, May 1918.
7. Fitzroy, op. cit., p. 159.
8. Knox, op. cit., vol. 1, pp. 362-3.
9. E.I., Report XII, 16 April 1917, Fawcett Library.
10. Ibid.
11. *History of The Times, 1912-1920*, p. 254.
12. Private information, Miss Hedges.
13. E.I. to Miss Palliser, 18 April 1917, Fawcett Library.
14. E.I., Report XII, 16 April 1917, Fawcett Library.
15. Ibid.
16. See Appendix.
17. E.I. to Miss Palliser, 18 April 1917, Fawcett Library.
18. E.I., Report XII, 16 April 1917, Fawcett Library.
19. E.I. to Eve Simson, 18 April 1917, Inglis Papers.
20. E.I., Report XII, 16 April 1917, Fawcett Library.
21. Fitzroy, op. cit., p. 144.

Chapter 23

1. *Blackwood's Magazine*, May 1918; Fitzroy, op. cit., pp. 137-8.

2. Dr Inglis's medal ribbons are preserved in the Imperial War Museum.
3. Photograph in Inglis Papers.
4. E.I. to Eve Simson, 28 July 1917, Inglis Papers.
5. E.I., Report XIII, 27 May 1917, Fawcett Library.
6. Fitzroy, op. cit., p. 140.
7. Meriel Buchanan, *Ambassador's Daughter*.
8. E.I., Report XIII, 27 May 1917, Fawcett Library.
9. Fitzroy, op. cit., p. 142.
10. E.I. to Miss Palliser, 27 March 1917, Fawcett Library.
11. Fitzroy, op. cit., p. 144.
12. E.I., Report XIII, 27 May 1917, Fawcett Library.
13. E.I. to Miss Palliser, 11 May 1917, Fawcett Library.
14. Ibid.
15. McLaren, *Elsie Inglis*, p. 70.
16. Knox, op. cit., vol. 1, p. 335.
17. E.I., Report XIII, 27 May 1917, Fawcett Library.
18. E.I. to Miss Palliser, 11 May 1917, Fawcett Library.
19. E.I. to Miss Palliser, 27 August 1917, Fawcett Library.
20. Foreign Office Papers, F.O. 372/1035/10026.
21. Foreign Office Papers, F.O. 371/2993/83817.
22. Foreign Office Papers, F.O. 371/2993/100068.
23. Foreign Office Papers, F.O. 371/2993/104037.
24. Foreign Office Papers, F.O. 371/2993/114470.

Chapter 24

1. Meriel Buchanan, *Ambassador's Daughter*, p. 172.
2. E.I., Report XIV, June 5 1917, Fawcett Library.
3. E.I. to Miss Palliser, June 5 1917, Fawcett Library.
4. E.I. to Miss Palliser, June 12 1917, Fawcett Library.
5. E.I. to Miss Palliser, June 5 1917, Fawcett Library.
6. E.I., Report XIV, June 5 1917, Fawcett Library.
7. *The Times*, 29 November 1917.
8. General Hunter Leggatt, quoted Edmonds, op. cit.
9. E.I. to Miss Palliser, 11 May and 5 June 1917, Fawcett Library.
10. E.I. to Miss Palliser, 27 August 1917, Fawcett Library.
11. E.I. to Miss Palliser, 12 June 1917, Fawcett Library.
12. E.I. to Miss Palliser, 5 June 1917, Fawcett Library.
13. E.I. to Miss Palliser, 12 June 1917, Fawcett Library.
14. *Common Cause*, 30 November 1917.
15. E.I. to Miss Palliser, 12 June 1917, Fawcett Library.
16. Foreign Office Papers, F.O. 371/2993/84976 and 371/2993/109678.
17. E.I. to Miss Palliser, 12 June 1917, Fawcett Library.
18. Foreign Office Papers, F.O. 371/2889/131892.
19. E.I. to Miss Palliser, June 24 1917, Fawcett Library.
20. Ibid.
21. Personal information, Mrs Sherry.
22. E.I. to Mrs Simson, 24 June 1917, Inglis Papers.
23. Balfour, op. cit., p. 83.

24. Ibid., p. 230.
25. *Blackwood's Magazine*, May 1918.
26. Foreign Office Papers, F.O. 371/2993/76115.
27. Foreign Office Papers, F.O. 371/2889/133164.
28. E.I. to Miss Palliser, July 15 1917, Fawcett Library.
29. Knox, op. cit., vol. 2, pp. 632-52.
30. Knox, op. cit., vol. 2, pp. 537-66.
31. Ibid., p. 666.
32. Ibid., p. 669.
33. Foreign Office Papers, F.O. 371/2889/14408.
34. Foreign Office Papers, F.O. 371/2889/144408.
35. Foreign Office Papers, F.O. 371/2889/148849.
36. E.I. to Mrs Kinnell, 28 July 1917, Fawcett Library.
37. See Chapter 20.
38. E.I. to Mrs Kinnell, 28 July 1917, Fawcett Library.
39. Foreign Office Papers F.O. 371/2993/149250.
40. Foreign Office Papers, F.O. 371/2889/154525.
41. Ibid., F.O. 371/2993/154909 et. seq.
42. E.I. to Mrs Kinnell, 28 July 1917, Fawcett Library.
43. E.I. to Miss Palliser, 28 July 1917, Fawcett Library.

Chapter 25

1. Foreign Office Papers, F.O. 371/2889/165539.
2. E.I., Report XV, 20 August 1917, Fawcett Library.
3. E.I., August 15, 1917, quoted Balfour, op. cit., p. 230.
4. E.I. to Miss Palliser, 27 August 1917, Fawcett Library.
5. Butler, *Paper Boats*, p. 66.
6. Ibid., p. 67.
7. Ibid., p. 69.
8. Foreign Office Papers, F.O. 371/2889/157367.
9. Foreign Office Papers, F.O. 371/2993/161161.
10. Balfour, op. cit., p. 230.
11. Foreign Office Papers, F.O. 371/2889/165429.
12. Knox, op. cit., vol. 2, p. 669.
13. Preserved in showcase at Imperial War Museum.
14. E.I. to Mrs Simson, quoted Balfour, op. cit., p. 231.
15. E.I., Report XV, 20 August 1917, Fawcett Library.
16. Box 1915, S.W.H. Records, Fawcett Library.
17. Foreign Office Papers, F.O. 371/2889/169949.
18. E.I. to Miss Palliser, 27 August 1917.
19. Ibid.
20. See photograph in McLaren, *History of the Scottish Women's Hospitals.*
21. Personal information, Miss Holme.
22. Foreign Office Papers, F.O. 371/2889/198581/17.
23. Foreign Office Papers, F.O. 371/2889/198581.

Chapter 26

1. E.I. to Miss Palliser, 1 October 1917, Fawcett Library; *Blackwood's Magazine,* May 1918.
2. E.I. to Miss Palliser, 1 October 1917, Fawcett Library.
3. Personal information, Miss Hedges and Miss Arbuthnot.
4. Personal information, Dr G. Ward.
5. Foreign Office Papers, F.O. 371/2889/172869.
6. McLaren, *History of the Scottish Women's Hospitals,* p. 217.
7. Knox, op. cit., vol. 2, pp. 632 and 669 et seq.
8. Foreign Office Papers, F.O. 371/2889/173029.
9. Foreign Office Papers, F.O. 371/2889/175379.
10. Foreign Office Papers, F.O. 371/2889/177536.
11. Knox, op. cit., vol. 2, p. 669.
12. Butler, *Daylight in a Dream,* generally.
13. *Blackwood's Magazine,* May 1918.
14. Ibid.
15. E.I. to Miss Palliser, 1 October 1917, Fawcett Library.
16. Foreign Office Papers, F.O. 371/2889/183540.
17. Foreign Office Papers, F.O. 371/2889/193370.
18. Personal information, Miss Holme.
19. Balfour, op. cit., p. 233.
20. *Blackwood's Magazine,* May 1918.
21. Knox, op. cit., vol. 2. Diary entry for October 12.
22. *Blackwood's Magazine,* May 1918.
23. E.I. to Miss Onslow, 22 October 1918, Fawcett Library.
24. *Blackwood's Magazine,* May 1918.
25. Ibid.
26. E.I., Report XVI, 29 October 1917, Fawcett Library.
27. Foreign Office Papers, F.O. 371/2889/222192 and F.O. 371/2889/233191.
28. Personal information, Miss Hedges.

Chapter 27

1. Personal information, Dr G. Ward.
2. Personal information, Miss Arbuthnot.
3. *Blackwood's Magazine,* May 1918.
4. Dr G. Ward. Letter to the writer.
5. Foreign Office Papers, F.O. 371/2889/173029.
6. *Blackwood's Magazine,* May 1918.
7. Falls, *The First World War,* p. 276.
8. Foreign Office Papers, F.O. 371/2889/28?7047 (stamp obscure) and F.O. 317/2889/210602.
9. Balfour, op. cit., p. 241.
10. Butler, *Paper Boats,* pp. 74-6.
11. Meriel Buchanan, *Ambassador's Daughter,* p. 189.
12. Butler, *Paper Boats,* pp. 74-6.
13. *Blackwood's Magazine,* May 1918.
14. Box 1915, S.W.H. Records. Fawcett Library.
15. *Daily Chronicle,* 28 November 1917.

16. *Blackwood's Magazine,* May 1918.
17. Preserved with E.I.'s belongings at Imperial War Museum.
18. *Blackwood's Magazine,* May 1918.
19. Personal information, Miss Arbuthnot.
20. Personal information, Mrs Sherry and others.
21. *Blackwood's Magazine,* May 1918.
22. Personal information, Miss Arbuthnot
23. Balfour, op. cit., p. 242.
24. The Seton Watson Papers.
25. Personal information, Dr G. Ward.
26. Balfour, op. cit., p. 245.
27. Personal information, Miss May Simson.
28. Balfour, op. cit., p. 246.
29. Personal information, Miss Arbuthnot.
30. *Blackwood's Magazine,* May 1918.
31. Mrs Haverfield, *Evening News,* 28 November 1917.
32. Balfour, op. cit., p. 246.
33. E.I. to Miss Palliser, 26 November 1917, Fawcett Library.
34. Personal information, Mrs Sherry and others.
35. Balfour, op. cit., p. 246.
36. See E.I.'s belongings preserved at the Imperial War Museum.
37. *Edinburgh Evening Despatch,* 27 November 1917.
38. See files of the newspapers quoted, and many others, for 28 and 29 November 1917; *The Lancet,* 8 December 1917.
39. Photographs in *Daily Mirror,* 1 December 1917.
40. This was first mentioned in the *Manchester Guardian,* very briefly, 19 February 1918.
41. *Scots Pictorial,* 8 December 1917.
42. Typescript note in Inglis Papers.

INDEX

Abbott, Mrs, 89, 90, 179
Aberdeen Free Press, 280
Abinger, 3rd Lord, 25
Ackermann, 268
Albania, Retreat through, 145-51 161-3, 168, 280
Alexander III of Russia, 187(n)
Alexander, Crown Prince of Serbia (later Alexander III of Yugoslavia), 123(n), 132, 145, 174, 179, 221, 246
Alexeyev, 19
Allahabad, 31
Anderson, Dr Elizabeth Garrett, 35, 36, 38, 52, 53, 61-3, 65, 75, 97
Anderson, Elizabeth Garrett, Hospital, *see* New Hospital for Women
Anderson, Dr Louisa Garrett, 97, 104
Anglo-Russian Hospital, Petrograd, 238
Antitch, Col. Tcholah, 150, 279
Arbuthnot, Miss E., 181, 260, 264, 272, 278
Archangel, 24, 184, 252, 253, 257, 258, 263, 265, 267, 269, 270(n), 271, 273, 275, 277
Argyll, 8th Duke of, 54(n)
Ascot, 102
Ashmore, Lady, 186, 198, 200, 210, 214
Asquith, H. H. (Earl of Oxford & Asquith), 88, 94-6, 140, 160, 207
Asquith, Mrs (Margot), 54(n)

Bagge, Mr (later Sir) John Picton, 244
Balfour, Col. Eustace, 54(n)
Balfour, Lady Frances, 54
Balkan War, First, 104
Barbour, Dr Hugh, 74
Barclay, Sir George, 200, 226, 265
Bareilly, 32
Baring-Gould, Rev. S., 118
Barnardo, Dr, 71
Barrie, Sir J. M., 52
Barker, General, 252, 265, 266
Beale, Dorothea, 39, 50
Beatson, Sir George, 99
Belgrade, 141, 142, 144, 171
Bengal, 30
Bengal Sporting Magazine, 30
Bennett, Dr Agnes, 179
Bergmann, Capt., 217, 225, 226
Berlin, 255
Berthelot, General, 267
Bevan, Capt. (later Commodore), 185, 273, 274
Boer War, 25, 75, 77, 98
Bombay, 31
Bouchier, J. D., 188(n)
Boykett, Sister, 112, 132
Braila, 194-7, 199, 202, 205, 206, 208, 209, 220
British Govt., 137, 150, 169, 207
Broadbent, Miss, 233
Brook, Dr, 120
Brown, Ford Madox, 65
Browning, Robert, 276
Bruntsfield Hospital, 73-6, 79, 86, 87 127, 162
Brusilov Offensive, 17
Bryson, Capt., 187, 190, 191, 204
Buchanan, Sir George, 240, 242, 251, 258, 259
Bucharest, 199, 200, 203, 204, 206
Bulbul Mic, 189, 202
Burke, Miss Kathleen, 117, 118, 179
Butler, Professor E. M., 47, 255, 256, 269, 274, 275
Butler, Josephine, 64

Cadell, Dr Georgina, 53, 54, 55
Cadell, Dr Grace, 53, 54, 55, 73, 75, 84, 117
Calais, 104, 105
Calcutta, 31, 32, 33
Caledonian Medical Journal, 75
Cambridge, women's colleges, 102

Caromarat, 27, 190
Cartonerts, Dr, 192, 193
Carson, Sir E., 140
Cascade School, Hobart, 39
Cavell, Edith, 104, 160
Cecil, Lord Robert, 258, 260, 261, 267
Central Midwives Board, 84
Chalmers Watson, Dr Mona, 75
Chamberlain, Sir Austen, 174-5
Chelmsford, Lord, 176-7
Cheltenham Ladies College, 39
Chesterton, G. K., 179
Chesney, Dr Lilian, 21, 22, 119, 127, 133, 149, 181, 189, 191, 202, 203, 206, 209, 218, 219, 220, 225, 238, 242, 250, 259, 266
Chicherin, 274
Christitch, Anny, 128
Churchill, Sir Winston, 106, 132
Ciulnitza, 204, 233
Clemaud, Dr, 197, 208, 220, 244
Clements, Capt., 126
Clive, Robert, 44
Cochrane-Shanks, Mrs E., 111
Common Cause, The, 100, 160
Constanza, 26, 190, 204
Corbett, Dr Catherine, 120, 148, 149, 152, 165, 166, 168, 169, 171, 181, 189, 196, 203, 209, 210, 217, 218, 225, 266, 268
Costinescu, Dr *see* Cartonerts
Cowdray, 1st Viscount, 252(n)
Cowdray, Viscountess, 110, 174, 176, 178, 180, 252, 257
Curcin, Dr Milan, 125, 126, 129, 138, 142, 144, 145, 150, 162, 174, 179, 180, 281
Cursiter, Mrs, 96
Curwen, Dame May, 183, 261
Czar, s.s., 273
Czaritza s.s., 273

Daily Express, 128
Daily Mail, 81, 124
Daily News, 21, 179
Daily Sketch, 280
Danials, 144, 150
Danube, 113, 139, 142, 145, 186, 187, 191, 192, 193, 194, 195, 196, 203, 212, 215, 216, 217, 225, 228
Darwin, Charles, 93
Davidson, Emily, 95
Day, Mr, 247
Decies, Gertrude, Lady, 266
Derby, 17th Earl of, 241, 261, 267
d'Esperey, Gen. Franchet, 29
de Tourcy, Gen., 117
Dickson, Miss Emily, 67
Dobruga, Battles and Retreats, 17, 20, 21, 22, 23, 24-8, 29, 189, 203, 208, 216, 252
Dolgourokoff, Prince, 230
Dolling, Mrs Alina, 181
Dwight, John S., 259
Dwinsk, s.s., 273

East Grinstead, 102
East India Company, 30, 32
Eastman Co., 47
Ecroyd, 239
Edinburgh, 43, 44, 50, 54, 55, 58, 65, 66, 68, 71, 73, 75, 79, 84, 86, 87, 96, 103, 104, 108, 111, 115, 116, 117, 124, 162, 182, 183, 278, 280
Edinburgh Castle, 98
Edinburgh Hospital for Women and Children, *see* Bruntsfield Hospital
Edinburgh Institution, 43
Edinburgh School of Medicine for Women, 51, 53, 68, 117
Edinburgh University, 66, 72, 73, 84
Edmunds, Mr, 45
Edwards, Sister, 195, 198, 200
Eglinton, Countess of, 76
Elmy, Mrs Wolstenholme, 64, 65, 88
Emslie, Dr Isobel (Lady Hutton), 103
Englishwoman, 158
Erskine, Dr Marion, 75
Eton College, 31, 38
Evans, Sir Arthur, 179

Faurei, 205
Fawcett, Henry, 63
Fawcett, Mrs (later Dame Millicent), 63, 71, 80, 95, 98, 100, 101, 244
Federation of Scottish Suffrage Societies, 77, 82
Fettes College, 48
Fitzroy, Miss Yvonne, 196, 207, 209, 210, 211
Franz Ferdinand, Archduke of Austria, 97
Fraser, Miss Madge Neil, 103, 115, 116
French, Mr, 239

French, Sir John, 103
Fry, Elizabeth, 107

Galatz, 20, 22, 24, 189, 190, 191, 192, 195, 196, 205-9, 211-13, 215, 220, 224, 227, 238, 239, 245
Galicia, 113
Gallipoli, 41
Gambetta, Leon, 47
Garrett, Elizabeth, *see* Anderson, Elizabeth Garrett
Garrett, Newson, 38
Gaza, Battle of, 248
Genge, Miss, 242, 243, 266
Gentitch, Col. Lazar, 125, 135, 137, 151
Geographical Statistical Atlas, 221(n)
George V, King, 95
George Square Hospital, 74
Geraitch, Col., 221, 222, 223, 284
Ghersova, 191, 192, 202, 209
Gibson, Dr George, 54, 57
Gladstone, W. E., 48
Glasgow Bulletin, 173, 280
Glasgow Herald, 58, 88
Glasgow Suffrage Society, 111
Gordon Brown, Miss, 46
Goüin, Mme, 101
Gregory, Cdr. Reginald, 209, 211, 212, 213, 214, 233, 244
Grey, Sir Edward, 81
Griffiths, Col. Norton, M.P., 206, 209
Grouitch, Mme, 101
Grutskoffsky, General, 187
Guardian, 277(n) (see also *Manchester Guardian*)

Hadji Abdul, 259, 264, 271
Hadjitch, Col., 22, 188, 203
Haileybury, 30
Hamilton, Miss Cicely, 103
Harberton, Viscountess, 46
Hardinge of Penshurst, 1st Lord, 176
Harley, Mrs, 103, 239
Hartsoff, Col., 192
Hastings, Warren, 30, 44
Haverfield, Hon. Mrs, 21, 22, 23, 25, 118, 119, 126-9, 133, 143, 151, 152, 157, 165, 167, 169, 170, 171, 173, 179, 181, 182, 187, 189, 197, 198, 199, 216-19, 220, 225, 243
Hedges, Miss Geraldine, 181, 193, 260, 264, 269
Henderson, Miss Mary, 239, 240, 244, 246, 247, 248
Hertslet, Sir Cecil, 172
Herzfeld, Miss Gertrude, 59(n)
History of the Scottish Women's Hospitals, 127
Holbourn, Marion, 92(n)
Hollway, Dr Edith, 106, 110, 120(n), 143, 146, 151, 153
Hollway, Sister, 120
Holme, Miss Vera, 134, 141, 170, 181, 259, 261, 262, 263, 267, 283
Hoover, Herbert, 165
Hope, Anthony, 112
Hospice, The, 77-9, 84, 87, 96, 104, 117, 183
Houldsworth, Miss Margaret, 87
Hunter, Col. William, 116, 125-9, 134, 243, 279
Hutchison, Dr Alice, 77, 78, 104, 105, 118, 121, 125, 126, 127, 131, 142, 143, 150, 161, 166, 173, 175
Huxley, T. H., 93

Ilneachenko, 204, 208, 211, 215
Indian Civil Service, 32, 36
Indian Mutiny, 31
Inglis, Amy (later Simson), sister of E. I., 31-8, 77, 97, 106, 124, 151, 182, 188, 195, 196, 248, 259, 279
Inglis, Cecil, brother of E. I., 38, 40, 41
Inglis, Elsie
  description of, 18, 19, 52, 77, 78, 256
  birth and early life, 29-37
  education, 34, 35, 39, 43-7
  family in Tasmania, 38-40
  moves to England, 41-2
  self-criticism, 50-1
  character of, 18-19, 27, 32, 42, 47, 70, 81-2, 89-95
  medical training, 51-3, 54, 56-9, 66-8
  and Medical College for Women, 55-6
  at New Hospital for Women, 61-6
  work for women's suffrage, 62-5, 67, 68, 79-84, 87-9, 96, 97, 99, 122, 244, 248
  home life, 85-6
  politics of, 51, 64, 67, 81-2, 179-80, 182
  attitudes to money, 51, 69, 76, 100, 200, 240

Inglis, Elsie—*Cont.*
attitudes to men, 48, 62, 63, 93-4, 124
makes nutritional survey, 78
practises in Edinburgh, 70-2, 77-9, 84-5, 96
sets up hospital, 73-7
relationships with patients, 71-2, 77
appointment at Bruntsfield Hospital, 79, 84, 86-7
lecturer at Edinburgh University, 84
amalgamation of The Hospice and Bruntsfield Hospital, 86-7
attempts to help war work, 97-100
founds Scottish Women's Hospitals, 19, 100-3
S.W.H. in France, 104-7
and Joan of Arc, 107-10, 182
work in Britain for S.W.H., 110-17
goes to Serbia, 118-19
at Kragujevatz, 119-20, 124, 132-7, 140-1, 144-8
and typhus epidemic, 123, 125
and health problems of Serbia, 124-7, 133-6
opens Mladanovatz hospital, 128
opens Valjevo hospital, 131-2
unveiling fountain at Mladanovatz, 138
opens Lazaravatz hospital, 139
retreats to Krushevatz, 145, 146, 148
hospital at Krushevatz, 149-57, 165-9
prisoner of war, 153-5, 158-64
repatriated, 170-3
receives Order of White Eagle, 174, 280
and Mesopotamia, 175-8
and fund raising, 76, 100, 102, 117-18, 179-80
leaves for Russia, 19, 183-5
work in Dobruga, 19-28, 186-92
at Ghersova, 192-3
at Braila, 194-203, 205
at Galatz, 205-14
in Reni, 187, 215-18, 225-46, 248-9, 256, 258-63
in Odessa, 185-6, 218-24, 246-8, 249-53, 257-8
in Bucharest, 202
at Ciulnitza, 204-5
and Russian Revolution, 229-30, 237-8, 242, 274-5
charged with spying, 231-5
staff problems, 84, 132-4, 197-200, 218-20, 240-1, 242-6, 247
efforts to remove Serbian Divs. from Russia, 251-63, 268-70
returns to England, 271-8
illness and death, 96, 166, 182, 264-5, 266, 268, 269, 270, 272-9
obituaries, funeral and memorial service, 280-1
Inglis, Ernest, brother of E. I., 31, 41, 69, 93
Inglis, Eva (later McLaren), sister of E. I., 31-4, 36-8, 42, 43, 49, 51, 69, 70, 74, 78, 88, 91, 107, 108, 119, 127, 158, 172, 176, 182, 198, 211, 212, 279
Inglis, George, brother of E. I., 40
Inglis, Harriet (*née* Thompson), mother of E. I., 30-6, 38, 46-50, 93
Inglis, Herbert, brother of E. I., 34, 40
Inglis, Horace, brother of E. I., 31, 32, 36, 39, 48
Inglis, Hugh, brother of E. I., 38-41
Inglis, John, father of E. I., 30-41, 46-52, 55, 56, 58, 62, 64, 65, 67, 68-71, 74, 81, 82, 85, 86, 89, 91, 92, 107, 112, 169, 174, 198, 231, 235
Inglis, Katherine, 85
Inglis, Louisa, sister-in-law of E. I., 40
Irish Daily Independent, 67
Irving, Sir Henry, 65
Ivens, Miss Frances, 103, 105, 119

Jambrishak, Dr, 261, 283, 286
Jassy, 203, 210, 223, 268
Jellicoe, Admiral Lord, 181
Jex-Blake, Dr Sophia, 35, 36, 43, 44, 51-6, 61, 68, 70, 71, 73-5, 79, 87, 128
Jivkovitch, Gen. Mihailo, 142, 180, 185, 186, 234, 249, 251, 253, 255, 262, 280(n)
Johnson, Mr Arthur, 277(n)
Juckes, Dr, 53

Kenney, Annie, 81
Kerensky, Alexander, 238, 250, 255, 256, 262(n), 265, 270, 273

Kimens, Mr, 240, 242, 256, 259
King Lear, 65
King, Olive Kelso, 103
King's Own Scottish Borderers, 248
Kinnell, Mrs Gertrude, 252, 253, 260
Kitchener of Khartoum, Lord, 98, 99, 122, 152, 158, 178, 184
Knott, Miss, 39, 41
Knott, Miss Fanny, 39
Knox, Gen. Sir Alfred, 188, 230, 251, 265(n)
Kolesnikoff, Sister Vera, 230, 231, 232, 235, 274(n)
Kornilov, General, 250, 265
Kostitchi, Dr, 25, 26, 27, 190, 191, 192, 198
Kragujevatz, 111, 114-16, 119, 121, 123, 132, 134-7, 139, 140, 141, 143-6, 166, 168, 174, 193, 212, 280
Kruger, Rayne, 121(n)
Krushevatz, 143, 148, 149, 155, 158, 160, 161, 171, 208, 231

Labour Party, 81
Lady's Pictorial, 181
Laird, Dr Janet, 120, 126, 149, 181, 225, 227, 250
Lancet, The, 280
Lang, Andrew, 108
Language problems, 103, 125, 167, 168, 256-7
Latrobe, Tasmania, 40
Launceston, Tasmania, 39
Laurie, Mrs, 99
Lawrence, John (1st Baron Lawrence), 30, 34, 37
Lawrence, Samuel, 52
Lazaravatz, 134, 138, 139, 141, 143
Leith Hospital, 53, 55
Lewis, Miss, 22
Lewis, C. S., 83(n)
Liberal Party, 46, 64, 81
Liberal Women's Association, 64
Lichtenstein, Mr, 45
Lipovschak, Lieut, 286
Littlejohn, Dr (later Sir Henry), 66
Lloyd George, David (later 1st Earl Lloyd George), 132, 140, 158, 207
London School of Medicine, 52, 54(n), 61
London University, 43
Lossiemouth, 88
Lucknow, 31, 32
Lytton, 1st Earl of, 37, 112
Macdonald, Flora, 76
MacEwen, Sir William, 56, 57, 58, 59
MacGregor, Dr Beatrice, 127, 128, 137, 138, 142, 143, 145, 150, 161, 162
MacGregor, Dr Jessie, 53, 68, 69, 70, 73, 75, 79
McIlroy, Dr (later Dame) Louise, 179
Mackensen, Field Marshal, 142, 203
McLaren, Amy (Mrs Maddox), 85
McLaren, Eva, *see* Inglis, Eva
McLaren, John Shaw, brother-in-law of E. I., 74
McLaren, Mr Moray, 81(n)
MacNicol, Dr Mary, 55
MacPhail, Dr Katharine, 103
M'Vea, Dr, 120
Mair, Miss Sarah, 100, 111, 149, 150
Malta Chronicle, 121
Manchester Guardian, 280
Marie Pavlovna, Grand Duchess of Russia, 186
Marie, Sister, 208, 217
Marx, Miss Margaret, 243, 244, 245, 250, 253, 254, 255, 259, 260
Mary, H.M. Queen, 87, 112, 279
Maude, General, 175
Medical College for Women, 55, 56, 66, 73, 179
Medical Education of Women, Scottish Assoc. for, 55
Medical women, education of, 35-6, 51-9, 66, 183
Mesopotamia, 173-8, 246
Mesopotamia Report, 174-5, 178
Methuen, 3rd Baron, 121, 127
Mihailovitz, Col., 137
Mills, Wallis, 122
Milne, Mrs Mary, 205, 221, 249, 266, 268, 273, 276, 278
Milotinovitch, Col., 260, 268, 279
Mladanovatz, 125, 126, 127, 128, 132, 137, 139, 142
Monastir, 239
Morgan Brothers, 40
Morning Post, 280
Moscow, 273
Motor ambulances, 101, 182, 189, 209
Muir, Sir William, 32, 66, 72, 181, 264
Murphy, Miss Agnes, 231, 232, 233
Murray, Prof. Gilbert, 102

Naini Tal, 29, 31, 32, 33, 36

Napier of Magdala, 1st Baron, 32
Nation, The, 179
Nevinson, Henry, 179
New Hospital for Women, 61, 63, 66
Nicholas II, Czar of Russia, 187(n), 222, 228, 251, 284
Nicolayevitch, Col., 126, 128, 129, 130
Nicolitch, Major, 153, 155, 156, 165
Nightingale, Florence, 50, 61, 64, 107, 114, 135, 143, 175, 178, 195, 244
Nish, 126-7, 136, 140, 158

Odessa, 184, 185, 193, 206, 209, 215-18, 220-3, 227, 232, 238, 240, 243, 244, 245, 248, 249, 252, 253, 254, 257, 261, 265, 268, 271, 273, 283, 284, 285, 286
Old Dominion, 276
Oliphant, Mr (later Sir Lancelot), 266
Oliphant, Mr (school director), 45
Onslow, Miss Alexandrina, 26, 191, 198, 250, 265, 266, 268, 278
Orkney Isles, 80, 102

Padham, Capt., 175-7
Paget, Lady (Dame Leila), 120, 136
Paget, Sir Ralph, 127, 128, 140, 142, 150, 151
Palliser, Miss Edith, 110, 220, 224, 225, 235, 239, 242, 245, 246, 247, 249, 250, 253, 260, 267, 279
Pankhurst, Christabel, 81
Pankhurst, Emmeline, 88
Pares, Miss G., 139
Paris, 46, 47
Parnell, Charles Stewart, 54
Pashitch, Prime Minister of Serbia, 174, 176, 179, 180
Perry, Miss, 53, 54
Pétain, Marshal, 118
Peter, King, of Serbia, 113, 123
Pethick-Lawrence, Emmeline, 80, 118, 182
Pethick-Lawrence, Frederick (later Lord), 80, 118, 182
Petrie, Mrs Flinders, 110
Petroff, 274
Petrograd, 184, 188, 200, 217, 228, 229, 234, 238, 239, 240, 249, 252, 256, 259, 265
Ploesti, 204
Popovitch, Lt.-Col., 167, 198, 203
Porto, s.s., 273-7
Potter, Dr Lena, 181, 195, 209, 210, 218, 223, 225
Protitch, Major, 120, 124, 144, 146
Punch, 48, 122
Putnik, Vojvode (Marshal), 112, 131
Pygmalion, 199

Ransome, Arthur, 21
Rattenbury, Mrs, *see* Dolling, Alina
Red Cross, 99, 185, 197, 199, 202, 204, 208, 212, 215, 216, 220, 222, 244, 245, 246, 257
Religion, 138, 179, 230, 239
Reni, 214, 215, 218-20, 223, 225-7, 232-3, 237, 248-50, 253, 255-9, 261, 267
Review of Reviews, 45, 46
Richardson, Mary, 95
Ristitch, 134
Robertson, Graham, 65(n)
Robinson, Miss Frances, 259, 261, 262, 263, 267, 283, 286
Rollitt, Sir A., 63
Rotunda Hospital, Dublin, 66, 69
R.A.M.C., 97, 98
Royal Navy, 144
R.N.A.S. Armoured Cars, 209, 210, 212, 213, 214, 224, 227, 233, 237, 239, 244
Royaumont, S.W.H. Unit at, 105-7, 179
Royden, Maude, 80, 82, 83
Russell, Dr Beatrice, 84
Russell, General, 175-7
Russian Revolution, 228-9, 238, 240, 254, 284, 285

Sackville-West, V., 109
Salisbury, 3rd Marquess of, 37
Sandhurst Military Academy, 41
Sarajevo, 52, 97, 112
Sarrail, General, 143
Scharlieb, Mrs (later Dame Mary), 61, 62, 65, 66
Scotsman, The, 40, 71, 280
Scots Pictorial, The, 280
Scott, Surgeon-Lieut Maitland, 209 210, 212, 213
Scottish Association for the Medical Education of Women, 55
Scottish Women's Hospitals, 18, 19, 21, 23, 24, 59, 98, 100-7, 110, 111, 114-16, 118-20, 123, 125,

Scottish Women's Hospitals—*Cont.* 127, 129, 130, 133, 142, 146, 155, 163, 169, 173, 176-8, 195, 202, 203, 208, 209, 217, 218, 222, 231, 237, 239, 240, 241, 244, 249, 254, 257, 259, 264, 265, 266, 270, 271, 274, 275
Scutari, 135, 195
Selbourne, Viscountess, 252
Serbia, appeals to Allies, 139
casualties in, 102
divisions in Russia, 180, 183-6, 188, 194, 203, 220-2, 247, 249, 251-5, 257, 258, 260, 262, 265-9, 270, 283-6
government of, 104, 105
history of, 112, 113
overrun, 161, 165
people and customs, 123-4, 126, 127, 131, 132-6, 144, 164, 165
politics, 179-80
religion, 128
retreat through Albania, 145-51, 161-3, 168, 280
S.W.H. unit in, 106, 118, 119-21, 138-9, 142, 143, 144-51, 163
and Yugoslav Committee, 246, 261
Serbian Relief Fund, 113, 134(n), 162, 180
Serbian Society, 182
Seton Watson, R., 104, 105, 113, 114, 116, 166, 180, 182, 252, 277
Shaw, George Bernard, 90
Shetland Isles, 80
Simla, 31
Simson, Amy, *see* Inglis, Amy
Simson, Evelyn, 77, 207, 217, 248, 278
Simson, Sir Henry J. F., 33(n)
Simson, Major James, 248, 279
Simson, Miss May, 82, 98
Simson, Robert, 33
Sinclair, Miss, 54
Six Sincere Students Society, 51
Skoplje, 136, 140, 152, 158
Smith, William, 106, 145, 146, 149, 151, 161
Smyth, Dr (later Dame) Ethel, 88
Snowden, Ethel, 80
Snowden, Philip (later Viscount Snowden), 80
Sofia, 242
Soltau, Dr Eleanor, 103, 106, 111, 115, 117
Somme, Battle of the, 17
Spectator, 48
Stanley, The Hon. Arthur, 241
Stanojevitch, Dr S., 189, 197
Stead, W. T., 45
Stephen, Alice, 39, 43
Stevenson, Robert Louis, 71, 93
Stobart, Mrs, 162
Stoney, Miss Edith, 103, 179
Strachey, Lytton, 128
Strange, Sister, 157
Sturmer, 284
Subotic, General, 120
Suffrage Movement, 19, 25, 46, 62, 63, 64, 67, 68, 72, 79, 80-3, 87-9, 110, 118, 183, 199
Sydney, Australia, 40
Szarderry, Mayor, 195, 196

Tecuci, 250
Terry, Ellen, 65
Thompson, George, grandfather of E. I., 30, 91
Thompson, Harriet, *see* Inglis, Harriet
Times, The, 54, 83(n), 113, 129, 175, 178, 179, 182, 188(n), 257, 279, 280
Todd, Dr Margaret, 79
Toughill, Mrs Caroline, 161, 162, 190
Trajan's Wall, 24
Trevelyan, G. M., 113
Trotsky, 274, 275
Troyes, S.W.H. Unit at, 117, 121, 163, 169, 179
Tulcea, 216
Typhus, 114, 115, 116, 119, 123, 125, 149, 157, 226-7

Uppingham, 31, 38

Valjevo, 127, 131, 132, 134, 136, 143
Vaughn, 239
Vernon, Rev. Edward, 163
Victoria, Queen, 35, 61
Vienna, 112
Vindictive, H.M.S., 275
Visolskin, Admiral, 187, 232, 234
Vizard, Matron, 225, 232, 237, 268, 272
Voluntary Health Visitors Association, 84
Vrinjatcha Banja, 143

Walcot, Baillie, 66

Ward, Dr Gillian, 250, 266, 272, 278, 279
Wardle, Miss, 156
Warwick, Australia, 40
Watson, Mr, 200
Watson, J. B., 40
Webb, Mrs Beatrice, 83
Webb, Dr Helen, 63, 64
Wells, H. G., 93
West, Dame Rebecca, 29
Westminster Gazette, The, 280
Whitehead, Miss, 157
Whyte, Sir Frederick, 180
Wilkins, Mr, 65
Williams, Dr Ethel, 278, 279
Williamson, Rev. Wallace, D.D., 86, 279
Women's Liberal Federation, 51
Women's suffrage movement, *see* Suffrage
Women's Suffrage Societies, National Union of, 102(n), 119, 252
Wright, Sir Almroth, 83(n)

Zourikoff, General, 234